Diagnostic Imaging for the General Surgeon

Guest Editors

THOMAS H. COGBILL, MD
BENJAMIN T. JARMAN, MD

SURGICAL CLINICS OF NORTH AMERICA

www.surgical.theclinics.com

Consulting Editor
RONALD F. MARTIN, MD

February 2011 • Volume 91 • Number 1

SAUNDERS an imprint of ELSEVIER, Inc.

W.B. SAUNDERS COMPANY

A Division of Elsevier Inc.

1600 John F. Kennedy Blvd., Suite 1800, Philadelphia, PA 19103-2899

http://www.theclinics.com

SURGICAL CLINICS OF NORTH AMERICA Volume 91, Number 1
February 2011 ISSN 0039–6109, ISBN-13: 978-1-4557-0509-2

Editor: John Vassallo, j.vassallo@elsevier.com
Developmental Editor: Jessica Demetriou

Surgical Clinics of North America (ISSN 0039–6109) is published bimonthly by Elsevier Inc., 360 Park Avenue South, New York, NY 10010-1710. Months of publication are February, April, June, August, October, and December. Business and Editorial Offices: 1600 John F. Kennedy Blvd., Suite 1800, Philadelphia, PA 19103-2899. Periodicals postage paid at New York, NY and additional mailing offices. Subscription prices are $311.00 per year for US individuals, $532.00 per year for US institutions, $152.00 per year for US students and residents, $381.00 per year for Canadian individuals, $661.00 per year for Canadian institutions, $429.00 for international individuals, $661.00 per year for international institutions and $210.00 per year for Canadian and foreign students/residents. To receive student/resident rate, orders must be accompanied by name of affiliated institution, date of term, and the *signature* of program/ residency coordinator on institution letterhead. Orders will be billed at individual rate until proof of status is received. Foreign air speed delivery is included in all *Clinics* subscription prices. All prices are subject to change without notice. POSTMASTER: Send address changes to *Surgical Clinics*, Elsevier Health Sciences Division, Subscription Customer Service, 3251 Riverport Lane, Maryland Heights, MO 63043. **Customer Service (orders, claims, online, change of address): Telephone: 1-800-654-2452 (U.S. and Canada); 314-447-8871 (outside U.S. and Canada). Fax: 314-447-8029. E-mail: journalscustomerservice-usa@elsevier.com (for print support); journalsonline support-usa@elsevier.com (for online support).**

Reprints. For copies of 100 or more, of articles in this publication, please contact the Commercial Reprints Department, Elsevier Inc., 360 Park Avenue South, New York, New York 10010-1710. Tel. (212) 633-3812, Fax: (212) 462-1935, e-mail: reprints@elsevier.com.

The Surgical Clinics of North America is also published in Spanish by McGraw-Hill Interamericana Editores S.A., P.O. Box 5-237 06500 Mexico D.F. Mexico; and in Portuguese by Interlivros Edicoes Ltda., Rua Comandante Coelho 1085, CEP 21250, Rio de Janeiro, Brazil; and in Greek by Paschalidis Medical Publications, Athens Greece.

The Surgical Clinics of North America is covered in *MEDLINE/PubMed (Index Medicus)*, *EMBASE/Excerpta Medica, Current Contents/Clinical Medicine*, *Current Contents/Life Sciences, Science Citation Index*, and *ISI/BIOMED*.

Printed and bound by CPI Group (UK) Ltd, Croydon, CR0 4YY

Transferred to Digital Print 2011

Contributors

CONSULTING EDITOR

RONALD F. MARTIN, MD
Staff Surgeon, Department of Surgery, Marshfield Clinic, Marshfield, Wisconsin; Clinical Associate Professor, University of Wisconsin School of Medicine and Public Health, Madison, Wisconsin; Colonel, Medical Corps, United States Army Reserve

GUEST EDITORS

THOMAS H. COGBILL, MD, FACS
Program Director Emeritus, General Surgery Residency, Department of General and Vascular Surgery, Gundersen Lutheran Health System, La Crosse, Wisconsin

BENJAMIN T. JARMAN, MD
Program Director, General Surgery Residency, Department of General and Vascular Surgery, Gundersen Lutheran Health System; Department of Medical Education, Gundersen Lutheran Medical Foundation, La Crosse, Wisconsin

AUTHORS

WILLIAM BATES, MD, FACR
Associate Professor of Radiology, Director of Cardiovascular CT Imaging, Medical College of Georgia, Augusta, Georgia

WALTER L. BIFFL, MD, FACS
Director, Surgery/Trauma Outreach, Department of Surgery, Denver Health Medical Center; Associate Professor of Surgery, University of Colorado School of Medicine, Denver, Colorado

JAMES G. BITTNER IV, MD
Resident in Surgery, Medical College of Georgia, Augusta, Georgia

KAREN BRASEL, MD, MPH
Professor of Surgery, Division of Trauma and Critical Care, Medical College of Wisconsin, Milwaukee, Wisconsin

LOWELL W. CHAMBERS, MD, FACS
Associate Program Director, Mount Carmel Surgical Residency; Medical Director, Mount Carmel West SICU, Columbus, Ohio

THOMAS H. COGBILL, MD, FACS
Program Director Emeritus, General Surgery Residency, Department of General and Vascular Surgery, Gundersen Lutheran Health System, La Crosse, Wisconsin

CLAY COTHREN BURLEW, MD, FACS
Director, Surgical Intensive Care Unit, Department of Surgery, Denver Health Medical Center; Associate Professor of Surgery, University of Colorado School of Medicine, Denver, Colorado

CLARK A. DAVIS, MD, FACS
Department of General and Vascular Surgery, Gundersen Lutheran Health System, La Crosse, Wisconsin

MICHAEL A. EDWARDS, MD, FACS
Associate Professor of Surgery; Director, Virtual Education and Simulation Laboratory; Surgical Director, Adrenal Center, Medical College of Georgia, Augusta, Georgia

DAVID C. HAN, MD, MS, FACS
Associate Professor of Surgery and Radiology, Penn State Hershey Heart and Vascular Institute; Vice Chair for Educational Affairs, Department of Surgery, Penn State Hershey Medical Center, Penn State College of Medicine, Hershey, Pennsylvania

BRUCE HARMS, MD, FACS
Professor of Surgery, Chief, Section of Colorectal Surgery, Department of General Surgery, University of Wisconsin-Madison, Madison, Wisconsin

BENJAMIN T. JARMAN, MD
Program Director, General Surgery Residency, Department of General and Vascular Surgery, Gundersen Lutheran Health System; Department of Medical Education, Gundersen Lutheran Medical Foundation, La Crosse, Wisconsin

STEVEN W. KHOO, MD
Fellow in Vascular Surgery, Penn State Hershey Heart and Vascular Institute, Penn State Hershey Medical Center, Penn State College of Medicine, Hershey, Pennsylvania

JULIAN KIM, MD, FACS
Charles Hubay Professor of Surgery, Case Western Reserve University; Chief, Division of Surgical Oncology, University Hospitals Case Medical Center, Cleveland, Ohio

SHANU N. KOTHARI, MD, FACS
Director of Minimally Invasive Bariatric Surgery, Department of General and Vascular Surgery, Gundersen Lutheran Health System, La Crosse, Wisconsin

JEFFREY LANDERCASPER, MD
Co-Director, Norma J. Vinger Center for Breast Care, Attending Surgeon, Department of Surgery, Gundersen Lutheran Health System, La Crosse, Wisconsin; Associate Clinical Professor of Surgery, Department of Surgery, University of Wisconsin School of Medicine and Public Health, Madison, Wisconsin; Chairman, Patient Quality Committee, American Society of Breast Surgeons, Columbia, Maryland

JARED H. LINEBARGER, MD
Department of Medical Education, Gundersen Lutheran Health System, La Crosse, Wisconsin

MEGHAN G. LUBNER, MD
Assistant Professor, Department of Radiology, University of Wisconsin-Madison, Madison, Wisconsin

JOHN D. MELLINGER, MD, FACS
Professor of Surgery, Chair of General Surgery, Residency Program Director, Southern Illinois University, Springfield, Illinois

DAVID J. MILIA, MD
Assistant Professor of Surgery, Division of Trauma and Critical Care, Medical College of Wisconsin, Milwaukee, Wisconsin

NANCY A. PARKS, MD
Surgical Critical Care Fellow, Department of Surgery, University of Tennessee Health Science Center, Memphis, Tennessee

NIRAV Y. PATEL, MD, FACS
Department of General and Vascular Surgery, Gundersen Lutheran Health System, La Crosse, Wisconsin

ANCIL K. PHILIP, MD
Department of General Surgery, University of Wisconsin-Madison, Madison, Wisconsin

JAMES T. QUANN, MD
Department of Surgical Education, Iowa Methodist Medical Center, Des Moines, Iowa

STEVEN REITZ, MD
Chief Surgery Resident, Department of Medical Education, Mount Carmel Health System, Columbus, Ohio

MELANIE L. RICHARDS, MD, MHPE
Professor of Surgery, Division of Gastroenterologic and General Surgery, Department of Surgery, Mayo Clinic, Rochester, Minnesota

JODY M. RIHERD, MD
Department of Diagnostic Radiology, Gundersen Lutheran Health System, La Crosse, Wisconsin

THOMAS J. SCHROEPPEL, MD
Assistant Professor of Surgery, Department of Surgery, University of Tennessee Health Science Center, Memphis, Tennessee

RICHARD A. SIDWELL, MD
Trauma Surgeon and Program Director of General Surgery Residency, Iowa Methodist Medical Center, Des Moines, Iowa; Adjunct Clinical Associate Professor, Department of Surgery, University of Iowa Carver College of Medicine, Iowa City, Iowa

KRISTINE SLAM, MD
Metropolitan Surgery, Columbus, Ohio

BIANCA J. VAZQUEZ, MD
Division of Gastroenterologic and General Surgery, Department of Surgery, Mayo Clinic, Rochester, Minnesota

ANTHONY VISIONI, MD
Surgery Resident, Department of Surgery, University Hospitals Case Medical Center, Case Western Reserve University, Cleveland, Ohio

HADYN T. WILLIAMS, MD, FACNM
Associate Professor of Radiology, Chief, Section of Nuclear Medicine, Medical College of Georgia, Augusta, Georgia

KURT J. ZIEGELBEIN, MD
Department of Radiology, Gundersen Lutheran Health System, La Crosse, Wisconsin

Contents

Computed tomography scanners now use multidetector row technology with contrast-delayed imaging for quicker and more accurate imaging. Magnetic resonance imaging with cholangiopancreatography can more clearly delineate liver lesions and the biliary and pancreatic ducts, and can diagnose pathologic conditions early in their course. Newer technologies, such as single-operator cholangioscopy and endoscopic ultrasonography, have sometimes shown superiority to traditional modalities. This article addresses the literature regarding available imaging techniques in the diagnosis and treatment of common surgical hepatobiliary and pancreatic diseases.

Radiological techniques are important in evaluating patients with gastrointestinal bleeding. Scintigraphic, computed tomographic angiographic, and enterographic techniques are sensitive tools in identifying the source of bleeding and may be useful in identifying patients likely to have a benign course and in selecting patients for therapeutic intervention. Angiography plays a key role in bleeding localization, and modern embolization techniques make this a viable therapeutic option. With the refining developments in body imaging and related reconstructive techniques, it is likely that radiological interventions will play an expanding and critical role in evaluating patients with gastrointestinal hemorrhage in the future.

There is a variety of options available to image the small bowel depending on the clinical scenario. This article describes multiple imaging options and focuses on several clinical scenarios common to general surgeons.

This article provides basic information about computed tomographic colonography (CTC) and reviews the preparation, methods, and tools required for the procedure. The clinical uses for CTC (screening/diagnosis of colon cancer and colonic obstruction) are outlined, and its accuracy and validity are compared with other diagnostic methods. A summary of the benefits and risks of the test are presented and the current practicalities for implementation are addressed.

Acute appendicitis is a common surgical emergency and the diagnosis can often be made clinically; however, many patients present with atypical findings. For these patients, there are multiple imaging modalities available to aid in the diagnosis of suspected appendicitis in an effort to avoid a negative appendectomy. Computed tomography is the test of choice in most patients in whom the diagnosis is not certain. Ultrasonography is particularly useful in children and pregnant women. Magnetic resonance imaging is recommended when ultrasonography is inconclusive. Appropriate use of these imaging studies avoids delays in treatment, prolonged hospitalization, and unnecessary surgery.

This article reviews the use of radiological imaging in the post–gastric bypass patient. A thorough understanding of the reconstructed anatomy is critical to interpret imaging abnormalities, when present. Radiological imaging can help guide the surgeon's management in this specific patient population.

While the use of duplex ultrasound (DUS) in the diagnosis of vascular disease has been established, its role in vascular procedures continues to expand. More powerful and portable technology has helped to overcome real and perceived barriers to the use of DUS. Familiarity with Doppler and ultrasound physics is helpful to understand the potential roles and limitations of DUS. Use of real-time imaging allows the surgeon to obtain central venous and peripheral arterial access, as well as place vena cava filters and treat iatrogenic arterial pseudoaneurysms with a greater degree of patient safety, comfort, and overall success.

Computed tomography (CT) is useful in the detection and diagnosis of abdominal aortic aneurysms (AAA). Rupture risk can be assessed by accurately measuring diameter, tortuosity, thrombus extent, and wall stress. CT can aid in accurately determining anatomic variants as well as AAA etiology. Evaluation for surgical intervention is made by close examination of AAA morphology and specific anatomic features.

Focused assessment with sonography for trauma (FAST) is an invaluable adjunct in the management of trauma patients for detection of free intra-abdominal and pericardial fluid. Over the past 2 decades, the use of this technique has increased significantly. This article reviews the clinical application and future direction of FAST.

Cervical spine injury can be excluded by clinical examination, without the need for radiographic study, in many patients. For those who require study, computed tomography of the cervical spine with sagittal and coronal reconstruction is the best modality for both screening and diagnosing cervical spine injury. Optimal evaluation of the obtunded patient remains controversial.

Originally thought to be a rare occurrence, blunt cerebrovascular injuries (BCVIs) are now diagnosed in approximately 1% of blunt trauma patients. Early imaging of patients has resulted in the diagnosis of BCVIs during the asymptomatic phase, thus allowing prompt treatment. Although the ideal regimen of antithrombotic therapy has yet to be determined, treatment with either antiplatelet agents or anticoagulation has been shown to markedly reduce BCVI-related stroke rate. BCVIs are rare, potentially devastating injuries; appropriate imaging in high-risk patients should be performed and prompt treatment initiated to prevent ischemic neurologic events.

From its beginnings as a time consuming and an inefficient imaging modality with no place in the evaluation of traumatically injured patients, computed axial tomographic (CT) scanners have evolved to yield rapid, highly sensitive images, revolutionizing trauma management protocols. This article describes the fundamentals of CT and the imaging protocols and discusses the use of CT in diagnosing injuries to various regions, such as abdomen, liver, spleen, pancreas, kidney, and chest.

Functional imaging using radiolabeled probes that specifically bind and accumulate in target tissues has improved the sensitivity and specificity of conventional imaging. Fluorodeoxyglucose (FDG)-positron emission tomography (PET) has shown improved diagnostic accuracy in differentiating benign from malignant lesions in the setting of solitary pulmonary nodules. FDG-PET has become useful in preoperative staging of patients with lung cancer, and is being tested with many other malignancies for its ability to change patient management. This article provides an overview of the current status of FDG-PET and presents the challenges of moving toward routine use.

THE CLINICS ARE NOW AVAILABLE ONLINE!
Access your subscription at:
www.theclinics.com

Foreword

Diagnostic Imaging for the General Surgeon

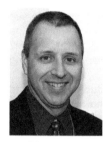

Ronald F. Martin, MD
Consulting Editor

My former chairman, Dr Carl E Bredenberg, would frequently make the teaching point that we only see what we look for. Over many years it became clear to me that he meant that in many ways. Among his many interests was a passion and absolute talent for photography. We both shared an interest in creating images but he really excelled at it. Nonetheless, we spent many hours talking about photography over the years and many more hours talking about surgery—sometimes in the hospital, sometimes at meetings, and sometimes over scotch whiskey, preferably Lagavulin.

One thing one learns in this business (either the easy way or the hard way) is that if one slows their usual frenetic pace a bit and listens to experts, one will learn something. The converse is true as well. However, one really has to listen to what experts say and then one has to think and study independently. Many of my conversations with my former boss about photography had fairly little to do with the image we were looking at but were more about how one went about making something look the way we wanted it to appear rather than the way it actually looked. Much of the conversation would dwell on the mechanics of cameras, lenses, filters, the properties of light, and how different types of film would react (yes, film). Usually something would come up that would prompt one or both of us to further study up on some subject. After a while it became clear that getting better images was mostly a process of reverse engineering the image one wanted out of what subject was available.

Medical imaging isn't all that much different from creative photography in some ways. Most of the images we use don't really look like the real subject at all. Livers aren't some Hounsfield gray color. Pulmonary arteries don't have bright white blood running through them. Yet, we get used to looking at these images and making the translation in our minds. Even though current imaging devices are far more sophisticated in terms of digital manipulation of the acquired data, the images are still shadows of reality. To really understand what these shadows mean, one has to do

Surg Clin N Am 91 (2011) xiii–xiv
doi:10.1016/j.suc.2010.11.001
0039-6109/11/$ – see front matter

two things: understand the process by which the images are created and compare a lot of images to the gold standard of reality.

The constant fractation of care has divided the medical community into two nonequal groups: those who look at the images they request and those who read the reports. Perhaps one of my most annoying professional disappointments is when someone calls me about a patient and tells me what the "report" of an imaging study states without having looked at the images, even when the person calling requested the study be performed. One night on call, I was asked by a calling physician to see a patient because "the CT said (sic) the patient had a bowel obstruction." I asked if he had seen the images of the patient he was calling me about. He replied, "Why should I? I am not a radiologist." It turned out he had not seen the patient either—disappointing on many levels.

To get the best out of imaging, we need to choose imaging studies wisely and interpret them correctly. In order to do that, we have to understand the power and limitations of imaging and its applications, especially how these studies complement clinical evaluation instead of replacing the history and physical exam. Drs Cogbill and Jarman, along with their colleagues, have assembled a collection of articles that will give the reader a much better foundation upon which to improve their understanding of imaging. Still, practice will be required in order to refine these skills. One will only see what one looks for but only if one actually looks.

Ronald F. Martin, MD
Department of Surgery
Marshfield Clinic
1000 North Oak Avenue
Marshfield, WI 54449, USA

E-mail address:
martin.ronald@marshfieldclinic.org

Preface

Diagnostic Imaging for the General Surgeon

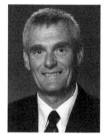 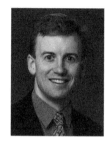

Thomas H. Cogbill, MD   Benjamin T. Jarman, MD
Guest Editors

The role of imaging in the diagnosis and treatment of conditions encountered by general surgeons has dramatically expanded with recent advancements in both technology and applications. It is essential that general surgeons have an excellent working knowledge of the indications for these techniques along with the relative advantages and risks. A radiologist is not always available for interpretation of important studies and general surgeons possess unique information about clinical settings that may enhance the accuracy and application of results.

In an effort to provide a single source update on diagnostic imaging, we have included 16 reviews on both common and cutting-edge techniques likely to be ordered by general surgeons.

The first article includes a review of the basic principles behind computed tomography, magnetic resonance, and ultrasound. Subsequent articles provide contemporary discussions of the diagnostic and therapeutic applications of imaging for conditions in endocrine, hepatobiliary/pancreatic, gastrointestinal, vascular, trauma, and oncologic surgery. In each area, the authors have included representative images to illustrate their use.

We would like to thank each of the authors for their excellent contributions. We would also like to express our appreciation to Ronald Martin, MD for the opportunity to act as guest editors for this issue of *Surgical Clinics of North America* and to the outstanding editorial assistance we received from the staff at Elsevier.

Surg Clin N Am 91 (2011) xv–xvi
doi:10.1016/j.suc.2010.10.019
0039-6109/11/$ – see front matter © 2011 Elsevier Inc. All rights reserved.

surgical.theclinics.com

Thomas H. Cogbill, MD
Gundersen Lutheran Health System
Department of General and Vascular Surgery
1836 South Avenue, C05-001
La Crosse, WI 54601, USA

Benjamin T. Jarman, MD
Gundersen Lutheran Health System
Department of General and Vascular Surgery
1900 South Avenue, C05-001
La Crosse, WI 54601, USA

E-mail addresses:
thcogbil@gundluth.org (T.H. Cogbill)
btjarman@gundluth.org (B.T. Jarman)

Computed Tomography, Magnetic Resonance, and Ultrasound Imaging: Basic Principles, Glossary of Terms, and Patient Safety

Thomas H. Cogbill, MD[a],*, Kurt J. Ziegelbein, MD[b]

KEYWORDS

- Computed tomography principles
- Magnetic resonance imaging physics • Ultrasound principles
- Radiation-induced malignancy
- Contrast-induced nephropathy • Nephrogenic systemic fibrosis

Imaging studies have become commonplace for the evaluation, preoperative planning, and follow-up of surgical patients in elective and emergency settings. Computed tomography (CT), magnetic resonance (MR), and ultrasound (US) have emerged as the 3 modalities most often relied on by general surgeons. General surgeons must be knowledgeable concerning the indications for each technique and be comfortable interpreting these studies. Radiologists are not always immediately available for consultation and the surgeon may have anatomic or clinical information that may make interpretation more accurate or pertinent. In this article, the basic principles underlying CT, MR, and US are reviewed to promote better understanding of their applications and limitations. The risks of each of these techniques are summarized along with strategies to improve patient safety. A glossary of frequently used terms for each imaging technique is provided to serve as a quick reference for nonradiologists.

The authors have nothing to disclose.

[a] Department of General and Vascular Surgery, Gundersen Lutheran Health System, 1900 South Avenue, La Crosse, WI 54601, USA

[b] Department of Radiology, Gundersen Lutheran Health System, 1900 South Avenue, La Crosse, WI 54601, USA

* Corresponding author.

E-mail address: THCogbil@gundluth.org

Surg Clin N Am 91 (2011) 1–14

doi:10.1016/j.suc.2010.10.006

0039-6109/11/$ – see front matter © 2011 Elsevier Inc. All rights reserved.

CT

Basic Principles

Image generation by CT scanners is based on the same physical principles as conventional radiographs (x-rays). X-rays are a type of penetrating electromagnetic radiation that travels in a straight line at the speed of light. X-ray paths are not changed by electrical or magnetic fields. The degree of x-ray penetration depends on their energy and the characteristics of the material through which they pass. X-ray radiation possesses enough energy to ionize matter and can therefore damage living cells. For conventional radiographs, x-rays are generated by directing a stream of high-velocity electrons at a target material; x-rays are emitted from that source. X-rays are then directed as a beam through a body area. All tissues differ in their ability to absorb x-rays, thus differentially affecting the penetration of x-rays and their ability to pass through the subject. X-ray films are radiation-sensitive materials in a thin emulsion that record the x-ray radiation that reaches them. In this way, an image is developed that records the differential x-ray penetration based on the relative absorption of x-rays by tissues through which they pass.

CT scanners were developed in the early 1970s. These early machines consisted of an x-ray source and a single detector, which were interconnected at the gantry and rotated around the patient (**Box 1**). A tomographic (cross-sectional) image or slice was created by computer integration of data from a large series of two-dimensional x-ray images taken around a single axis of rotation. The early generations of CT scanners acquired a single anatomic cross section before the patient was moved a given distance, stopped, and the next slice obtained. Spiral or helical CT scan technology uses continuous movement of the patient through the gantry combined with continuous rotation of the x-ray source/detector system, creating a helical volume of data that can then be reconstructed at slice thicknesses specified by the user to create traditional axial image sets (**Fig. 1**). Modern spiral scanners with multiple rows of x-ray detectors (called multislice scanners, multirow scanners, or multirow detector scanners) allow image reconstruction of the CT volume data in other anatomic planes (eg, sagittal, coronal) and create a set of data that can be manipulated to produce complex three-dimensional images (**Fig. 2**).[1] This property is especially useful for depicting anatomic structures such as blood vessels that may span a long length or possess complex geometry, limiting the amount of information that can be obtained from traditional axial CT images. Rapid scanning minimizes motion artifact and allows acquisition of images in multiple phases of contrast enhancement (eg, arterial and portal venous phases in the liver).

The digital nature of CT scan data permits many sophisticated uses. These data can be easily transmitted from one location to another and digitally remastered. Magnified views, accurate measurements, and three-dimensional reconstructions are possible. Measurements of relative tissue density can be calculated for each pixel and numerically represented as Hounsfield units for comparison with reference tissues. Specific organs can be highlighted by variations in the gray tone scale in the processes known as windowing and leveling (**Fig. 3**). CT scans are often performed after administration of gastrointestinal contrast or with timed doses of intravascular contrast media to enhance the differences between adjacent structures.

CT imaging has tremendous diagnostic applications. CT scanning can also be a valuable therapeutic adjunct because it allows for precise three-dimensional targeting for invasive procedures such as percutaneous drainage, tube thoracostomy, and percutaneous biopsies.

Box 1
CT glossary of useful terms

Collimation

Process of controlling the size and shape of the x-ray beam that emerges from the x-ray tube or source

Detector

Portion of CT scanner at gantry that detects radiation that has penetrated the object being scanned

Gantry

Donut-shaped portion of CT scanner that contains both the x-ray source and detector(s)

Helical CT

Synonymous with spiral CT. Modern CT scanners in which the rotating x-ray beam traces a helical or spiral path around the patient as the CT table moves continuously through the gantry during scanning, in distinction to earlier scanners, in which the table stepped incrementally as each slice was obtained. All multislice or multirow detector scanners scan helically, although the first helical scanners contained only a single row of detectors and hence were single-slice machines.

Hounsfield Unit (HU)

Numeric information contained in each pixel of a CT image. This arbitrary unit is used to represent the x-ray attenuation capacity of tissue depicted by each pixel. By definition, water has a value of 0 HU, with other substances scaled relative to the attenuating capacity of water. For example, bone has Hounsfield values greater than 300.

Multidetector CT

Machine making simultaneous use of multiple rows of detectors that allow acquisition of a volume of data in a single gantry rotation such that multiple slices can be reconstructed from the data acquired in that single rotation. Synonymous with multirow detector CT and multislice CT.

Multiplanar reconstruction

Process of reformatting CT images in multiple planes based on data analysis of a volume of CT data obtained helically. This process is practical only with multislice scanners that have the necessary longitudinal (z-axis) resolution to allow distortion-free reconstruction. Reconstruction is possible in any anatomic plane that might be useful to visualize the anatomy of interest, although standard coronal and sagittal planes are most commonly used.

Phase

A set of CT images obtained during a single passage of the patient through the scanner, usually after the administration of contrast media

Pitch

Term used in spiral CT scanning to describe the distance that the patient table travels during one 360° rotation of the gantry divided by the collimated width of the x-ray beam. Pitch = 1 when the entire patient surface area is scanned without overlap or gap in the x-ray beam.

Slice

Single tomographic reconstruction of an anatomic cross section

Windowing

Process of determining the contrast and brightness levels assigned to CT image data. The optimal window level and width vary according to the tissue of interest (eg, lung vs soft tissue).

X-ray source

Synonymous with x-ray tube. Portion of CT scanner located within the gantry that generates penetrating electromagnetic radiation.

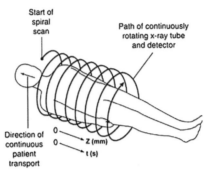

Fig. 1. Helical CT scan illustrating the spiral path traced around the patient as the table continuously moves through the gantry. (*Reprinted from* Mahesh M. The AAPM/RSNA Physics Tutorial for Residents: search for isotropic resolution in CT from conventional through multiple-row detector. Radiographics 2002;22:955; with permission.)

Patient Safety

The use of diagnostic CT scans has increased by as much as 20 times in the United States in the past 20 years.[2,3] The number of CT scans performed in the United States during 2007 was estimated at 70 million.[4] This dramatic trend has led to recent concern about the cumulative radiation exposure and associated lifetime attributable risk of radiation-induced cancers from CT scanning.[2–8] The most common radiation-induced cancers include thyroid cancer, breast cancer in women, lung cancer, and leukemia.[4] More than 90% of the collective population dose of radiation from diagnostic radiographs comes from a few high-dose procedures, including CT scans, interventional radiology studies, and barium enemas.[2] The risk of malignancy from a given radiation exposure is greater in young children and women.[4,8] Radiation exposure risks decrease with increasing age in both sexes.[8] Of all CT scans, those focused on the abdomen and pelvis impart the greatest radiation exposure, particularly when multiple acquisition phases are used.[3,4]

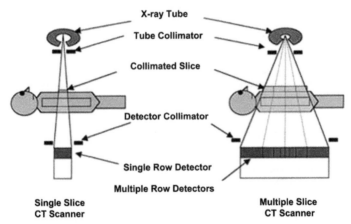

Fig. 2. Comparison of single-slice CT scanner (*left*) with a multiple-row detector unit (*right*). (*Reprinted from* Mahesh M. The AAPM/RSNA Physics Tutorial for Residents: search for isotropic resolution in CT from conventional through multiple-row detector. Radiographics 2002;22:958; with permission.)

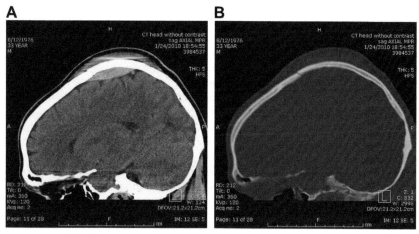

Fig. 3. CT scan of the head performed in a trauma patient. (*A*) Soft-tissue (cerebral) window shows hyperdense, lenticular fluid collection consistent with epidural hematoma. (*B*) Bone window clearly shows the associated, nondisplaced parietal bone fracture.

Using risk models based on organ-specific radiation doses and the biologic effects of ionizing radiation, one group estimated that 29,000 future cancers were related to CT scans performed in the United States during 2007 alone.[4] One-third of these projected cancers were attributed to CT scans performed in patients from 35 to 54 years old and 66% were in women.[4] In a study of trauma patients undergoing CT scans in an emergency department, the mean radiation dose was 22.7 mSv measured by dosimeters placed at the neck, chest, and groin.[7] These investigators extrapolated that the measured doses of radiation would result in 190 additional cancer deaths in a population of 100,000 receiving similar exposure.[7] In another study, the cumulative radiation exposure from 190,712 CT scans performed in 31,462 patients over a 22-year period was estimated.[6] Five percent of these patients underwent between 22 and 132 CT scans. CT scan radiation exposure was estimated to produce 0.7% of total expected cancer incidence and 1% of total cancer deaths in the entire study group. In a study of emergency department patients undergoing diagnostic CT scans over a 7.7-year period, the lifetime attributable risk of malignancy was calculated to be 1 in 82 patients.[5] Findings from these studies must be considered when determining the risk/benefit ratio of diagnostic CT imaging.

There are many strategies to mitigate the lifetime attributable risk of radiation-induced malignancies associated with CT scanning. Most important, the number of unnecessary scans must be reduced.[2,6–8] The number of routine follow-up CT scans should be limited to those that are clearly indicated.[5,6] Alternative imaging modalities should be used whenever possible. Institutions should standardize protocols that minimize the radiation dose for a given examination.[3] Methods to reduce the radiation dose delivered to a patient include reducing the milliampere-seconds value, increasing the pitch, using wider x-ray beam collimation (for multirow detector scanners), varying the milliampere-seconds value according to patient size, and lowering the beam energy.[9] The number of phases per study should be minimized.[3] Reconstructions using existing accessible data should be generated in lieu of additional scans or phases. In selected cases, CT scans can be limited to only those levels needed to image a single organ (eg, appendix or kidney). The increased risk of radiation exposure in young children and women should receive special consideration when CT scans are contemplated.[4,8]

Contrast-induced nephropathy (CIN) is the term used to describe nephrotoxicity associated with the use of intravascular iodinated contrast media. The pathophysiology of CIN involves contrast-induced reductions in renal perfusion and renal tubular flow resulting in an acute reduction in glomerular filtration rate (GFR).[10] Risk factors include preexisting chronic kidney disease (CKD) and diabetes.[10,11] The incidence of CIN after CT scanning in patients with CKD has been quantified at 2.5% despite pretreatment with intravenous fluid and N-acetyl cysteine.[11] N-acetyl cysteine is rapidly metabolized to intracellular glutathione, a powerful natural antioxidant. The incidences of CIN in this study were 0, 2.9%, and 12.1% in patients with estimated GFR of 45 to 59, 30 to 44, and less than 30 mL/min/1.73 m^2, respectively.[11] The development of CIN was associated with poor long-term kidney survival. Strategies to prevent CIN include use of intravenous fluid hydration before and after a CT scan with contrast and ordering alternative imaging tests that do not use radiographic iodinated contrast.[12] Although pretreatment of patients with renal impairment using N-acetyl cysteine has been controversial, the results of 2 recent meta-analyses support its use for prevention of CIN in high-risk patients.[13,14] The administration of N-acetyl cysteine decreased the incidence of CIN more than hydration alone at low cost and with few side effects.[13,14]

MR
Basic Principles

MR imaging (MRI) is based on the magnetic properties of hydrogen nuclei in human tissue. Hydrogen nuclei act as tiny magnets that spin in random directions until subjected to an externally applied magnetic field. When an outside source of strong magnetic energy is applied, the magnetic fields of the hydrogen atoms align themselves parallel to the direction of the external magnetic field, along an axis parallel to the length of the patient called the longitudinal axis or z-axis (**Figs. 4** and **5**).[15] The spinning hydrogen atoms each contain a tiny magnetic field that precesses about the externally applied magnetic field, much as a spinning top precesses about its axis (**Fig. 6**).[15] A radiofrequency (RF) pulse is then applied that is specifically targeted to hydrogen atoms. The pulse frequency is chosen such that it is equal to the frequency

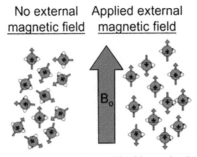

No external   Applied external
magnetic field   magnetic field

B$_0$

"Net Magnetization"

Fig. 4. The effect of a strong external magnetic field on hydrogen nuclei. On the left, hydrogen nuclei are oriented randomly in the absence of a magnetic field. On the right, hydrogen nuclei align themselves parallel to a strong magnetic field. (*Reprinted from* Pooley RA. AAPM/RSNA Physics Tutorial for Residents: fundamental physics of MR imaging. Radiographics 2005;25:1089; with permission.)

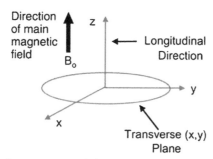

Fig. 5. In MRI, the coordinate system is defined with the longitudinal (z) axis aligned with the main magnetic field. The transverse plane lies perpendicular to the z-axis. (*Reprinted from* Pooley RA. AAPM/RSNA Physics Tutorial for Residents: fundamental physics of MR imaging. Radiographics 2005;25:1089; with permission.)

of precession of the tiny magnetic field of each hydrogen atom. This special RF pulse results in the efficient absorption of energy by the hydrogen atoms known as resonance, causing the hydrogen atoms (or more accurately their magnetic fields) to tip and assume a new orientation of precession. For example, a 90° pulse causes precessing hydrogen atoms to tip, changing the precession from the longitudinal axis to the transverse axis. When the RF pulse is terminated, the precessing hydrogen atoms return to their baseline alignment, releasing RF energy that can be detected and converted into an image.[16] This emitted RF energy is the echo measured in so-called spin-echo MRI pulse sequences. The frequency of the spinning protons or hydrogen atoms, and hence the frequency of the RF pulse needed for resonance, is determined by the Larmor equation (**Box 2**).[16]

Tissue contrast in MRI is related to differences in rates of magnetization decay and repolarization within specific tissues (so-called T1 and T2 constants, which vary in different tissues) as well as the proton content of different tissues. These differences in T1 and T2 constants can be exploited by selecting scan parameters that highlight these characteristics. T1-weighted images use short intervals between application of RF pulses (short TR) and short intervals between pulse application and signal acquisition (short TE). T2-weighted images emphasize differences in the T2 time constant of various tissues by using long TR and long TE.[17]

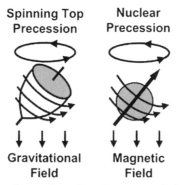

Fig. 6. Precession. Similar to the motion of a spinning top (*left*), precession describes the motion of hydrogen nuclei within an externally applied magnetic field (*right*). (*Reprinted from* Pooley RA. AAPM/RSNA Physics Tutorial for Residents: fundamental physics of MR imaging. Radiographics 2005;25:1090; with permission.)

Box 2
MR glossary of useful terms

Diffusion MRI

MRI that measures the diffusion of water molecules in different tissues. This is a highly sensitive study for the diagnosis of acute ischemic stroke.

Gadolinium

Element with paramagnetic properties that is used as an intravenous contrast agent in MRI

Gradient magnets

Three paired coils each oriented along one of the orthogonal axes, designed to produce gradients within the main magnetic field. These gradients allow spatial encoding of points within the image.

Larmor equation

Equation describing the relationship between an externally applied magnetic field and the frequency of precession of nuclei in that field

Pulse sequences

A preselected set of defined RF pulses and magnetic field gradient applications used to produce MR images

RF pulse

Electromagnetic signal emitted to cause resonance of hydrogen nuclei in the magnetic field. This process leads to the eventual release of RF energy, which is measured and used to create the MR image.

Relaxation

The process that occurs after termination of the RF pulse. The system of precessing nuclei relax, going from a higher energy state to a lower energy state and releasing RF energy, which is detected and converted to the MR image.

T1 relaxation

Also called spin-lattice relaxation. This process is regrowth of longitudinal magnetization as the spinning nuclei realign with the external magnetic field. The rate of this regrowth is tissue specific, and described by the T1 time constant of various tissues.

T1-weighted images

Images obtained using short intervals, or repetition times (TR), between application of RF pulses. The time to echo (TE), or the time at which the emitted RF signal caused by relaxation is measured, is also short. Using short TR and TE produces images in which tissue contrast is produced primarily by differences in the T1 time constant of various tissues.

T2 relaxation

Also called spin-spin relaxation. Decay of magnetization in the transverse plane after the RF pulse is terminated. The rate of this decay is tissue specific, and described by the T2 time constant of various tissues.

T2-weighted images

Images obtained using long intervals, or TR, between application of RF pulses. The TE, or the time at which the emitted RF signal caused by relaxation is measured, is also long. Using long TR and TE produces images in which tissue contrast is produced primarily by differences in the T2 time constant of different tissues.

Tesla

International unit of magnetic field strength or degree of magnetic induction

Time-of-flight

Technique using flow-related enhancement to generate images of blood vessels without the use of contrast media

Contrast media containing gadolinium can be administered intravenously to high-light differences seen in tissues on MR images. Gadolinium is a rare earth element (atomic number 64) that has paramagnetic properties. Administration of gadolinium causes a significant magnetic response in a well-perfused organ or blood vessel, making it strongly visible on MRI (gadolinium has a long T1 time constant relative to most tissues and is therefore bright on T1-weighted images). Contrast-enhanced MR angiography is often used to more accurately image arteries.

T1- and T2-weighted imaging form the basis of modern MRI sequences; however, new imaging sequences are continually being developed that exploit differences in the way various tissues respond to the complex manipulation of external magnetic fields and RF pulse delivery. For example, diffusion MRI has been developed to measure the diffusion of water molecules in certain tissues.[16] This study is highly sensitive for the diagnosis of acute ischemic strokes (**Fig. 7**).

The advantages of MRI include the absence of ionizing radiation and the infre-quent need for contrast media. MRI has been especially useful for the diagnosis

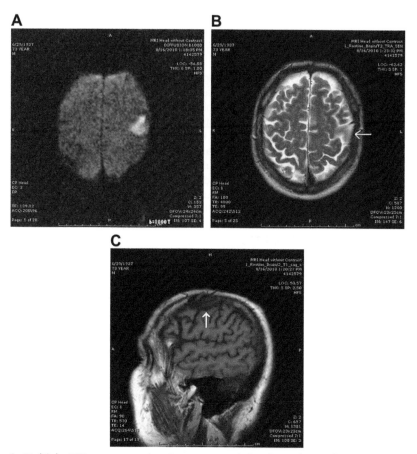

Fig. 7. Multiple MRI sequences showing an acute ischemic stroke in the middle cerebral artery territory of the left frontal lobe. (*A*) Diffusion-weighted sequence illustrates the bright, high signal lesion. (*B*) T2-weighted image shows more subtle high-signal lesion (*arrow*). (*C*) T1-weighted image shows subtle low signal lesion (*arrow*).

of multiple sclerosis, brain neoplasms, soft-tissue masses, bone masses, spinal injuries, joint injuries, and infections of the brain, joints, spine, and soft tissues. It also remains the most accurate imaging modality for the early diagnosis of ischemic stroke. Disadvantages include high cost, limited availability in certain locations, inability to scan patients with some implants (eg, pacemakers), long scan times, susceptibility to metallic and motion-related artifacts, and need for sedation in claustrophobic patients.

Patient Safety

There are no known biologic hazards to humans from exposure to magnetic fields or the RF pulses used in current MRI.[16] However, there are significant risks from the effects of the powerful magnets on metallic objects within the MR suite or within potential patients. MRI is contraindicated in patients with permanent cardiac pacemakers, metallic fragments within the eyes, and ferromagnetic intracranial aneurysm clips. If the metallic implants are strongly incorporated, they are not at risk for deflection in the magnetic field. For example, patients with total joint prostheses are not at risk for dislodgement because of the strength of cement and bony incorporation. Also, metals without iron are not affected by the magnets. Therefore, patients with intravascular stents made of a nickel-titanium alloy may safely undergo MRI. A list of MR-safe and MR-unsafe devices is available online at http://www. mrisafety.com/.

The use of gadolinium-based contrast agents for MRI has recently been shown to have risks in selected patients. Anaphylactic reactions to these agents are rare. However, an association between gadolinium-based contrast media given for MRI and the development of nephrogenic systemic fibrosis (NSF) in patients with CKD has been described.[18–21] NSF develops in patients with severe, end-stage renal disease after exposure to gadolinium-based contrast in a dose-dependent and time-dependent fashion.[18] Since several public health warnings about this association were issued by the US Food and Drug Administration, one study has documented a 71% decrease in the number of gadolinium-enhanced MR studies used in patients with GFR less than 30 mL/min/1.73 m^2.[20] If contrast imaging is necessary in patients with CKD, the risk of NSF must be balanced against the risks of alternative procedures, such as CIN with CT imaging.[21]

US
Basic Principles

Conventional US is based on the pulse-echo principle in which sound waves are transmitted through a medium and reflected back.[22] US machines consist of a transducer that both emits the ultrasonic sound waves and detects the echo. The frequency of sound waves used is more than the auditory limit of 20 kHz or 20,000 cycles/s.[22] The piezoelectric crystals within the transducer both convert electrical energy into acoustic waves and reverse the process when returning sound waves are received (**Box 3**).[22] The echo signals reflecting off the many structures lying along the path of the pulse are then analyzed and displayed as a cross-sectional tomographic image.[23] For B-mode US, the brightness of each pixel corresponds to the amplitude of the reflected sound wave.[23] Hyperechoic structures appear brighter and hypoechoic tissues are darker than surrounding tissues. The strength of an echo is determined by the differential acoustic impedance between adjacent structures.[23]

Images can be made clearer by changing the angles of the transducer, increasing piezoelectric crystal size, changing the US frequency, or focusing the sound beam.

Box 3
US glossary of useful terms

Acoustic impedance

Property of tissue defined as the product of the tissue density multiplied by the velocity of sound waves traveling through the tissue. The strength of an echo is determined by the difference in impedance between adjacent tissues.

Acoustic intensity

Power of a US pulse per unit of cross-sectional area

Attenuation

Loss of US signal strength as it passes through tissue as a result of absorption and scattering

B-mode

Brightness mode US. Brightness of each pixel corresponds to amplitude of the reflected sound wave.

Color-flow Doppler

US image in which flow (typically blood flow) is color coded for motion toward or away from the transducer. The image produced is a hybrid combining anatomic information from a B-mode image as well as pulsed Doppler analysis.

Continuous-wave Doppler

Device with separate transmitting and receiving probes that allows for continuous transmission of sound waves. Used to detect flow within blood vessels.

Doppler US

Device that uses Doppler shift effect of sound reflected off a moving object. The magnitude of the frequency shift can be used to calculate the velocity of moving objects such as red blood cells.

Duplex US

US using both B-mode imaging and Doppler waveform analysis

Echogenic

Capable of producing echoes. Various structures may be more (eg, gallstones) or less (eg, fluid) echogenic.

Gain

Amplification of the returning US signal

Hyperechoic

Image echoes are brighter than surrounding tissues

Hypoechoic

Image echoes are darker than surrounding tissues

Intensity

Magnitude or strength of US signal

Piezoelectric property

Material property by which mechanical motion or deformation is converted into electrical current, and vice versa.

Pulsed-wave Doppler

Transmission of sound waves in pulses. Transmission and reception are performed by the same transducer. The depth of a tissue echo can be measured and therefore localized in 3 dimensions.

Doppler spectrum

The range of frequencies (or, more accurately, frequency shifts) measured over time, which is converted by the US unit to velocity measurements. When velocity (y-axis) is plotted versus time (x-axis), the result is the characteristic waveform seen when interrogating a blood vessel. Flow velocity is related to vessel stenosis. Synonymous with Doppler waveform.

Transducer

Device from which US waves are emitted and echoes are detected

As US frequency is increased to improve axial resolution, the depth of tissue penetration is decreased.[23] This property makes US especially well suited for evaluating superficial structures such as the thyroid, breast, and carotid artery. Machine gain can be adjusted to increase the volume of echoes. The US beam is usually directed to the depth of the anatomic structure for which US images are most desired. Contemporary US technology allows for multiple areas of beam focusing on the same image.[24]

In addition to the visual images created in B-mode US, Doppler US is a useful adjunct for interrogating moving objects, such as red blood cells within blood vessels. Using the Doppler shift effect of sound reflecting off a moving object, the velocity of the object can be calculated by analysis of the frequency changes. Spectral analysis of these reflected frequencies is used to calculate the flow velocity within a blood vessel. Increases in velocity are then related to stenoses in the involved vessel. Color flow Doppler US equipment color codes for the direction of flow within a vessel (**Fig. 8**).[22] Duplex US refers to the use of both B-mode images and Doppler waveform analysis in diagnostic studies.

US has both diagnostic and therapeutic applications. Its real-time capability and mobility of the equipment makes this modality ideal as an adjunct for numerous bedside or operating-room procedures. Specialized probes have enhanced use in transvaginal, transrectal, and endoscopic settings. The lack of ionizing radiation makes US-associated techniques safer for both patients and operators.

Patient Safety

Although US energy has the potential for inducing temperature increases and cavitation of tissues as well as triggering an inflammatory response, these effects have not been reported to occur at the US output power levels used by current diagnostic machines. Human injury has never been attributed to the clinical practice of US as long as it is used within well-established standards of output power.[23] Precise definitions of US energy characteristics, output power measurement procedures, and labeling requirements have helped ensure the safety of this diagnostic modality.

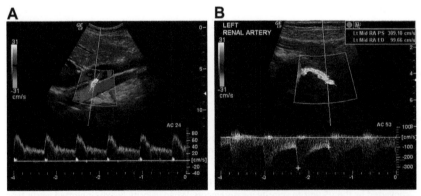

Fig. 8. Color flow duplex US images of renal arteries. (*A*) Normal left renal artery with uniform red color, indicating laminar blood flow in a single direction. Peak systolic velocity = 80 cm/s, which is consistent with less than 40% stenosis. (*B*) Left renal artery with a variety of colors, indicating turbulent blood flow in multiple directions. Peak systolic velocity = 309 cm/s, which is consistent with more than 70% stenosis.

REFERENCES

1. Mahesh M. Search for isotropic resolution in CT from conventional through multiple-row detector. Radiographics 2002;22(4):949–62.
2. Hall EJ, Brenner DJ. Cancer risks from diagnostic radiology. Br J Radiol 2008; 81(965):362–78.
3. Smith-Bindman R, Lipson J, Marcus R, et al. Radiation dose associated with common computed tomography examinations and the associated lifetime attributable risk of cancer. Arch Intern Med 2009;169(22):2078–86.
4. Berrington de Gonzalez A, Mahesh M, Kim KP, et al. Projected cancer risks from computed tomographic scans performed in the United States in 2007. Arch Intern Med 2009;169(22):2071–7.
5. Griffey RT, Sodickson A. Cumulative radiation exposure and cancer risk estimates in emergency department patients undergoing repeat or multiple CT. AJR Am J Roentgenol 2009;192(4):887–92.
6. Sodickson A, Baeyens PF, Andriole KP, et al. Recurrent CT, cumulative radiation exposure, and associated radiation-induced cancer risks from CT of adults. Radiology 2009;251(1):175–84.
7. Tien HC, Tremblay LN, Rizoli SB, et al. Radiation exposure from diagnostic imaging in severely injured trauma patients. J Trauma 2007;62(1):151–6.
8. Mayo JR. Radiation dose issues in longitudinal studies involving computed tomography. Proc Am Thorac Soc 2008;5(9):934–9.
9. McNitt-Gray MF. AAPM/RSNA Physics Tutorial for Residents: topics in CT. Radiation dose in CT. Radiographics 2002;22(6):1541–53.
10. Feldkamp T, Kribben A. Contrast media induced nephropathy: definition, incidence, outcome, pathophysiology, risk factors and prevention. Minerva Med 2008;99(2):177–96.
11. Kim SM, Cha RH, Lee JP, et al. Incidence and outcomes of contrast-induced nephropathy after computed tomography in patients with CKD: a quality improvement report. Am J Kidney Dis 2010;55(6):1018–25.
12. Ellis JH, Cohan RH. Prevention of contrast-induced nephropathy: an overview. Radiol Clin North Am 2009;47(5):801–11.
13. Kelly AM, Dwamena B, Cronin P, et al. Meta-analysis: effectiveness of drugs for preventing contrast-induced nephropathy. Ann Intern Med 2008;148(4):284–94.
14. Trivedi H, Daram S, Szabo A, et al. High-dose N-acetylcysteine for the prevention of contrast-induced nephropathy. Am J Med 2009;122(9):874, e9–15.
15. Pooley RA. AAPM/RSNA Physics Tutorial for Residents: fundamental physics of MR imaging. Radiographics 2005;25(4):1087–99.
16. Bitar R, Leung G, Perng R, et al. MR pulse sequences: what every radiologist wants to know but is afraid to ask. Radiographics 2006;26(2):513–37.
17. Horowitz AL. MRI physics for radiologists: a visual approach [etc]. New York: Springer; 1995.
18. Abujudeh HH, Kaewlai R, Kagan A, et al. Nephrogenic systemic fibrosis after gadopentetate dimeglumine exposure: case series of 36 patients. Radiology 2009;253(1):81–9.
19. Broome DR. Nephrogenic systemic fibrosis associated with gadolinium based contrast agents: a summary of the medical literature reporting. Eur J Radiol 2008;66(2):230–4.
20. Kim KH, Fonda JR, Lawler EV, et al. Change in use of gadolinium-enhanced magnetic resonance studies in kidney disease patients after US Food and

Drug Administration warnings: a cross-sectional study of Veterans Affairs Health Care System data from 2005–2008. Am J Kidney Dis 2010;56(3):458–67.

21. Saab G, Abu-Alfa A. Nephrogenic systemic fibrosis–implications for nephrologists. Eur J Radiol 2008;66(2):208–12.

22. Case TD. Ultrasound physics and instrumentation. Surg Clin North Am 1998; 78(2):197–217.

23. Hangiandreou NJ. AAPM/RSNA Physics Tutorial for Residents. Topics in US: B-mode US: basic concepts and new technology. Radiographics 2003;23(4): 1019–33.

24. Smith RS, Fry WR. Ultrasound instrumentation. Surg Clin North Am 2004;84(4): 953–71.

Imaging of the Thyroid and Parathyroid Glands

Bianca J. Vazquez, MD, Melanie L. Richards, MD, MHPE*

KEYWORDS

- Thyroid ultrasound • Parathyroid imaging • Thyroid nodule
- Hyperparathyroidism • Thyroid imaging

The development of highly advanced and modern imaging techniques played a critical evolutionary role in the surgical management of thyroid disorders. Historically, the surgery for thyroid disease was limited to cases of impending death and even then was met with reluctance because of the prohibitive mortality and morbidity.[1,2] In combination with advances in asepsis, anesthesia, and surgical instrumentation, the development of ultrasonography (US) during the twentieth century provided the platform to continue the rapid acceleration of thyroid and parathyroid surgery.

With a better understanding of thyroid and parathyroid anatomy and physiology, a multimodal approach can be offered to thyroid disorders, starting with a focused clinical history, physical examination, biochemical studies, and possible fine-needle aspiration (FNA). This article presents an overview of the modern imaging techniques available to supplement this evaluation, including high-resolution US, nuclear scintigraphy, thin-section CT, MRI, and combination modalities, such as fludeoxyglucose F 18 positron emission tomography (FDG PET) and single-photon emission computed tomography (SPECT).

THYROID GLAND

In patients with thyroid disorders, clinical examination by an experienced clinician with appropriate laboratory values is the initial diagnostic protocol of choice. When assessing the morphology of the thyroid, a systematic approach should be undertaken to document thyroid volume, texture, number and location of lesions, and a thorough description of nonthyroidal anatomy. Most thyroid nodules are nonpalpable lesions found as incidental findings (incidentalomas) during imaging for unrelated pathologic condition. Numerous studies suggest an overall prevalence of 2% to 6% with

The authors have nothing to disclose.
Division Gastroenterologic and General Surgery, Department of Surgery, Mayo Clinic, 200 First Street SW, Rochester, MN 55905, USA
* Corresponding author.
E-mail address: richards.melanie@mayo.edu

Surg Clin N Am 91 (2011) 15–32
doi:10.1016/j.suc.2010.10.015
0039-6109/11/$ – see front matter © 2011 Elsevier Inc. All rights reserved.

palpation, 19% to 35% with US, and 8% to 65% in autopsy data.[3,4] Despite the high prevalence of nonpalpable thyroid nodules in the population, thyroid cancer is found in approximately 5% to 10% of these patients with nonpalpable thyroid nodules[5] and many have subcentimeter microcarcinomas that are often of no clinical significance. Approximately 37,200 new cases of thyroid cancer were expected to be diagnosed in 2009 and 1630 patients were expected to die of the disease.[6] The prevalence of cancer in patients with solitary lesions is similar to that in those with multinodular disease (approximately 15%).[7]

US

Ultrasound evaluation and ultrasound-guided FNA biopsy are critical for the diagnosis and treatment of patients with thyroid nodular disease.[8] US of the neck remains the most useful imaging technique in the evaluation of the thyroid gland for patients with a confirmed or suspected thyroid nodule on physical examination. It is safe, noninvasive, relatively inexpensive, and easily available for point-of-care evaluation in the clinic or the operating room. The portable equipment provides an immediate 2-dimensional gray scale image of the neck through high resolution and frequency transducers. Although the technique accurately identifies nonpalpable lesions, it should not be considered a screening tool but rather a diagnostic aid in the evaluation of diffuse thyroid disease and suspected thyroid nodules or to assess for metastatic thyroid cancer in the neck.

High resolution and frequency (7–13 MHz) linear US can detect lesions as small as 3 mm and distinguish cystic versus solid lesions. Scanning should occur in the transverse and longitudinal planes. The patient should be in supine position with neck extension. A patient with a thicker neck may benefit from lower frequencies (6 MHz) because this improves the image depth. Qualitative features, such as contents, calcifications, borders, shapes, echotexture, and vascularity, when evaluated, in combination, can provide information about the malignancy potential of thyroid lesions and should be documented.

A normal thyroid gland appears homogeneous with lack of internal architecture and with multiple small vessels within and adjacent to the gland on color Doppler.[8] US for diffuse thyroid disease is limited by its lack of specificity. Hashimoto thyroiditis can be identified as a diffusely heterogeneous gland filled with millimeter-sized hypoechoic nodules separated by echoic septation and without evidence of normal thyroid parenchyma. Depending on the stage and duration of the disease, the size of the thyroid gland may appear normal, enlarged, or small.[9] US findings that are consistent with Graves disease are a diffusely hypoechoic gland with lobulations.

Ultrasound-guided FNA is the initial diagnostic procedure of preference to evaluate suspicious thyroid nodules with a higher likelihood of nondiagnostic cytology (>25%–50% cystic component) or sampling error (difficult to palpate or posterior location).[10] The American Thyroid Association (ATA) recommends ultrasound guidance when repeating the FNA procedure for a nodule with initial nondiagnostic cytology results.[10] To obtain an accurate biopsy with the lowest risk of nondiagnostic cytology the authors recommend using ultrasound guidance with all FNA biopsies. When compared with conventional FNA biopsy performed with palpation, ultrasound guidance provides diagnosis with higher sensitivity (91.8% vs 97.1%), specificity (68.8% vs 70.9%) and accuracy (72.6% vs 75.9%).[11]

Despite low sensitivity and positive predictive value, certain ultrasonography findings, when appearing together, can suggest an increased risk of malignancy in a thyroid lesion (**Fig. 1**).[5,10–14] A cystic nodule with a large solid component and microcalcifications may represent papillary cancer and should prompt biopsy. Hypoechoic

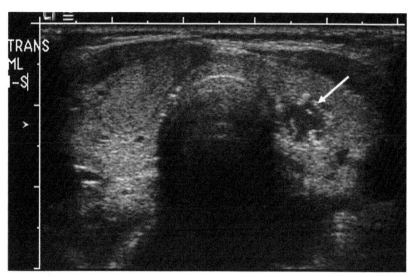

Fig. 1. Neck US, transverse view, showing left suspicious thyroid nodule (*white arrow*). On FNA, papillary thyroid cancer was found to be harbored.

nodules and elongated shape (AP to transverse ratio >1) are features considered suspicious for malignancy. These US findings differ from those, typical of benign nodules and not of concern, such as: well-defined borders; punctuated hyperechogenicity; comet-tail artifact; spongiform appearance; or coarse, large, scattered, or peripheral (eggshell) calcifications.[8,15,16] Spiculated, nodular borders and hypervascularity on color Doppler ultrasonography concern papillary thyroid cancer invading surrounding tissues. Follicular carcinoma, Hürthle cell carcinoma, and the follicular variant of papillary cancer do not exhibit the classic malignant sonographic features. Follicular cancer is most likely to appear as a hyperechoic nodule, with thick irregular halo and no microcalcifications.[17] Sillery and colleagues[18] found that the sonographic features of follicular adenoma and follicular carcinoma are very similar, but the lack of a sonographic halo and hypoechoic appearance and absence of cystic change may suggest a follicular carcinoma. Within the follicular carcinoma subgroup, Hürthle cell variant of follicular carcinoma was more often seen in older patients with nodules having a heterogeneous appearance and lacking internal calcifications.[18]

The use of preoperative ultrasonography for the diagnosis of metastatic or locally advanced disease in patients with known thyroid cancer has been shown to alter the planned operative procedure and guide the extent of lymphadenectomy by identifying suspicious cervical lymphadenopathy (**Fig. 2**). In a Mayo Clinic series, Stulak and colleagues[19] reviewed 709 patients with papillary thyroid carcinoma who underwent preoperative neck US. Sonography detected nonpalpable lymph node metastasis in 33% of patients, thereby altering the initial operative approach. The ATA and the American Association of Clinical Endocrinologists recommend preoperative neck US on all patients undergoing thyroidectomy for biopsy-proven malignancy.[10,20] These associations do not recommend the use of other routine imaging modalities (CT, MRI, or positron emission tomography [PET]), given their low sensitivities for detection of cervical lymph node metastasis.[10] The role of US in the postoperative surveillance and pregnancy setting has also been established; US is a beneficial alternative method to scintigraphy to evaluate the thyroid bed and local node basins without requiring thyroid hormone cessation[8] or radioactive agent exposure. Patients

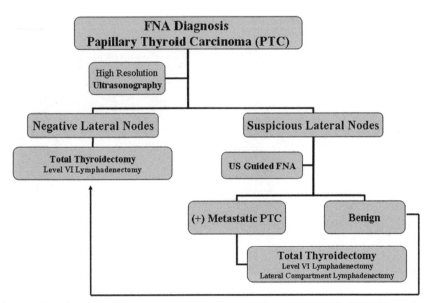

Fig. 2. Algorithm for locoregional nodal assessment in patients with FNA diagnosis of papillary thyroid carcinoma.

with thyroid cancer undergo routine neck US as part of their ongoing surveillance for recurrent disease. The ATA recommends cervical US to evaluate the thyroid bed and central and lateral cervical nodal compartments at 6 to 12 months and then periodically, depending on the patient's risk for recurrent disease and thyroglobulin status.[10]

Sonographic elastography has emerged as a new modality to characterize thyroid nodules by measuring tissue stiffness and deformity under external compression. Malignant tumors are harder than benign disease, and therefore it is suggested that they show less deformity than surrounding normal thyroid tissue. Rago and colleagues[21] presented a series of 92 consecutive cases in which the highest elasticity scores were invariably associated with malignancy with a minimal loss of sensitivity (specificity 100%, sensitivity 97%). Wang and colleagues[22] also reported promising results diagnosing papillary thyroid microcarcinomas with a sensitivity of 91%, a specificity of 89%, and an accuracy of 90%. These results show potential; however, further prospective studies are needed to establish this technique as routine in the diagnostic evaluation of patients with thyroid malignancies. Sample size, interobserver agreement, and usefulness in the diagnosis of all subtypes of thyroid malignancies are current issues to be addressed.

Scintigraphy

This nuclear medicine technique relies on the affinity of thyroid and parathyroid tissues for several different radioisotopes. Many of the tracers were initially used as myocardial perfusion agents; however, these tracers were found to be taken up by hyperfunctioning thyroid or parathyroid tissues. Scintigraphy is an important tool when evaluating an enlarged thyrotoxic gland and the patient with nodular thyroid disease and a suppressed thyroid-stimulating hormone (TSH) level.

Although its routine use has largely been abandoned, the role of scintigraphy in the evaluation of the dysfunctional thyroid gland has been established for years. Two radiotracers, sodium iodide I 123 and technetium Tc 99m pertechnetate, are used to outline the gland in patients with abnormal TSH levels. Thyroid activity can be established with a 5-minute technetium Tc 99m pertechnetate image,[23] providing physicians with a quick and sharp anatomic evaluation. Because sodium iodide I 123 is taken up and organified by the gland, it is preferred when evaluating thyroid function. Gamma camera–standardized protocols using pinhole and parallel hole collimator images allow for high spatial resolution and accurate tissue marking, respectively. Thyroid scintigraphy is limited by medications (ie, lithium) and dietary iodine intake. The technique requires cessation of thyroid supplementation for 3 to 4 weeks. Diffuse increased uptake is seen in Graves disease and early Hashimoto thyroiditis. Subacute Hashimoto or postpartum thyroiditis is present with diffused decrease radiotracer uptake. A solitary nodule with increased uptake is known as a "hot nodule" and is usually considered a benign finding representative of a hyperfunctioning adenoma. The risk of cancer is very low; therefore these patients can be managed medically. A hot nodule in a patient with a suppressed TSH can be treated with radioiodine, surgery, or antithyroid medications. A solitary nodule with decreased uptake is known as a "cold nodule" and most commonly represents a colloid cyst or adenoma. However, cancer risk is increased and further diagnostics, ie, FNA, may be required. The literature reports the risk of cancer to be 1% to 4% for a hot nodule and 15% to 25% for a cold nodule.[24]

Radioiodine has also been used as a radiotracer for whole body scans (WBSs) in patients with thyroid cancer to assess completeness of surgical resection, detect recurrence, or diagnose metastatic disease. WBS can be performed as a pretherapy, posttherapy, or diagnostic test after total thyroidectomy. Pretherapy WBS (before starting therapeutic dosage of radioactive iodine) has fallen out of favor because of its usual lack of effect on treatment plan and because of concerns of radiotracer-induced tissue stunning. Thyroid stunning is usually defined as the inhibition or suppression of iodine trapping by remnant thyroid tissue or by functioning metastases after a diagnostic dose of sodium iodide I 131.[25] If pretherapy WBS is performed, it should use sodium iodide I 123 or low-activity sodium iodide I 131 with the therapeutic activity optimally administered within 72 hours of the diagnostic activity to minimize risk of stunning.[10,26] Posttherapy WBS performed a week posttherapeutic dosage of radioactive iodine can help in predicting prognosis and identifying patients requiring additional workup.[27] This technique has a higher diagnostic value than pretreatment studies. Fatourechi and colleagues[28] presented a series of patients with posttherapy WBS in which 13% of patient scans demonstrated abnormal uptake that was not seen on pretherapy WBS, changing management strategy in 9% of patients. A diagnostic WBS is used to determine the need for further radioiodine treatment in the setting of metastatic disease or residual thyroid bed tissue in patients with a past history of radioactive iodine therapy. The follow-up of high- or intermediate-risk patients for persistent disease is the current indication for its use.[10] Radioiodine WBS offers limited anatomic landmarks because the tracer is taken up or secreted in various organs and in infected/inflamed tissues, limiting its sensitivity and increasing false-positive results.[29]

PET

A relatively new topic of interest is the incidental finding of thyroid nodules found on PET imaging done during the evaluation of other malignancies. About 1% to 2% of patients undergoing PET scan for unrelated reasons have thyroid incidentalomas discovered.[10,30–32] The risk of malignancy in these nodules has been reported to be 33% to 35% and is higher in young patients and when the malignancy harbors aggressive histopathologic features; therefore prompt evaluation is recommended.[10,30–32] In patients with recurrent thyroid cancer, PET scan may be of modest benefit. Grant and colleagues[33] presented the comparative value of PET versus US for localization of locoregional recurrence in patients reoperated for recurrent papillary thyroid cancer, demonstrating high false-negative rates (50%). The use of PET imaging added diagnostic value over US in only 10% of the patient population. FDG PET scan seems to have a high sensitivity for identifying malignant tissue, but its low specificity, high false-negative rates, and cost limit the use of this technique as a routine screening or surveillance tool.

CT

The role of CT imaging in thyroid disease is primarily limited to presurgical evaluation with a goal of assessing the extent of the disease, substernal components, or pathologic relationship with extrathyroidal structures, ie, trachea-esophageal or vascular involvement (**Fig. 3**). This modality can also be used in the evaluation of extrathyroidal manifestation of thyroid disorders. In patients with Graves orbitopathy, CT provides precise imaging of the osseous periorbital structures, making it an excellent method to plan CT-guided orbital decompression surgery.[34]

CT provides thin-section (3–5 mm) images by obtaining a series of radiographic projections in various angles and reconstructing them in a 2-dimensional fashion. Because of its high iodine content, the thyroid gland attenuates more than nearby soft tissues, appearing slightly brighter.[35]

If possible, CT should be performed without contrast because the iodine load received may delay treatment with radioiodine and may also lead to thyroid storm. When contrast is used, scintigraphy has to be delayed for approximately 4 to 6 weeks, given the cellular saturation with iodinated contrast agent.[36] Although CT scan is not as sensitive as ultrasonography and scintigraphy for the evaluation of intrathyroidal lesions, it can detect enlarged cervical lesions, tumor extension in the surrounding tissues,[8] and distant chest and abdominal metastases. Considering all compartments of the neck (level I-VI), contrast-enhanced CT scan can detect involved lymph nodes with a sensitivity of 35%, specificity of 96%, and diagnostic accuracy of 87%.[37]

SPECT/CT is a recently developed hybrid modality that combines nuclear medicine and CT technology to identify tissue nature and enhanced characteristics of large neck masses, especially if the tissues extend into the mediastinum. The CT portion provides the structural map to accurately localize the radiotracer uptake site. This technique

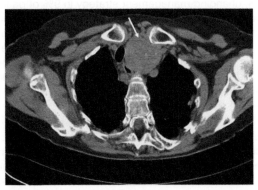

Fig. 3. An axial image of CT scan demonstrating a large thyroid goiter with substernal components (*white arrow*).

can be performed in a single session without moving the patient from the radiology suite. A recent study showed an incremental value of SPECT/CT over WBS in increasing diagnostic accuracy, reducing pitfalls, and modifying therapeutic strategies in patients with differentiated thyroid cancers.[38]

MRI

MRI is generally used for specific indications, including the evaluation of substernal goiters and their relation to other structures, assessment of the local extent of thyroid carcinomas, and localization of recurrent sites of thyroid neoplasia. MRI has also been used for the investigation of congenital disorders of the thyroid gland and the evaluation of diffuse thyroid diseases, such as Graves disease, Hashimoto and Riedel thyroiditis, and hemochromatosis.[39] Thyroid carcinomas are isointense or slightly hypointense lesions on T1-weighted images and hyperintense lesions on T2-weighted images compared with normal thyroid tissue.[40]

PARATHYROID GLANDS

A solitary parathyroid adenoma is the most common cause of primary hyperparathyroidism (HPT), the most common disorder of the parathyroid glands and the focus of this review. Historically, a bilateral cervical exploration to identify 4 parathyroid glands was the gold standard because of the presence of multiglandular disease in approximately 15% of patients. Without localization studies, the success of the bilateral exploration is approximately 98%. The advent of intraoperative parathyroid monitoring brought about advances in parathyroid imaging and allowed surgeons to perform a focused exploration with equivalent success to a bilateral exploration. This transition from an operation that required no preoperative imaging to an operation that depended on imaging has led to the development of new techniques in parathyroid imaging.

Scintigraphy

Although multiple modalities have been used to image the parathyroid glands, the most clinically relevant is scintigraphy. Technetium Tc 99m sestamibi, technetium Tc 99m tetrofosmin, and thallous chloride Tl 201 are the parathyroid tissue–localizing agents. The most common agent used is technetium Tc 99m sestamibi. Because of a lack of specificity for parathyroid tissue, these radiotracers can be used in combination with specific thyroid agents, such as sodium iodide I 123. The sestamibi are taken up by thyroid and parathyroid tissue; however, abnormal parathyroid tissue takes up the tracer more avidly and retains it for a longer period of time.[41] Therefore, initial grayscale 2-dimensional planar views show both glands, with areas of more intense uptake corresponding to hyperfunctional parathyroid tissue (**Figs. 4** and **5**). Images that are limited to the neck can overlook ectopic glands. Therefore, images should extend from the base of the jaw to the apex of the heart (**Fig. 6**).[42] Once the tissues are visualized, the thyroid scan done with sodium iodide I 123 can be digitally subtracted, allowing better visualization of suspicious parathyroid tissue. Delayed sestamibi images (2 hours later) confirm these findings. When the suspected tumor is ectopically located, intrathyroidal or in deeper tissues of the neck, an immediate SPECT 3-dimensional image (**Fig. 7**) can be obtained for increased resolution and improved anatomic characterization and surgical planning.[43] Pinhole or parallel hole SPECT collimator images can be obtained. A pinhole collimator can detect parathyroid pathology with a higher sensitivity (87%) than parallel hole SPECT (82%) in patients with primary HPT.[44]

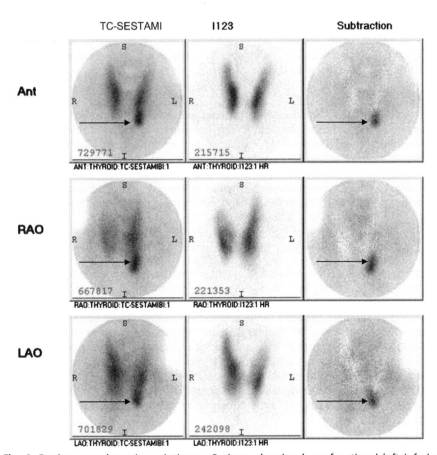

Fig. 4. Dual-tracer subtraction scintigram, 3 views, showing hyperfunctional left inferior parathyroid gland (*black arrows*). Ant, anterior; HR, hour; I, inferior; L, left; LAO, lateral anterior oblique; R, right; S, superior.

Parathyroid scintigraphy with technetium Tc 99m sestamibi can identify a single adenoma, double adenomas, and multiglandular hyperplasia with sensitivities of 88%, 29.9%, and 44%.[45] A technetium Tc 99m sestamibi–sodium iodide I 123 parathyroid subtraction scan is the authors' localization study of choice in patients with primary HPT who are being evaluated for surgery. Combining this technique with SPECT has been shown to increase sensitivity to 96% for single hyperfunctional adenoma, 83% for double adenomas, and 45% for multiglandular disease, for an overall sensitivity of 87%.[46]

The decision to use parathyroid scintigraphy in patients with secondary or tertiary HPT is surgeon dependent. Even when a bilateral exploration is planned, parathyroid scintigraphy may aid the surgeon in identifying ectopic or extranumerary parathyroid glands. In a retrospective review of the Mayo Clinic database from 2000 to 2004, scintigraphy correctly identified both the number and locations of all hyperplastic glands in only 28% of the patients with secondary or tertiary HPT.[47]

Imaging is mandatory before reoperation for parathyroid disease, and scintigraphy results should, ideally, be confirmed with a second technique (**Fig. 8**).[48] Parathyroid reexplorations, in the past, had been associated with increased failure rates, incidence of permanent hypocalcemia greater than 10%, and 5-fold increased recurrent

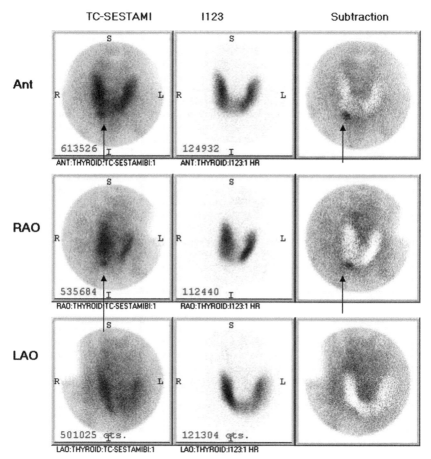

Fig. 5. Dual-tracer subtraction scintigram, 3 views, showing hyperfunctional right inferior parathyroid gland (*black arrows*). Ant, anterior; HR, hour; I, inferior; L, left; LAO, lateral anterior oblique; R, right; S, superior.

laryngeal nerve injury rate.[49] To improve these outcomes, a localizing study becomes critical in the decision to proceed with reoperations for HPT. Detection of recurrent or persistent parathyroid disease with both sestamibi subtraction and neck US allows the surgeon to confidently predict the precise location of the involved parathyroid gland.[49] Combined imaging clearly improves diagnostic accuracy and parathyroid localization and aids in surgical planning. Curative surgery has been reported in up to 89% of patients, with permanent hypoparathyroidism as low as 3%.[49]

US

On US, a parathyroid adenoma appears as a homogeneous, hypoechoic, and well-demarcated mass contrasting with a hyperechoic thyroid gland (**Fig. 9**).[48] These adenomas are usually found on the posterior aspect of the thyroidal lobes with a tendency to migrate in a downward direction.[48] The current role of US in parathyroid disease is limited to localization and delineation rather than diagnostics, and US is usually used as a complement to scintigraphy in the evaluation of patients with a diagnosis of HPT.

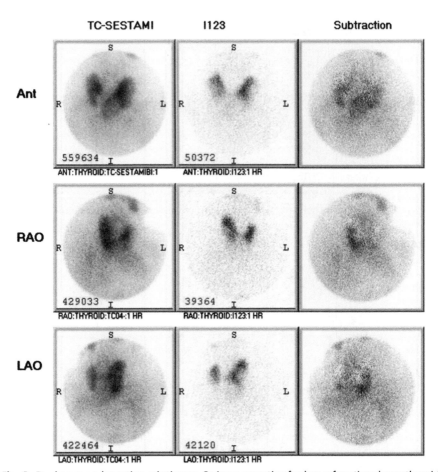

Fig. 6. Dual-tracer subtraction scintigram, 3 views, negative for hyperfunctional parathyroid glands. Ant, anterior; HR, hour; I, inferior; L, left; LAO, lateral anterior oblique; R, right; S, superior.

The ultrasound technique is similar to that of thyroid gland evaluation with longitudinal (**Fig. 10**) and transverse views of the neck from the carotid to the midline and from the hyoid region to the sternal notch. Deeply located retroclavicular inferior glands can be visualized by having patients swallow under real-time observation.[50] However, sonography is limited in patients with ectopic glands, especially those glands located in the mediastinum. When used as the initial localizing technique, surgeon-performed US can identify all abnormal parathyroids with a sensitivity of 77%.[51] The authors' experience in the localization of parathyroid glands has found US to have a sensitivity of 61% compared with a sensitivity of 86% for dual-isotope parathyroid scintigraphy.[52] When used in combination with scintigraphy, US localizes pathologic glands with a sensitivity as high as 95%.[41] The technique is particularly helpful in the reoperative setting in which concordant findings on 2 imaging studies are associated with an improved outcome.[53]

US is clearly an advantageous technique, readily available without patient morbidity. However, US is limited by low sensitivity and operator dependency. In combination with other diagnostic and imaging modalities, the technique may provide physicians with invaluable information.

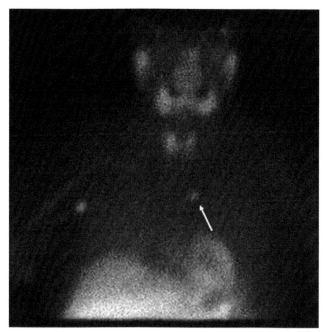

Fig. 7. A SPECT view depicting ectopic parathyroid adenoma in the thoracic cavity (*white arrow*).

CT

Thin-cut, contrast-enhanced, axial CT from the base of the skull to the mediastinum can be used in the setting of conflicting initial studies secondary to altered anatomy or after failed exploration. The sensitivity of CT for the detection of abnormal parathyroid glands depends on the size of the lesions and has been reported to range from 46% to 87%.[35,39]

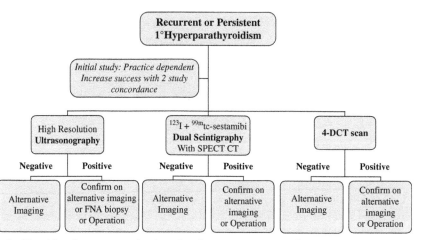

Fig. 8. Algorithm for preoperative imaging for recurrent or persistent primary HPT.

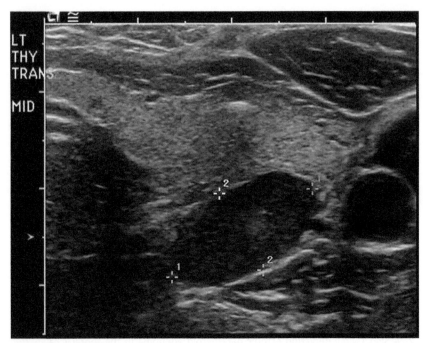

Fig. 9. High-resolution neck US image, transverse view, depicting a left parathyroid adenoma (*white crosses*).

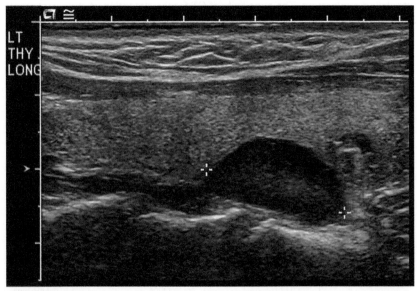

Fig. 10. High-resolution neck US image, longitudinal view, depicting a left parathyroid adenoma (*white crosses*).

Density measurements can assist in differentiating adenomas from lymph nodes and normal thyroid tissue. The spontaneous attenuation of parathyroid adenomas is lower than 80 hounsfield units (HU), whereas the density of normal thyroid tissue is greater than 80 HU. Forty-five seconds after contrast injection, adenomas have a density greater than 130 HU, whereas lymph nodes have a density lesser than 130 HU. Furthermore, between 45 and 70 seconds after injection, the attenuation of parathyroid adenomas decreases (>20 HU), whereas the attenuation of lymph nodes increases.[54]

The sensitivity of SPECT/CT (**Fig. 11**) to identify solitary parathyroid adenomas can be increased with the addition of US; a recent series reported 90% sensitivity for SPECT/CT alone, which was increased to 95% (91% accuracy) with concomitant sonography.[55] However, given the high cost associated with redundant testing, some surgical communities have advocated US as the sole study for parathyroid imaging,[51,55] recommending the use of SPECT/CT for selective cases with equivocal sonographic findings.[56]

An emerging technique in the evaluation of initial, recurrent, or persistent primary HPT is 4-dimensional CT (4D CT) (**Fig. 12**). The sensitivity of 4D CT for high-precision localization has been reported to be as high as 88%[57,58] in the reoperative setting. Recent reports indicate a higher sensitivity for identifying multiglandular disease when compared with sestamibi and high-resolution sonography.[57,58] Although 4D CT may be comparable or even superior to sestamibi for the detection of abnormal parathyroid tissue, further cost analysis and large sample studies are needed to recommend it as the imaging modality of choice in the setting of primary HPT.

MRI

The role of MRI is limited to parathyroid localization in the setting of persistent disease or recurrence. The sensitivity in the reoperative setting was found to be comparable to that of sonography and scintigraphy. In a series of 98 consecutive patients with bio-chemically proven persistent or recurrent HPT, Gotway and colleagues[59] reported sensitivity and positive predictive values of 82% and 89%, respectively. When used

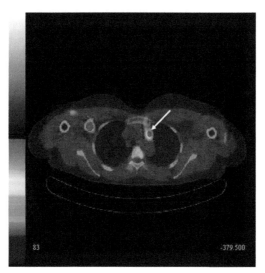

Fig. 11. A SPECT/CT image, axial view, depicting an ectopic left parathyroid adenoma near the aortic arch (*white arrow*).

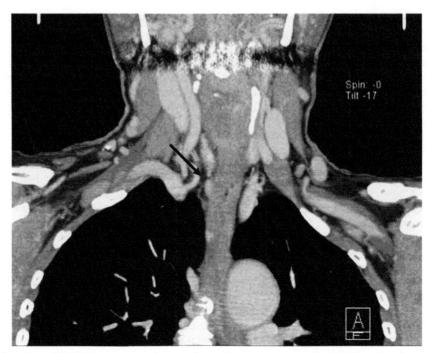

Fig. 12. A 4D CT image, coronal view, diagnosing a right superior parathyroid adenoma (tracheoesophageal grove) in the setting of persistent primary HPT (*black arrow*).

in combination with technetium Tc 99m 2-methoxy-isobutyl-isonitrile scintigraphy, the reported sensitivity was 94% and positive predictive value was 98%.[59] Multiplanar images, 3 to 5 mm thick, are obtained from the hyoid bone to the thoracic inlet, and in cases of suspicion for ectopic disease, the axials can be extended into the mediastinum. The characteristic signals are low intensity on T1-weighted sequences and high intensity on T2-weighted sequences. The addition of gadolinium-enhanced T1-weighted images can increase sensitivity in patients with high intensity on T2 sequences. For evaluation of ectopic adenomas in the mediastinum, MRI with gadolinium and fat suppression is the modality of choice.[35,60] A consideration of the lack of radiation exposure, superior anatomic detail without need for contrast administration, and minimal artifact effect on surrounding tissues make MRI superior to thin-cut CT. However, 4D CT has localization advantage over MRI because it pertains to sensitivity (88% vs 82%) and the level of detail seen and interpreted.[57]

SUMMARY

Overall advances in diagnostic radiology have played an immense role in the success of thyroid and parathyroid surgery. These advances have allowed in many instances, a reduction in morbidity and failure rates. US and ultrasound-guided biopsy remain the most accurate and cost-effective and the safest diagnostic tools in the evaluation of thyroid nodules and should be available routinely in the initial evaluation of the thyroid gland. Scintigraphy remains the most sensitive test for hyperfunctional thyroid/parathyroid tissue and remains the authors' imaging modality of choice for the initial localization of parathyroid lesions.

Reoperations in the setting of recurrence of persistent HPT represent a challenge for even the most experienced surgeons. Combining imaging modalities decreases failure rates and morbidity. New modalities, such as 4D CT and SPECT/CT, represent alternatives and options for patients with equivocal imaging studies, with diagnostic uncertainty, and in the reoperative setting. However, more data are needed before these modalities become routine practice.

REFERENCES

1. Sakorafas GH. Historical evolution of thyroid surgery: from the ancient times to the dawn of the 21st century. World J Surg 2010;(8):1793–804.
2. Becker WF. Pioneers in thyroid surgery. Ann Surg 1977;185:493–504.
3. Dean DS, Gharib H. Epidemiology of thyroid nodules. Best Pract Res Clin Endocrinol Metab 2008;22(6):901–11.
4. Wang C, Crapo LM. The epidemiology of thyroid disease and implications for screening. Endocrinol Metab Clin North Am 1997;26:189–218.
5. Papini E, Guglielmi R, Bianchini A, et al. Risk of malignancy in nonpalpable thyroid nodules: predictive value of ultrasound and color-Doppler features. J Clin Endocrinol Metab 2002;87(5):1941–6.
6. Jemal A, Siegel R, Ward E, et al. Cancer statistics, 2009. CA Cancer J Clin 2009; 59(4):225–49.
7. Frates MC, Benson CB, Doubilet PM, et al. Prevalence and distribution of carcinoma in patients with solitary and multiple thyroid nodules on sonography. J Clin Endocrinol Metab 2006;91(9):3411–7.
8. Hopkins CR, Reading CC. Thyroid and parathyroid imaging. Semin Ultrasound CT MR 1995;16(4):279–95.
9. Sheth S. Role of ultrasonography in thyroid disease. Otolaryngol Clin North Am 2010;43(2):239–55.
10. Cooper DS, Doherty GM, Haugen BR, et al. Revised American Thyroid Association management guidelines for patients with thyroid nodules and differentiated thyroid cancer. Thyroid 2009;19:1167–214.
11. Danese D, Sciacchitano S, Farsetti A, et al. Diagnostic accuracy of conventional versus sonography-guided fine-needle aspiration biopsy of thyroid nodules. Thyroid 1998;8:15–21.
12. Lew JI, Rodgers SE, Solorzano CC. Developments in the use of ultrasound for thyroid cancer. Curr Opin Oncol 2010;22(1):11–6.
13. Mendez W, Rodgers SE, Lew JI, et al. Role of surgeon-performed ultrasound in predicting malignancy in patients with indeterminate thyroid nodules. Ann Surg Oncol 2008;15:2487–92.
14. Jabiev AA, Ikeda MH, Reis IM, et al. Surgeon performed ultrasound can predict differentiated thyroid cancer in patients with solitary thyroid nodules. Ann Surg Oncol 2009;16(11):3140–5.
15. Ahuja A, Chick W, King W, et al. Clinical significance of the comet-tail artifact in thyroid ultrasound. J Clin Ultrasound 1996;24(3):129–33.
16. Bonavita JA, Mayo J, Babb J, et al. Pattern recognition of benign nodules at ultrasound of the thyroid: which nodules can be left alone? AJR Am J Roentgenol 2009;193(1):207–13.
17. Jeh SK, Jung SL, Kim BS, et al. Evaluating the degree of conformity of papillary carcinoma and follicular carcinoma to the reported ultrasonographic findings of malignant thyroid tumor. Korean J Radiol 2007;8:192–7.

18. Sillery JC, Reading CC, Charboneau JW, et al. Thyroid follicular carcinoma: sonographic features of 50 cases. AJR Am J Roentgenol 2010;194(1):44–54.
19. Stulak JM, Grant CS, Farley DR, et al. Value of preoperative ultrasonography in the surgical management of initial and reoperative papillary thyroid cancer. Arch Surg 2006;141(5):489–94.
20. Gharib H, Papini E, Paschke R, et al. American Association of Clinical Endocrinologists, Associazione Medici Endocrinologi, and EuropeanThyroid Association medical guidelines for clinical practice for the diagnosis and management of thyroid nodules. Endocr Pract 2010;16(Suppl 1):1–43.
21. Rago T, Santini F, Scutari M, et al. Elastography: new developments in ultrasound for predicting malignancy in thyroid nodules. J Clin Endocrinol Metab 2007;92(8): 2917–22.
22. Wang Y, Dan HJ, Dan HY, et al. Differential diagnosis of small single solid thyroid nodules using real-time ultrasound elastography. J Int Med Res 2010;38(2):466–72.
23. Smith JR, Oates E. Radionuclide imaging of the thyroid gland: patterns, pearls, and pitfalls. Clin Nucl Med 2004;29(3):181–93.
24. Price DC. Radioisotopic evaluation of the thyroid and parathyroids. Radiol Clin North Am 1993;31:991–1015.
25. Leger AF, Pellan M, Dagousset F, et al. A case of stunning of lung and bone metastases of papillary thyroid cancer after a therapeutic dose (3.7 GBq) of 131I and review of the literature: implications for sequential treatments. Br J Radiol 2005;78:428–32.
26. Morris LF, Waxman AD, Braunstein GD. The nonimpact of thyroid stunning: remnant ablation rates in 131I scanned and nonscanned individuals. J Clin Endocrinol Metab 2001;86:3507–11.
27. Wong KT, Choi FP, Lee YY, et al. Current role of radionuclide imaging in differentiated thyroid cancer. Cancer Imaging 2008;10(8):159–62.
28. Fatourechi V, Hay ID, Mullan BP, et al. Are post-therapy radioiodine scans informative and do they influence subsequent therapy of patients with differentiated thyroid cancer? Thyroid 2000;10:573–7.
29. Shapiro B, Vittoria R, Ayman J, et al. Artifacts, anatomical and physiological variants, and unrelated diseases that might cause false-positive whole-body 131-I scans in patients with thyroid cancer. Semin Nucl Med 2000;30: 115–32.
30. Shie P, Cardarelli R, Sprawls K, et al. Systematic review: prevalence of malignant incidental thyroid nodules identified on fluorine-18 fluorodeoxyglucose positron emission tomography. Nucl Med Commun 2009;30(9):742–8.
31. Bogsrud TV, Karantanis D, Nathan MA, et al. The value of quantifying 18F-FDG uptake in thyroid nodules found incidentally on whole-body PET-CT. Nucl Med Commun 2007;28:373–81.
32. Are C, Hsu JF, Ghossein RA, et al. Histological aggressiveness of fluorodeoxyglucose positron-emission tomogram (FDG-PET)-detected incidental thyroid carcinomas. Ann Surg Oncol 2007;14:3210–5.
33. Grant CS, Thompson GB, Farley DR, et al. The value of positron emission tomography in the surgical management of recurrent papillary thyroid carcinoma. World J Surg 2008;32(5):708–15.
34. Kirsch E, Hammer B, von Arx G. Graves' orbitopathy: current imaging procedures. Swiss Med Wkly 2009;139(43–44):618–23.
35. Reading CC, Gorman CA. Thyroid imaging techniques. Clin Lab Med 1993;13(3): 711–24.

36. Weber AL, Randolph G, Aksoy FG. The thyroid and parathyroid glands. CT and MR imaging and correlation with pathology and clinical findings. Radiol Clin North Am 2000;38(5):1105–29.
37. Jeong HS, Baek CH, Son YI, et al. Integrated 18F-FDG PET/CT for the initial evaluation of cervical node level of patients with papillary thyroid carcinoma: comparison with ultrasound and contrast-enhanced CT. Clin Endocrinol (Oxf) 2006;65(3):402–7.
38. Chen L, Luo Q, Shen Y, et al. Incremental value of 131I SPECT/CT in the management of patients with differentiated thyroid carcinoma. J Nucl Med 2008;49(12): 1952–7.
39. Gotway MB, Higgins CB. MR imaging of the thyroid and parathyroid glands. Magn Reson Imaging Clin N Am 2000;8(1):163–82.
40. Mihailović J, Stefanović LJ, Prvulovic M. Magnetic resonance imaging in diagnostic algorithm of solitary cold thyroid nodules. J BUON 2006;11(3):341–6.
41. Johnson NA, Tublin ME, Ogilvie JB. Parathyroid imaging: technique and role in the preoperative evaluation of primary hyperparathyroidism. AJR Am J Roentgenol 2007;188(6):1706–15.
42. Smith JR, Oates ME. Radionuclide imaging of the parathyroid glands: patterns, pearls, and pitfalls. Radiographics 2004;24(4):1101–15.
43. Lorberboym M, Minski I, Macadziob S, et al. Incremental diagnostic value of preoperative 99mTc-MIBI SPECT in patients with a parathyroid adenoma. J Nucl Med 2003;44(6):904–8.
44. Carlier T, Oudoux A, Mirallié E, et al. 99mTc-MIBI pinhole SPECT in primary hyperparathyroidism: comparison with conventional SPECT, planar scintigraphy and ultrasonography. Eur J Nucl Med Mol Imaging 2008;35(3):637–43.
45. Ruda JM, Hollenbeak CS, Stack BC Jr. A systematic review of the diagnosis and treatment of primary hyperparathyroidism from 1995 to 2003. Otolaryngol Head Neck Surg 2005;132(3):359–72.
46. Civelek AC, Ozalp E, Donovan P, et al. Prospective evaluation of delayed technetium-99m sestamibi SPECT scintigraphy for preoperative localization of primary hyperparathyroidism. Surgery 2002;131(2):149–57.
47. Pham TH, Sterioff S, Mullan BP, et al. Sensitivity and utility of parathyroid scintigraphy in patients with primary versus secondary and tertiary hyperparathyroidism. World J Surg 2006;30(3):327–32.
48. Hindié E, Ugur O, Fuster D, et al. 2009 EANM parathyroid guidelines. Eur J Nucl Med Mol Imaging 2009;36(7):1201–16.
49. Richards ML, Thompson GB, Farley DR, et al. Reoperative parathyroidectomy in 228 patients during the era of minimal-access surgery and intraoperative parathyroid hormone monitoring. Am J Surg 2008;196(6):937–42.
50. American Institute of Ultrasound in Medicine. AIUM practice guideline for the performance of a thyroid and parathyroid ultrasound examination. J Ultrasound Med 2003;22:1126–30.
51. Solorzano CC, Carneiro-Pla DM, Irvin GL 3rd. Surgeon-performed ultrasonography as the initial and only localizing study in sporadic primary hyperparathyroidism. J Am Coll Surg 2006;202(1):18–24.
52. Richards ML, Grant CS. Current applications of the intraoperative parathyroid hormone assay in parathyroid surgery. Am Surg 2007;73(4):311–7.
53. Thompson GB, Grant CS, Perrier ND, et al. Reoperative parathyroid surgery in the era of sestamibi scanning and intraoperative parathyroid hormone monitoring. Arch Surg 1999;134(7):699–704.

54. Ernst O. Hyperparathyroidism: CT and MR findings. J Radiol 2009;90(3 Pt 2): 409–12.
55. Patel CN, Salahudeen HM, Lansdown M, et al. Clinical utility of ultrasound and 99mTc sestamibi SPECT/CT for preoperative localization of parathyroid adenoma in patients with primary hyperparathyroidism. Clin Radiol 2010;65(4):278–87.
56. Tublin ME, Pryma DA, Yim JH, et al. Localization of parathyroid adenomas by sonography and technetium Tc 99m sestamibi single-photon emission computed tomography before minimally invasive parathyroidectomy: are both studies really needed? J Ultrasound Med 2009;28(2):183–90.
57. Mortenson MM, Evans DB, Lee JE, et al. Parathyroid exploration in the reoperative neck: improved preoperative localization with 4D-computed tomography. J Am Coll Surg 2008;206(5):888–95.
58. Rodgers SE, Hunter GJ, Hamberg LM, et al. Improved preoperative planning for directed parathyroidectomy with 4-dimensional computed tomography. Surgery 2006;140(6):932–40.
59. Gotway MB, Reddy GP, Webb WR, et al. Comparison between MR imaging and 99mTc MIBI scintigraphy in the evaluation of recurrent of persistent hyperparathyroidism. Radiology 2001;218(3):783–90.
60. Kang YS, Rosen K, Clark OH, et al. Localization of abnormal parathyroid glands of the mediastinum with MR imaging. Radiology 1993;189(1):137–41.

Contemporary Breast Imaging and Concordance Assessment: A Surgical Perspective

Jeffrey Landercasper, MD[a,b,c,]*, Jared H. Linebarger, MD[d]

KEYWORDS

- Surgeons • Breast • Ultrasonography
- Magnetic resonance imaging • Mammography • Concordance
- Quality measures

Disease conditions of the breast and the surgery to treat them are common. The lifetime risk for a woman to develop breast cancer is 12%.[1] Silverstein and colleagues[2] estimated that 1.7 million breast biopsies are performed annually in the United States, and the American Cancer Society estimates that 209,000 new cases of invasive breast cancer will be identified in 2010.[1] Nearly all of these patients will undergo breast imaging for screening or diagnostic evaluation. The aim of this article is to discuss contemporary methods of breast imaging along with their applicability and use by surgeons. From the surgeon's perspective, breast imaging never occurs in a vacuum; rather, imaging occurs in the context of a patient history, family history, clinical examination, and sometimes a prior image-guided core needle biopsy (CNB). Given this information, it is a surgeon's responsibility to perform patient risk and concordance assessment, and then establish a working diagnosis and action plan.

In this review, the modalities of mammography, breast ultrasonography (US), and breast magnetic resonance imaging (MRI) are discussed. The content of this report

---

The authors have nothing to disclose.
[a] Norma J. Vinger Center for Breast Care, Department of Surgery, Gundersen Lutheran Health System, 1900 South Avenue, Mailstop: EB1-002, La Crosse, WI 54601, USA
[b] Department of Surgery, University of Wisconsin School of Medicine and Public Health, 750 Highland Avenue, Madison, WI 53705, USA
[c] Patient Quality Committee, American Society of Breast Surgeons, 5950 Symphony Road, Suite 212, Columbia, MD 21044, USA
[d] Department of Medical Education, Gundersen Lutheran Health System, 1900 South Avenue, Mailstop: C01-005, La Crosse, WI 54601, USA
* Corresponding author. Norma J. Vinger Center for Breast Care, Department of Surgery, Gundersen Lutheran Health System, 1900 South Avenue, Mailstop: EB1-002, La Crosse, WI 54601.
E-mail address: jlanderc@gundluth.org

Surg Clin N Am 91 (2011) 33–58
doi:10.1016/j.suc.2010.10.003
0039-6109/11/$ – see front matter © 2011 Elsevier Inc. All rights reserved.

and its recommendations are based on literature review and the authors' experience, and is not meant to represent an official policy or position statement regarding author affiliations to the American Society of Breast Surgeons (ASBrS) or other professional organizations.

MAMMOGRAPHY

Mammography is used for both screening and diagnostic purposes. The history of screening mammography in the United States dates back approximately 50 years. The first breast cancer screening trial began in 1963 when women aged 40 to 64 years who were enrolled in the Health Insurance Plan (HIP) of Greater New York were randomly assigned to study and control groups.[3] The study group was invited for an initial screening, consisting of clinical breast examination and 2-view film mammography (cephalocaudal and lateral), with 3 subsequent annual reexaminations. At 18 years, for women ages 40 to 49 and 50 to 59 at the time of entry, a reduction in breast cancer mortality of approximately 25% was reported.[3] Following initial reports in the late 1960s and early 1970s of a reduction in breast cancer mortality from invited mammographic screening, the Breast Cancer Detection Demonstration Project (BCDDP) was implemented in 1973 and continued through 1980. The BCDDP was initially a method to disseminate breast cancer screening to the public and to medical professionals, but a Data Management Center was added just months following initial enrollment.[4,5] The BCDDP study was sponsored by the American Cancer Society (ACS) and the National Cancer Institute (NCI) and enrolled 283,222 women, 35 to 74 years old, at 29 centers across the United States. Women in the study received 5 annual physical examinations with 2-view mammography. Four thousand two hundred and seventy-five women were diagnosed with breast cancer during the course of this study. In 1997, 96% 20-year follow-up data were available for analysis. In retrospect, a high proportion of the cancers were diagnosed by imaging alone (43.7% for women 40–49 years old and 49.6% for women 50–59 years old). Ninety-five percent of diagnoses involved 2-view mammography, and 28.6% were smaller than 1.0 cm. The overall adjusted survival rate was 80.5%, though it was 90.2% for cancers smaller than 1.0 cm.[6] Meanwhile, outside the United States, the Swedish Two-County Trial, another early landmark randomized controlled breast cancer screening trial that began enrollment in 1977, resulted in a 32% reduction in breast cancer–related mortality at 20-year follow-up.[7,8] Additional long-term follow-up of these studies is available in the literature.[9–12]

Current breast cancer screening recommendations by many professional organizations for women at average risk for breast cancer are relatively similar to screening protocols of the earliest breast cancer screening trials. The American College of Radiology (ACR), ACS, ASBrS, and National Comprehensive Cancer Network (NCCN) have issued similar recommendations for screening mammography.[13–18] Screening mammograms for women should begin at age 40 and should be continued for as long as they remain in good health,[16] or until a decision to stop routine mammography has been reached through an informed decision between the woman and her physician.[13] The ACR recommends 2-view imaging to include craniocaudal (CC) and mediolateral oblique (MLO) views, with additional views as required for optimal or complete visualization.[13] According to the ACS, women should be advised regarding the potential benefits (detection) and risks (false positives) of breast self-examination (BSE) and choose, themselves, whether to perform BSE regularly, intermittently, or not at all.[16] Clinical breast examination by a health care professional is recommended every 3 years for women 20 to 39 years old, and then annually, and screening mammography should occur at the same age as initiation of yearly breast examinations by a health care professional.[18] The NCCN reiterates many of these recommendations, endorsing yearly mammography with clinical breast examination and breast awareness, facilitated by "periodic, consistent breast self-examination" beginning at 40 years of age.[17]

Producing stark contrast to the screening protocols of the HIP and BCDDP studies as well as current screening recommendations of the ACS, ACR, ASBrS, NCBC, and NCCN, the United States Preventive Services Task Force (USPSTF) amended its breast cancer screening recommendations in 2009 for asymptomatic women at average risk for breast cancer.[19] This task force was composed of a panel of primary care physicians and epidemiologists funded, staffed, appointed by the Agency for Health care Research Quality (AHRQ). One major departure in the USPSTF guidelines is a recommendation against routine screening mammography in women 40 to 49 years old. Screening in women younger than 50 years has been a point of controversy since the original breast cancer screening studies, with potential risks and benefits well described in the literature.[20-25] Furthermore, the USPSTF has concluded that there is insufficient available evidence to assess the benefits and harms of clinical breast examination by a health care provider. The USPSTF makes no recommendation for clinical breast examination in addition to screening mammography for women older than 40 years and, beyond this, the task force currently recommends against clinicians teaching women how to perform BSE. For women 50 to 74 years of age, the USPSTF endorses biennial screening mammography, while cautioning that the decision to begin screening should be individualized by patient context, including "the patient's values regarding specific benefits and harms." Finally, the USPSTF has concluded that there is insufficient information to assess the risks and benefits of screening mammography in women older than 74 years. These recommendations represent a departure from previous recommendations, continue to be a source of debate, and are only applicable to asymptomatic women of average risk for breast cancer. The task force does not deviate in advice for the use of mammography in the evaluation of a breast symptom or complaint, such as a mass.

For women at high risk for breast cancer, recommendations are naturally different than those proposed for the general population. Various models exist for estimation of lifetime breast cancer risk and include the Gail model, the Claus model, and the Tyrer-Cuzick model. The ACS defines "high risk" as an estimated lifetime cancer risk of 20% to 25% or greater, as well as any woman with a known BRCA1 or BRCA2 gene mutation; a first-degree relative with a BRCA1 or BRCA2 gene mutation but no genetic testing, herself; a history of radiation to the chest between 10 and 30 years of age; or a personal history of Li-Fraumeni syndrome, Cowden syndrome, or Bannayan-Riley-Ruvalcaba syndrome, or first-degree relatives with one of these syndromes.[26] According to the ACS, these women should have a yearly mammogram and MRI for breast cancer screening purposes.[16,26] To the list of "high-risk" factors for breast cancer, the NCCN adds lobular carcinoma in situ (LCIS) or atypical hyperplasia, and while recommending mammography every 12 months, the NCCN endorses yearly MRI only as a consideration.[17] For women with a history of thoracic radiation, the NCCN recommends initiation of annual mammography and consideration of annual MRI at 25 years of age or 8 to 10 years after radiation (whichever is first), and for women with a strong family history or genetic predisposition, annual mammography and MRI are recommended beginning at age 25.[17] According to the ACS, women with a 15% to 20% estimated lifetime risk of breast cancer, a personal history of breast cancer, ductal carcinoma in situ (DCIS) or LCIS, or those with extremely dense beasts or breast that are unevenly dense on mammography are at moderate risk for breast cancer, and these women should discuss the benefits of adding yearly MRI to routine mammography with their health care providers.[16] In addition, the NCCN recommends that for women older than 35 years with a 5-year risk of cancer greater than 1.7%, annual mammography should be performed. Finally, the NCCN recommends risk reduction and breast awareness for many higher risk breast cancer categories.[17]

In contrast to screening mammography in asymptomatic women, diagnostic mammography is performed to address a specific clinical question. This radiography study is used to evaluate a breast complaint or an abnormality detected on physical examination or routine screening mammography. Diagnostic mammography is typically accomplished with additional views (beyond CC and MLO), magnification, or compression, and the study requires the direct supervision of an interpreting physician.[13] The ACR enumerates indications for diagnostic mammography to include women with a specific focus of clinical concern, a possible radiographic abnormality on screening mammography, recommended short interval follow-up of a probable benign lesion, examinations requiring direct involvement of the radiologist (special views, physical breast examination, or consultation), and any woman previously treated for breast cancer.[13,27] Furthermore, the ACR emphasizes that any woman with breast symptoms or a previous abnormality for which short-term follow-up was recommended is not a candidate for screening mammography.[13] The NCCN recommends diagnostic mammography as part of the initial evaluation of a dominant breast mass in any woman older than 30 years and yearly diagnostic mammography in patients with LCIS being followed clinically.[17] Additional uses of diagnostic mammography include tumor localization[28,29] and stereotactically guided percutaneous tissue acquisition.[29–32] Diagnostic mammography is also useful for image confirmation of the presence of target image detected abnormalities in biopsy or lumpectomy specimens,[30,33] and the ACR states that specimen mammography is the "standard of care" for needle-localized breast biopsy.[28]

Methods for differentiating benign versus malignant lesions on mammography have been described.[27] In simple terms mammographic findings of cancer can be divided into major, or conventional, signs of malignancy and supporting, or indirect, signs of malignancy.[34,35] One major sign of malignancy is spiculated margins, which represents fibrosis of peritumoral tissue strands from the desmoplastic response, and this finding is pathognomonic for breast cancer (**Fig. 1**). Clustered microcalcifications, defined as 5 or more calcifications less than 1 mm in diameter and within a tissue volume of 1 cm^3, is another major mammographic sign of malignancy; however, the distribution and morphology of the calcifications define their significance (**Fig. 2**).[36] Supporting signs of malignancy include a poorly defined mass, microlobulations (measuring a few millimeters), architectural distortion (without a visibly defined mass), asymmetric density (density greatest at the center and fading toward the periphery), nipple retraction, and axillary adenopathy. In 1997 the ACR Breast Imaging-Reporting and Data System (ACR BI-RADS) was introduced as a quality tool to standardize reporting of mammographic assessment and eliminate ambiguity in reporting.[37] Now in its fourth edition,[38] and expanded to include ultrasound and MRI, the efficacy of this reporting system for mammography has been well documented in the literature and sample images are available in the public domain.[39–44] The ACR BI-RADS system is summarized in **Box 1**.

Beyond the introduction of the ACR BI-RADS reporting system, advances in quality of image acquisition, detection, and reporting have continued since the initiation of the HIP study, the Swedish Two-County Trial, and the BCDDP. From the introduction of dedicated mammography machines in 1969, to xeroradiography in 1971 and screen-film systems in 1972, early advances in mammography coincided with the very first breast cancer screening studies.[6,45] Development of special x-ray tubes to

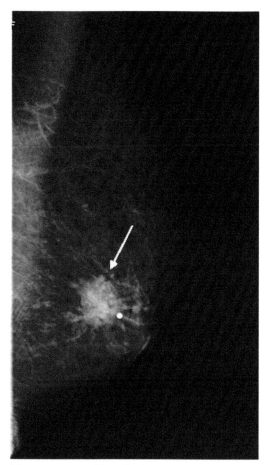

Fig. 1. Mammographic appearance of invasive breast cancer. A 92-year-old patient with an abnormal screening mammogram demonstrating a new mass in the breast (*arrow*) with an irregular, spiculated margin. Needle biopsy was positive for invasive ductal carcinoma.

optimize tissue penetration, special films and cassettes, and evolving film processing and film display are also among the advances in plain film mammography.[45] In 1987, the ACR developed the Mammography Accreditation Program to emphasize image quality and controlling radiation dose levels, and in 1992 the ACR Quality Control Manual was introduced, describing minimum standards for data reporting.[46,47] In 1994 the Mammography Quality Standards Act (MQSA) became law and required that a mammography facility be certified by the United States Food and Drug Administration (FDA).[48] At present, all interpreting physicians, medical physicists, and radiologic technologists working in mammography must meet the requirements of the MQSA.[46,48] In 2000, the FDA approved the first digital mammography unit for clinical use. These units use the same mammography machinery, but capture the images digitally for display and potential enhancement. The potential of digital mammography continues to be explored, and while optimization of this modality continues, some literature reports superior detection results.[45,49,50] Computer aided detection and diagnosis, telemammography, contrast uptake imaging, tomosynthesis, tissue

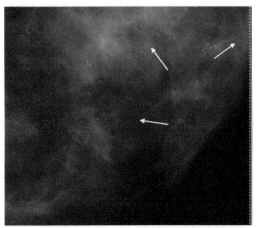

Fig. 2. Mammographic appearance of ductal carcinoma in situ. A 40-year-old patient with an abnormal screening mammogram demonstrating pleomorphic microcalcifications (*arrows*) in a segmental distribution in the lower inner quadrant of the breast. Stereotactic biopsy was positive for high-grade, comedo-type ductal carcinoma in situ.

characterization, and quantitative image analysis for future risk assessment have also been described.[45]

The application of advances in breast cancer detection, with a central focus on screening and diagnostic mammography, continues to be explored and debated. Suggested as a testament to the benefits of breast cancer screening and diagnostic evaluation, the introduction of screening mammography has been reported to have led not only to improved detection of breast cancer, but to detection of cancer at an earlier stage.[45] For example, before widespread use of screening mammography, DCIS was considered an uncommon lesion in isolation, accounting for approximately 0.85% to 5.0% of breast cancers.[51] However, since the introduction of screening mammography, DCIS accounts for 30% to 45% of all detected cancers.[52] Nonetheless, others have questioned the cost, morbidity, and reported benefit of screening practices, as referenced above.[21–25] To better understand many facets of these debates, the Breast Cancer Surveillance Consortium (BCSC) was established in 1994. The BCSC is a "research resource for studies designed to assess the delivery and quality of breast cancer screening and related patient outcomes in the United States" sponsored by the NCI.[53] The BCSC is a collaborative network of 7 mammography databases with links to pathology and/or tumor registries, which can be used to investigate population-based outcomes. The goal of the BCSC is to improve the understanding and performance of breast cancer screening practices in the United States and to understand the association between stage at diagnosis and breast cancer mortality.[53] For example, in 2006 Weaver and colleagues[54] reported a retrospective review of BSCS data from 1996 to 2001 to identify pathology specimens obtained within a year of mammography for women 40 to 89 years of age undergoing routine screening for breast cancer. The study represented 786,846 women undergoing 1,664,032 mammograms followed by 26,748 known biopsies (1.6%). Using results from this database, a 78% pathologic node-negative rate was reported for this screen-detected cancer population, compared with a 66% prevalence observed in the Surveillance Epidemiology and End Results (SEER) data during the same time period. In addition, proportional rates of invasive carcinoma (27%), DCIS (6%), and benign findings (67%) were able to be established among those who underwent biopsy, with higher percentages of carcinoma noted in older patients (81% benign findings for women 40 to 49 years old compared with 37% benign findings for those 80 to 89 years old).[54]

Mammography has been the cornerstone of programs for early detection of breast cancer around the world, and patients with screen detected cancers generally a have good prognosis.[55–57] Tabar and colleagues[55] report a greater than 95% breast cancer survival in patients with screen-detected cancers measuring less than 15 mm. Furthermore, specific mammographic findings, such as casting calcifications, add further prognostic value regarding patient outcome that is not currently accounted for in the American Joint Committee on Cancer (AJCC) TNM staging system.[55–58] Continued advances in technology are inevitable, and the context of continued research dedicated to understanding screening and diagnostic mammography will undoubtedly evolve and continue to be debated.

BREAST ULTRASONOGRAPHY

Of all available diagnostic breast imaging modalities, US is the most commonly employed by surgeons. The use of breast US is evolving, and changes have occurred since a recent review of this topic.[59,60] A simplistic explanation of ultrasound technology follows.[61,62] With US, a pulse of high-frequency sound waves is produced by a transducer placed on the breast. The transducer also functions to collect information that is reflected back by the breast tissue. The energy delivered to the breast by the transducer is absorbed, scattered, or reflected back. Tissue reflectors in the breast bounce the sound waves back toward the transducer, and computation of the duration of time elapsed from pulse-wave generation to reflection to subsequent return determine depth. Brightness of the ultrasound image depends on tissue type and is related to the strength of signal that returns to the transducer. Enough rapid-fire pulses and collections of sound waves occur that the accumulated information allows for real-time tissue images as the transducer moves over the breast. Most breast ultrasound imaging requires 7.5 MHz systems or higher to provide adequate resolution of imaging. US demonstrates the layers of the breast in an anterior to posterior direction. Skin, subcutaneous fat, fibroglandular parenchymal tissue, retromammary fat, pectoralis fascia, pectoralis muscle, pleura, and ribs are displayed from top to bottom. Different tissues display variable echogenicity. The echogenicity of fat in the breast serves as the standard to which other breast tissue is compared. Breast tissue or lesions that have similar echogenicity to fat are called isoechogenic and display the same amount of brightness as fat. Breast lesions that display brighter (whiter) or darker appearance are termed hyperechogenic or hypoechogenic, respectively. Lesions with no echogenicity (black) are called anechoic.

Breast US may be used for either screening or diagnostic evaluation. The use of US in asymptomatic women for breast cancer screening has not been fully defined. In contrast, the diagnostic use of breast US is well established. The primary role of diagnostic US is to help differentiate palpable lumps or nonpalpable mammographically detected abnormalities as cystic or solid and benign or malignant. The ACR, the ASBrS, and the NCCN provide information on indications for breast US.[63–65] Indications include evaluation of palpable lumps (or thickening), evaluation of nonpalpable mammographically detected abnormalities, and evaluation of focal breast symptoms such as pain, fullness, or nipple discharge. US is indicated for characterization of known cancers and for needle biopsy guidance of indeterminate abnormalities. US

Box 1
ACR BI-RADS ultrasound assessment categories

Assessment Categories

1. Assessment is Incomplete

   Category 0

   Need Additional Imaging Evaluation and/or Prior Mammograms for Comparison:

   In many instances, the ultrasonography completes the evaluation of the patient. If US is the initial study, other examinations may be indicated. An example would be the need for mammography if US were the initial study for a patient in her late twenties evaluated with US for a palpable mass that had suspicious sonographic features. Another example might be where mammography and US are nonspecific, such as differentiating between scarring and recurrence in a patient with breast cancer treated with lumpectomy and radiation therapy. Here, MRI might be the recommendation. A need for previous studies to determine appropriate management might also defer a final assessment.

2. Assessment is Complete—Final Categories

   Category 1

   Negative:

   This category is for sonograms with no abnormality, such as a mass, architectural distortion, thickening of the skin, or microcalcifications. For greater confidence in rendering a negative interpretation, an attempt should be made to correlate the ultrasound and mammographic patterns of breast tissue in the area of concern.

   Category 2

   Benign Finding(s):

   Essentially a report that is negative for malignancy. Simple cysts would be placed in this category, along with intramammary lymph nodes (also possible to be included in Category 1), breast implants, stable postsurgical changes, and probable fibroadenomas noted to be unchanged on successive ultrasound studies.

   Category 3

   Probably Benign Finding—Short-Interval Follow-Up Suggested:

   With accumulating clinical experience and by extension from mammography, a solid mass with circumscribed margins, oval shape, and horizontal orientation, most likely a fibroadenoma, should have a less than 2% risk of malignancy. Although additional multicenter data may confirm safety of follow-up rather than biopsy based on US findings, short-interval follow-up is currently increasing as a management strategy. Nonpalpable complicated cysts and clustered microcysts might also be placed in this category for short-interval follow-up.

   Category 4

   Suspicious Abnormality—Biopsy Should be Considered:

   Lesions in this category would have an intermediate probability of cancer, ranging from 3% to 94%. An option would be to stratify these lesions, giving them a low, intermediate, or moderate likelihood of malignancy. In general, Category 4 lesions require tissue sampling. Needle biopsy can provide a cytologic or histologic diagnosis. Included in this group are sonographic findings of a solid mass without all of the criteria for a fibroadenoma and other probably benign lesions.

   Category 5

   Highly Suggestive of Malignancy—Appropriate Action Should be Taken:

(Almost certainly malignant)

The abnormality identified sonographically and placed in this category should have a 95% or higher risk of malignancy so that definitive treatment might be considered at the outset. With the increasing use of sentinel node imaging as a way of assessing nodal metastases and also with the increasing use of neoadjuvant chemotherapy for large malignant masses or those that are poorly differentiated, percutaneous sampling, most often with imaging-guided CNB, can provide the histopathologic diagnosis.

BI-RADS US

Category 6

Known Biopsy-Proven Malignancy—Appropriate Action Should Be Taken:

This category is reserved for lesions with biopsy proof of malignancy before institution of therapy, including neoadjuvant chemotherapy, surgical excision, or mastectomy.

From American College of Radiology (ACR). ACR BI-RADS—4th Edition. ACR Breast Imaging Reporting and Data System, Breast Imaging Atlas; BI-RADS. Reston (VA): American College of Radiology; 2003; with permission. Reprinted with permission of the American College of Radiology. No other representation of this material is authorized without expressed, written permission from the American College of Radiology.

is also useful after breast operations. In these patients, US aids evaluation of breast swelling and tenderness by identifying seromas, hematomas, and abscesses. In addition, breast US facilitates the diagnosis and treatment of benign disease. If the specific characteristics of a simple cyst are identified on US, then selected patients may be followed without aspiration or biopsy. Ultrasound-guided aspiration, of course, is an option for symptomatic cysts and attempted aspiration, CNB or excision is indicated for complex or complicated cysts. Complicated cysts have most but not all elements of a simple cyst; they may contain debris, but have no solid mass or septa.[65] Complex cysts have a discrete solid component.[65] Abscesses in the breast may have ultrasound characteristics of complex cysts.

For women younger than 30 years presenting with a breast mass, NCCN guidelines recommend US as the preferred method of initial diagnostic evaluation of the mass.[65] For women 30 years or older, NCCN guidelines recommend both mammography and US as part of the initial diagnostic evaluation of a mass.[65] US is also a diagnostic adjunct for women presenting with persistent reproducible unilateral nipple discharge, asymmetric breast thickening, nodularity, and clinically suspicious skin changes of the breast.[65] The use of US by surgeons for all these indications has been well documented.[59]

Multiple investigators and professional organizations have detailed the specific ultrasound findings that aid in the differentiation of solid versus cystic and benign versus malignant lesions.[61,62,66,67] The ACR and the ASBrS recommend use of a specific lexicon of terms to describe the features of ultrasound-visible abnormalities.[64,67] The ACR's recommended categories of description for lesions able to be seen on US include the following.[67,68] For a space-occupying mass, the image should describe the shape, orientation, margin, boundary, echogenicity, posterior acoustic characteristics, and surrounding tissue. Calcifications, if visible, may also be characterized, and "special cases with a unique finding" such as complicated cysts, complex cysts, skin masses, foreign bodies, and lymph nodes are noted. The presence or absence and the degree of vascularity are also reported. The exact lexicon of specific descriptors is detailed in **Box 2**. The typical US characteristics of breast cysts, fibroadenomas, and breast cancer are detailed in **Table 1**.[61,62] See **Fig. 3** for the ultrasound image of a breast cancer.

Box 2
ACR BI-RADS US Lexicon classification form for description of mass[a]

Masses: A mass occupies space and should be seen in two different projections

Shape (select one) Description (oval, round, or irregular)

Orientation (select one) Description (parallel or not parallel)

Margin (select one) Description (circumscribed or not circumscribed)

Lesion Boundary (select one) Description (abrupt interface or echogenic halo)

Echo Pattern (select one) Description (anechoic, hyperechoic, hypoechoic, or complex)

Posterior Acoustic Features (select one) Description (enhancement, shadowing or none)

Surrounding Tissue Description (ie, skin thickening, architectural distortion, or other)

[a] **Box 2** is an abbreviated ACR US Lexicon. For full description, see Ref.[67]
From American College of Radiology (ACR). ACR BI-RADS—4th Edition. ACR Breast Imaging Reporting and Data System, Breast Imaging Atlas; BI-RADS. Reston (VA). American College of Radiology; 2003. Reprinted with permission of the American College of Radiology. No other representation of this material is authorized without expressed, written permission from the American College of Radiology.

After ultrasound assessment, the ACR BI-RADS system is used as a method of categorizing lesions based on their likelihood of malignancy.[37–39,66] Similar to mammography, the ACR BI-RADS reporting system for US standardizes the reporting of ultrasound interpretations (see **Box 1**). The authors endorse and the ASBrS includes the option of use of the ACR's BI-RADS reporting system in their guidelines for surgeon use of US.[64] The interobserver agreement with ACR BI-RADS categories using the ACR BI-RADS lexicon is good and has been validated.[68] After US, the

---

Table 1
Ultrasound characteristics of breast lesions[a]

	Cancer	Simple Cyst	Fibroadenoma
Shape	Irregular	Round or oval	Oval
Orientation	Not parallel	Parallel	Parallel
Margin	Not circumscribed	Circumscribed	Circumscribed
Echo pattern	Hypoechoic	Anechoic	Isoechoic to mildly hypoechoic
Posterior acoustic features	Shadowing	Enhancement	None or enhancement
Other	Architectural distortion	Compressible	Thin echogenic capsule

[a] Not all benign and malignant lesions have the characteristics detailed here. Needle aspiration and/or biopsy are usually indicated for indeterminate lesions that have any single malignant feature.
Data from Kopans DB. Breast imaging. 3rd Edition. Philadelphia: Lippincott Williams & Wilkins, a Wolters Kluwer Business; 2007. p. 555–606, 691–732, 783–888; and Stavros AT. Breast ultrasound. Philadelphia: Lippincott Williams & Wilkins, a Wolters Kluwer Business; 2004. p. 16–41, 276–350, 445–528, 528–96, 834–76.

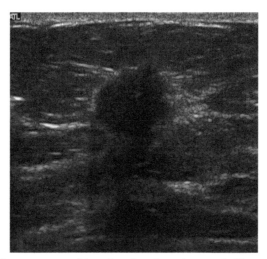

Fig. 3. Ultrasound appearance of invasive ductal carcinoma. A 62-year-old patient with a self-detected right breast mass. US demonstrates a hypoechoic mass with indistinct margins and posterior acoustic shadowing. Needle biopsy was positive for invasive ductal carcinoma.

patient's history, physical examination, and other imaging findings (if performed) are used to generate a differential diagnosis and action plan. Subsequent steps in diagnosis or treatment could be either reassurance (with no follow-up) or observation with a specific imaging follow-up schedule. In other patients, a CNB, surgery, or more imaging may be recommended. Assessment for concordance of all available data is essential and is emphasized later in this discussion.

Surgeons and radiologists both use breast US for image guidance to target and biopsy nonpalpable and palpable breast lesions. There is widespread acceptance of the superiority of image-guided CNB over open surgical excisional biopsies.[2,69–72] The ASBrS emphasized the importance of image-guided CNB by choosing it as one of their first three quality measures to include in their national quality initiative called the "Mastery Program."[73] Image guidance with ultrasound increases the accuracy of CNB of palpable lumps compared with CNB of the same lesion guided only by palpation. Other advantages of image-guided CNB over open biopsy include, but are not limited to, less pain, lower cost, improved cosmesis, and better planning for definitive oncologic procedures.[2,69,70,74,75] Preoperative diagnosis of cancer by CNB also increases one-step surgery success rate by improving the likelihood of negative lumpectomy margins and by allowing scheduling of axillary nodal surgery concurrent with breast surgery.[70,76] The accuracy of image-guided CNB has been established.[69,70] However, despite widespread endorsement, there is continued underutilization.[2,69–72] High rates of breast cancer diagnosis, exceeding 90%, are achievable by CNB.[77,78]

In the patient with breast cancer, US is a valuable aid for preoperative axillary assessment and for planning the surgical procedure.[59,60,64,79] Intraoperative uses of US include verification of location of nonpalpable image-detected tumors and optimization of the exact location of incision. For palpable tumors, US may also differentiate a post-CNB palpable hematoma from the adjacent palpable cancer. US often demonstrates the depth of cancer, improving decisions about whether to remove the skin overlying the cancer or the muscle fascia beneath it, thereby optimizing the goal of negative surgical margins in both lumpectomy and mastectomy patients. Furthermore, preoperative US of the axilla sometimes identifies enlarged or architecturally abnormal lymph nodes.[79,80] Such nodes can undergo image-guided fine needle aspiration (FNA) or CNB. If nodal positivity is verified histologically and preoperatively, these patients can be scheduled for axillary dissection without need for sentinel lymph node (SLN) mapping or biopsy. The sensitivity of preoperative axillary US to identify positive axillary nodes is variable, ranging from 30% to 70%, but the specificity is high.[79]

There are many different models of perioperative and intraoperative use of breast US and other breast imaging modalities. Historically, most nonpalpable breast lesions requiring resection have undergone excision inside the operating room (OR) after placement of localizing needle hookwires by radiologists, using ultrasound or stereotactic methods, outside the OR.[81] In the contemporary version of this model, a radiologist will have performed complete diagnostic imaging evaluation, image-guided needle biopsy, and concordance assessment before a surgical consultation.[78,82] If breast lumpectomy for a nonpalpable lesion is planned, the radiologist then aids the surgeon preoperatively by placing a needle hookwire through or adjacent to the lesion. The surgeon may or may not subsequently use US in the OR. Immediately after excision, the radiologist performs and both the radiologist and surgeon interpret specimen imaging of the resected specimen to determine whether the intended target was successfully removed. Two-view orthogonal images are obtained to assess margin status. Excellent results can be achieved with this model.[76,78] A different model of perioperative imaging occurs when breast surgeons perform diagnostic US and ultrasound image-guided CNB. After CNB and a cancer diagnosis, these surgeons then use ultrasound or stereotactic imaging to target nonpalpable lesions themselves inside or outside the operating room. Surgeons may choose to place a standard needle hookwire for intraoperative targeting, or may opt to simply use intraoperative US without a needle, to target the lesion.[59,60] If the surgeon accurately performs intraoperative lumpectomy localization, potential patient- and surgeon-centered advantages may occur, including increased opportunity to offer conscious sedation to select patients for needle localization. The likelihood of needle dislodgment during transportation from radiology to surgery is also decreased. More efficient patient and surgical scheduling may also occur. For surgeons who do not perform their own needle localizations of nonpalpable lesions, intraoperative US remains a valuable aid for defining the exact location for excision in those patients who have had their needle localization performed by their radiology partners. Surgeon use of intraoperative US in these patients identifies the trajectory of the wire and distance of the lesion to the hook. In some patients, needle hookwire dislodgment or pull-back secondary to patient transport or movement may have occurred. US can potentially identify this change in location. US will also identify "bending" of the needle that occasionally occurs after release of the breast from compression during a stereotactic location. If the trajectory of the needle hookwire is not identified by the surgeon, errors in surgical incision location can occur despite very accurate needle placement by radiologists. Surgeon use of intraoperative US as an adjunct to lumpectomy surgery has been demonstrated to be associated with lower reexcision lumpectomy rates in some studies, and is routinely employed by surgeons at the authors' hospital.[60,76,78] In the absence of randomized controlled trials to compare patient outcomes between the different models of lesion localization and perioperative imaging described herein, the authors recommend that all care providers, including radiologists and surgeons, audit their imaging performance to measure the quality of their imaging. See **Box 3** for a list of imaging performance metrics that measure the quality of imaging.

Multiple professional organizations provide certification criteria, accreditation criteria, or position statements regarding training or competency of care providers to practice breast US. These organizations include the ACR, the Society of Breast Imaging (SBI), the ASBrS, and the American Institute of Ultrasound Medicine (AIUM).[64,83–86] The ASBrS has developed "Performance and Practice Guidelines for Breast Ultrasound."[64,86] The ASBrS ultrasound guidelines include information regarding indications, equipment, surgeon sonographer qualifications, safety requirements, and quality assessment. Minimum standards for annotation, labeling, documentation, data reporting, concordance assessment, and quality improvement are also included. Moreover, the ASBrS guidelines detail specific educational, volume, and testing requirements for formal ASBrS certification in US. The ACR and AIUM have different requirements for certification or accreditation in breast US. The AIUM accepts ASBrS certification "as proof of sufficient training" for AIUM accreditation.[85] The ACR does not. The National Accreditation Program for Breast Centers (NAPBC) requires care providers practicing breast US in accredited centers to meet certification criteria from one of these organizations.[87] Certification criteria detail the minimum criteria to begin independent practice for breast US. Regardless of which certification criteria are sufficient or optimal, there is a need to assess ongoing actual performance. Measures of performance or quality are detailed in **Box 3**.

Box 3
Potential quality measures for surgeon use of US

1. For patients undergoing ultrasound image-guided biopsy
   - Sensitivity to detect cancer = TP/(TP+FN)
   - Specificity = TN/(TN+FP)
   - Positive predictive value = TP/(TP+FP)
   - Percentage of patients with documentation of imaging-pathology concordance after ultrasound image-guided biopsy

2. Interval cancer detection rate = percentage of patients with assessment of ACR BI-RADS 1, 2, or 3 (after surgeon clinical examination and US) who have cancer detected in ipsilateral breast within 1 year

3. Percentage of patients with correct lexicon for description of lesions visible on US as defined by ACR, ASBrS, or the American Institute of Ultrasound in Medicine (AIUM)

4. Percentage of patients with correct annotation and labeling of ultrasound images as defined by ACR, ASBrS, or AIUM

5. Percentage of patients with an upgrade or misses in diagnosis when an ultrasound image-guided biopsy demonstrating benign disease is followed by open surgical excision

6. Percutaneous procedure complication rate

7. Percentage of patients with documented follow-up within 6 months after cyst aspiration or image-guided biopsy with benign finding

8. Percentage of patients with documented clinical examination before image-guided biopsy

9. Surgeon ultrasound volume

Abbreviations: TP, true positive; FP, false positive; TN, true negative.

BREAST MAGNETIC RESONANCE IMAGING

The use of breast MRI for both screening and diagnostic evaluation has increased greatly during the last 20 years. During this time, breast MRI has evolved from being investigational to become a breast imaging modality that is routinely recommended for screening of BRCA-positive patients, and is selectively used for diagnostic evaluation of indeterminate lesions identified on mammography and US.[26,88,89] Furthermore, breast MRI is commonly used to complete the comprehensive imaging examination of newly diagnosed patients with breast cancer.[2,89,90]

Discrimination of malignant from benign breast conditions on MRI is improved by the intravenous injection of the dye gadolinium to search for "enhancement."[61,90,91] The technique of image "subtraction" of the precontrast image subtracted from the postcontrast image identifies only the breast tissue that contains contrast to be seen on the image. Fat contains little contrast, greatly reducing fat from the image. Most breast cancers enhance and become more visible after subtraction.[61] Gadolinium travels through the vascular system to small vessels and capillaries, including new microvascular beds that may have developed in response to tumor induced angiogenesis. Gadolinium also leaks out of the microvasculature. The term "washout" is used to describe the loss of visible gadolinium dye as it dilutes and leaks out of the microvasculature, disappearing over time. Gadolinium also alters tissue magnetic characteristics and produces a bright signal on T1-weighted images.[61] The kinetics of contrast uptake and washout by different tissues over time can be computed and displayed in graphic format as a "MRI washout or kinetic curve." The kinetic curves of benign and malignant tissue usually differ. Benign lesions most often have continuous gradual enhancement and no washout. Cancers have rapid uptake and rapid washout. A kinetic pattern of gradual uptake followed by a "plateau" is indeterminate. Both the morphologic and the kinetic analysis of lesions visible on breast MRI aid in determining the level of concern for cancer. The typical morphologic features of breast cancer on MRI are seen in mass lesions with irregular shapes and ill-defined or spiculated margins, similar to the morphology of the same mass on mammography or US (**Fig. 4**). Breast cancer commonly enhances on MRI, either uniformly or heterogeneously, and may exhibit "rim enhancement." Contrast enhancement characteristics may vary in premenopausal patients depending on when the scan is obtained during their menstrual cycle. Normal tissue may enhance significantly during the luteal phase, before menses, and during menses. MRI during this time interval may be difficult to interpret. The optimal timing for MRI is between days 7 and 14 of the menstrual cycle.[92]

Multiple professional organizations have provided recommendations for the use of MRI for screening and diagnostic evaluation.[26,88,89,93,94] The indications for screening asymptomatic patients for breast cancer with MRI have recently been published by the ACS.[26] The ACS recommendation is to consider annual bilateral breast MRI if the patient's personal lifetime risk of breast cancer exceeds 20% to 25%, based on breast cancer prediction models that are largely based on family history. The ASBrS, ACR, and NCCN all support this policy.[64,88,93] Furthermore, annual MRI for screening is recommended for women beginning at age 25 years if they have been identified as having BRCA mutations or other mutations known to confer high risk for future breast cancers.[26,88] Women who have received chest wall radiation for treatment of non-breast malignancy are also candidates for screening with MRI.[26,88] There are many indications for diagnostic breast MRI[94] including, but not limited to, evaluation of patients with breast cancer for eligibility for breast-conserving therapy (BCT) by aiding the assessment of focality and size and extent of cancer.[95,96] MRI in patients with

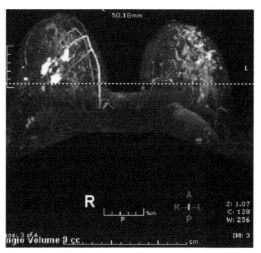

Fig. 4. MRI of mammographically occult contralateral breast cancer. A 43-year-old patient with biopsy-proven invasive and in situ ductal carcinoma of the left breast (identified by microcalcifications on mammography) underwent a preoperative MRI. The MRI demonstrates 3 separate foci of invasive cancer in the right breast that were not palpable on clinical examination. The right sided multifocal cancers were occult on mammography and US. The presence and extent of the known left breast cancer were not appreciated on MRI.

presumed unilateral breast cancer will also screen the contralateral breast and identify contralateral breast cancer in 2% to 5% of patients.[97] Other indications include identification of a primary breast cancer in patients who present with axillary metastases but no known breast cancer seen on conventional imaging with mammography and US.[98] Evaluation of breast implants for integrity is another indication for MRI. Finally, MRI is also indicated for guidance of CNB in patients with MRI-detected suspicious lesions not seen with other imaging modalities.

Despite major advancements in the technology and applicability of breast MRI, there remain valid concerns about the full scope of its use in patients with breast cancer insofar as its success in improving patient outcomes.[97,99] There are controversies as well as unresolved performance and cost issues associated with breast MRI, which have been detailed in recent publications.[97,99–104] One controversy is whether breast MRI should be routinely or selectively employed in the newly diagnosed patient with breast cancer. The argument for routine use is based on case studies in which MRI was used to identify extra ipsilateral cancer sites in patients who had presumed unifocal cancer after completion of their clinical examination and conventional imaging.[97,102] By meta-analysis, a median of 16% (range 11%–24%) of patients had upgrading from unifocal to multifocal or multicentric cancer when MRI was employed as part of their diagnostic examination.[97] The discovery of additional cancers can change the patient's eligibility for BCT. In addition, MRI sometimes identifies occult contralateral cancer. Houssami and Hayes,[97] in a review of 22 observational studies (3253 patients), reported a true positive contralateral breast cancer identification rate of 4% with MRI. Thus, there is general agreement that MRI improves the sensitivity of breast cancer detection. However, pertinent questions remain regarding the clinical significance of MRI to identify additional cancers and whether MRI's increased sensitivity justifies its routine use.[102–104] For example, would these extra cancers require later treatments if MRI had not been performed, and will patients have worse long-term local regional recurrence or disease-specific mortality? These questions are relevant because there is discordance between the number of extra cancers discovered by MRI and published contemporary ipsilateral breast tumor recurrence (IBTR) rates after BCT.[104] Published IBTR rates in BCT patients receiving postoperative radiation therapy are generally lower than 1% per year in contemporary reports.[76,105–107] In the Early Breast Cancer Trialists Collaborative Group analysis, the IBTR was 7% after 5 years of follow-up in patients treated with BCT.[108] Most of these patients would not have had breast MRI, given the calendar years in which they were treated, and one can infer that they had small extra sites of cancer that were not seen on conventional imaging, yet never recurred. Moreover, pathologic and clinical studies demonstrate that extra foci of cancer occur in patients with presumed unifocal cancer in 20% to 60% of cases.[109–111] In the 12-year follow-up of NSABP B06, the cohort of patients treated with lumpectomy without radiation had an IBTR of 35%.[112] The comparison group of patients undergoing lumpectomy with radiation had only 10% IBTR at 12-year follow-up, indicating that radiation treatment was effective treatment for small occult foci of cancer in the ipsilateral breast. MRI identifies these extra cancers in some, but not all cases. Even with MRI, some small cancer foci remain undetected in the breast in many patients, but these do not become clinically apparent in most patients as a recurrence, if the BCT patient received radiation. Two observational studies of local recurrence rates in patients who either had or did not have preoperative MRI demonstrated conflicting results.[113,114] To the authors' knowledge, there are no published reports of randomized controlled trials comparing long-term recurrence or survival rates for patients with breast cancer stratified by whether MRI was performed or not. It is unlikely that randomized controlled trials will be performed because many breast surgeons and breast centers, based on personal experience and anecdotal benefits, have already adopted either a selective or routine policy for MRI use. Anecdotal cases should not drive MRI policy decisions, but it is understandable why MRI influences changes in the usage policy of MRI. The patient in **Fig. 4** is an example. There is one published randomized controlled trial comparing reexcision lumpectomy rates between BCT patients stratified by preoperative MRI use. The COMICE trial did not demonstrate any improvement in reexcision lumpectomy rates with MRI.[115]

MRI may directly or indirectly influence other performance and practice issues regarding patients with breast cancer. In a meta-analysis of the MRI effect on changes in surgical planning, from less to more extensive surgery, the pooled estimate of change to more surgery averaged 11% and conversions from planned lumpectomy to mastectomy, after MRI, ranged from 4% to 33%.[97] Other statistical associations between the use of MRI and increased ipsilateral and contralateral mastectomy rates and delays in time to treatment have also been reported.[96,100,101,116,117] In addition to timeliness delays, MRI has also been associated with other detrimental patient-centered care issues, including cost, insurance denials, and differences in image quality due to different machines, magnet strengths, and performance protocols. In addition, there is no standard method to transport MRI images from one care provider to the next to assist in interdisciplinary care and second opinions. All of the aforementioned potentially contribute to increased patient anxiety, difficulties in concordance assessment of all imaging modalities with histology, the need for repeat MRI examinations at the breast center providing second opinion services, and time to treatment. Furthermore, some diagnostic MRIs are performed by centers without MRI biopsy capability, which is another cause of repeat MRI examinations. Finally, the specificity of MRI needs improvement. In an overview analysis of 19 studies (N = 2610 patients), the pooled estimate of true-positive to false-positive lesions seen on MRI was 1.9:1 and the positive predictive value was 66%.[96] This result means that 1 of 3 MRI lesions that are labeled suspicious for cancer is not cancer; hence the recommendations for not changing surgical treatment plans from BCT to mastectomy without biopsy confirmation of the suspicious lesion.[2,89]

CONCORDANCE TESTING

The concept of concordance testing is integral to incorporate breast imaging into clinical patient care. Breast surgeons intuitively process multiple levels and types of information during their care of a patient with breast cancer. Concordance assessment of all available information about the patients and their breast cancer is a term given to the intellectual process of deciding whether all the information "makes sense" and whether it is sufficient or lacking in content or clarity to identify the side, number, and site(s) of lesions, a necessity to plan correct treatment. If there is discordance in patient history, clinical examination, mammography, US, and MRI, or if there is discordance between the imaging findings and pathology of either CNB or surgical specimens, then the failure to recognize discordance may lead to delays or misses in breast cancer diagnosis or failure to remove or correctly target and excise all lesions. The importance of recognizing discordance is understood by radiologists, pathologists, and surgeons, and all must work together as a team to reconcile discordance, if it exists.[2,118,119] The lack of recognition of discordance is also recognized by the legal profession, and is a leading cause of successful litigation by plaintiffs.[120,121]

The risk of discordance exists whenever a patient's care crosses specialty lines. For example, a primary care provider discovers a palpable lateral right breast lump and orders a mammogram. The mammogram is interpreted by a radiologist as normal. If neither care provider recognizes or explains this discordance, nor orders further diagnostic evaluation, then a delay in the diagnosis of breast cancer may occur. If a mammogram and subsequent US in this same patient demonstrates a benign breast cyst at the upper midline, then discordance still exists because the palpable lump is at a different location from the image-detected cyst. Care providers must accept responsibility to correlate all available information to determine concordance. The importance of concordance continues through every step of patient evaluation. In a patient with a needle biopsy–confirmed nonpalpable upper outer quadrant cancer who arrives in the operating room with a needle inserted in a different quadrant, the surgeon must recognize and investigate this discordance to prevent surgery at the wrong site. Another patient with CNB-proven multifocal cancer in the same quadrant who has a lumpectomy pathology report return with confirmation of a single excised cancer also has discordance. In this latter example, 3 specialists (radiologist, surgeon, pathologist) must communicate with each other to reconcile discordance and develop an action plan for further investigation with postlumpectomy imaging, to ensure that no lesion was missed.

A common clinical scenario that requires concordance assessment is after CNB identifies benign disease. A critical next step is to correlate the image findings with CNB histology. If the mammogram and US findings suggest a fibroadenoma and the CNB demonstrates a fibroadenoma, then there is concordance. In this instance, it is unlikely that surgical excision will identify malignancy. By contrast, if image findings are suspicious, categorized an ACR BI-RADS 4 or 5, but CNB demonstrates normal breast tissue, then the imaging does not correlate with the histology and an action plan is necessary. The action plan may be to repeat a CNB, hoping for more accurate targeting, or to perform an excision. Some further attempt at tissue diagnosis is indicated. Some image-detected ACR BI-RADS 4 indeterminate lesions that undergo CNB are found to have a specific benign histologic condition. These lesions include, but are not limited to, papillary lesions, mucocele-like lesions, atypical ductal hyperplasia, lobular neoplasia (atypical lobular hyperplasia or LCIS), and radial scars (complex sclerosing lesions).[122] Assessment of imaging pathology concordance is complicated for these patients because their lesions may have variable and nonspecific imaging characteristics. Furthermore, there can be upgrades for each of these conditions to a malignant diagnosis in up to 5% to 30% of cases if the patient undergoes excisional surgical biopsy after CNB.[122] Pseudoangiomatous stromal hyperplasia, fibroepithelial lesions with a cellular stroma, and lesions with spindle cell or vascular histology identified on CNB also require careful concordance assessment to decide on which lesions to excise to prevent missed cancer, phyllodes tumor, and rare sarcoma and desmoid diagnoses. Who bears ultimate responsibility for correlation assessment in these complex situations? The answer is all of us; that is, any care provider participating in the patient's breast care. Surgeons can optimize their chance of making correct decisions about excision versus follow-up when they work effectively with their partners in radiology and pathology, soliciting their opinions.

The lack of adequate concordance assessment has been identified as a "gap" in contemporary breast cancer care by the American Society of Breast Disease.[123] The concept of appropriate concordance assessment has been endorsed by consensus conferences, professional organizations, and acknowledged breast cancer experts, and it is integral to the incorporation of breast imaging into the synthesis of care of the breast patient.[2,123] See **Boxes 4** and **5** for specific recommendations regarding methods of concordance testing during the continuum of care of the patient with breast cancer. All these methods are employed at the authors' breast center.

Box 4
Methods for concordance testing

1. Synoptic template reporting by clinical breast radiologists who record in the electronic medical record (EMR) their assessment of concordance after CNB

2. Weekly CNB imaging—pathology correlation assessment conference

3. Synoptic template reporting by breast surgeons who record in the EMR their assessment of concordance after CNB or surgical procedure

4. Presentation of complex cases at an interdisciplinary tumor board

5. Planned procedural pauses before commencement of either CNB or surgical procedures that include patient, site, and side verification

6. Staff surgeons provide the concordance document detailed in **Box 5** to surgical residents in training to emphasize its importance

7. Acknowledgment of the important roles that breast specialty nurses, medical assistants, and radiology technicians play in a systems approach to optimizing care. In other words, if nonphysician staff question any process of care regarding patient identification, annotation, site (or side) marking, or procedure, then a procedural pause occurs until there is reconciliation and mutual agreement

---

Box 5
Breast disease concordance testing over continuum of time: a document for education of surgical residents and fellows and a checklist for breast surgeons

Purpose

1. Prevent delayed diagnosis of breast cancer

2. Prevent "wrong" side and site procedures and surgery

3. Optimize technical performance of lumpectomy and mastectomy to achieve negative margins and low local regional recurrence rates

4. Global concordance evaluation after breast operation

Method: Clinical breast examination (CBE), imaging, and histology must be continuously assessed for concordance.

Side and site must be concordant for each of the following:

1. History (patient's report of location of palpable lump and complete chart review of any care provider's description of location of lump)

2. CBE—primary care provider and breast consultants

3. Imaging (mammogram, US, MRI, other imaging [eg, positron emission tomography])

4. Procedure (FNA site, CNB site, other minimally invasive biopsy site, incisional biopsy site, needle localized excisional biopsy site, skin biopsy site, lumpectomy site)

5. Procedure pathology report(s) (description of site location)

Location of breast index lesion and verification of removal is further determined by concordance of the following:

Radiologist description of location

Surgeon description of location in preoperative evaluation

Location of preoperative needle hookwire as seen in the OR

Location of breast lesion on intraoperative ultrasound

Operative report description of excision location

Specimen mammogram and/or US confirmation of lesion(s) and margins

Pathology description of location of lesion in pathology report

Confirmation of removal of a lesion that histologically is concordant with patient history, CBE and Imaging.

Failure to explain/account for discordance at any point along the care pathway may lead to missed lesions, delayed diagnosis of breast cancer, wrong side or site of surgery, inadequate surgery, positive margins, early breast recurrence, or recommendations for follow-up/observation when a lesion is still present in the breast.

In clinical practice, adherence to the principles discussed here means that the care provider who performs needle biopsy, needle localization, or surgery must review all of the aforementioned before performing the procedure.

SUMMARY

Further refinements and innovations in diagnostic and therapeutic breast imaging will undoubtedly occur. Our patients will be the beneficiaries of these changes. Surgeons are advised to keep up to date and to understand how imaging is incorporated into interdisciplinary breast care.

ACKNOWLEDGMENTS

The authors wish to thank Brooke De Maiffe for assistance in manuscript preparation.

REFERENCES

1. Jemal A, Siegel R, Xu J, et al. Cancer statistics 2010. CA Cancer J Clin 2010;60: 277–300. DOI: 10.1002/caac.20073.
2. Silverstein MJ, Recht A, Lagios MD, et al. Image-detected breast cancer: state-of-the-art diagnosis and treatment. J Am Coll Surg 2009;209:504–20.
3. Shapiro S. Periodic screening for breast cancer: the HIP Randomized Controlled Trial. Health Insurance Plan. J Natl Cancer Inst Monogr 1997;22:27–30.
4. Baker LH. Breast cancer detection demonstration project: five-year summary report. CA Cancer J Clin 1982;32:194–225.
5. Beahrs OH, Shapiro S, Smart CR. Report of the Working Group to review the National Cancer Institute-American Cancer Society Breast Cancer Detection Demonstration Projects. J Natl Cancer Inst 1979;62(3):639–709.
6. Smart CR, Byrne C, Smith RA, et al. Twenty-year follow-up of the breast cancers diagnosed during the Breast Cancer Detection Demonstration Project. CA Cancer J Clin 1997;47(3):134–49.
7. Tabar L, Vitak B, Chen HH, et al. Beyond randomized controlled trials: organized mammographic screening substantially reduces breast carcinoma mortality. Cancer 2001;91(9):1724–31.
8. Tabar L, Vitak B, Chen HH, et al. The Swedish Two-County Trial twenty years later: updated mortality results and new insights from long-term follow-up. Radiol Clin North Am 2000;38:625–51.
9. Byrne C, Smart CR, Chu KC, et al. Survival advantage differences by age. Evaluation of the extended follow-up of the Breast Cancer Detection Demonstration Project. Cancer 1994;74(Suppl 1):301–10.
10. Cunningham MP. The Breast Cancer Demonstration Detection Project 25 years later. CA Cancer J Clin 1997;47(3):131–3.
11. Duffy SW, Tabar L, Smith RA. The mammographic screening trials: commentary on the recent work by Olsen and Gotzsche. CA Cancer J Clin 2002;52(2):68–71.
12. Seidman H, Gelb SK, Silverberg E, et al. Survival experience in the Breast Cancer Detection Demonstration Project. CA Cancer J Clin 1987;37(5):258–90.
13. ACR Practice Guideline for the Performance of Screening and Diagnostic Mammography Res 24. 2008. Available at: www.acr.org/SecondaryMainMenu Categories/quality_safety/guidelines/breast/Screening_Diagnostic.aspx(ACR). Accessed June 21, 2009.
14. Position statement on USPSTF. Available at: http://www.breastcare.org. Accessed July 17, 2010.
15. Screening mammography indications. Available at: http://www.breastsurgeons. org. Accessed July 17, 2010.
16. Screening mammography indications. Available at: http://www.cancer.org/ docroot/CRI/content/CRI_2_4_3X_Can_breast_cancer_be_found_early_5.asp(ACS). Accessed July 17, 2010.
17. Breast cancer screening and diagnosis guidelines. Available at: http://www. nccn.org. Accessed July 17, 2010.
18. Smith RA, Cokkinides V, Brooks D, et al. Cancer screening in the United States, 2010: a review of current American Cancer Society guidelines and issues in cancer screening. CA Cancer J Clin 2010;60(2):99–119.

19. US Preventive Task Force. Screening for breast cancer: US Preventive Task Force Recommendation Statement. Ann Intern Med 2009;151(10):716–26.
20. Armstrong K, Moye E, Williams S, et al. Screening mammography in women 40 to 49 years of age: a systematic review for the American College of Physicians. Ann Intern Med 2007;146(7):516–26.
21. Djulbegovic B, Lyman GH. Screening mammography at 40-49 years: regret or no regret? Lancet 2006;368(9522):2035–7.
22. Keen JD, Keen JE. What is the point: will screening mammography save my life? BMC Med Inform Decis Mak 2009;9:18.
23. Kopans DB. Beyond randomized controlled trials: organized mammographic screening substantially reduces breast carcinoma mortality. Comment on: Cancer 2001;1;91(9):1724–3. Cancer 2002;94(2):580–1 [author reply: 581–3].
24. Moss SM, Cuckle H, Evans A, et al. Effect of mammographic screening from age 40 years on breast cancer mortality at 10 years' follow-up: a randomised controlled trial. Lancet 2006;368:2053–60.
25. Whitman GJ. The role of mammography in breast cancer prevention. Curr Opin Oncol 1999;11(5):414–8.
26. Saslow D, Boetes C, Burke W, et al. American Cancer Society guidelines for breast screening with MRI as an adjunct to mammography. American Cancer Society Breast Cancer Advisory Group. CA Cancer J Clin 2007;57(2):75–89.
27. Jackson VP. Diagnostic mammography. Radiol Clin North Am 2004;42(5): 853–70, vi.
28. Homer MJ, Berlin L. Radiography of the surgical breast biopsy specimen. AJR Am J Roentgenol 1998;171:1197–9.
29. Jackman RJ, Marzoni FA. Needle-localised breast biopsy: why do we fail? Radiology 1997;204:677–84.
30. ACR practice guideline for the performance of stereotactically guided breast interventional procedures (Revised) Res 28. 2009. Available at: http://www. acr.org/SecondaryMainMenuCategories/quality_safety/guidelines/breast.aspx. Accessed June 21, 2009.
31. Performance and practice guidelines for stereotactic breast procedures. Available at: http://www.breastsurgeons.org/statements/index.php. Accessed July 7, 2010.
32. Stomper PC, Budnick RM, Stewart CC. Use of specimen mammography-guided FNA (fine-needle aspirates) for flow cytometric multiple marker analysis and immunophenotyping in breast cancer. Cytometry 2000;42(3):165–73.
33. McCormick JT, Keleher AJ, Tikhomirov VB, et al. Analysis of the use of specimen mammography in breast conservation therapy. Am J Surg 2004;188(4): 433–6.
34. Popli MB. Pictorial essay: mammographic features of breast cancer. Indian J Radiol Imaging 2001;11:175–9.
35. Sickles EA. Mammographic features of 300 consecutive non-palpable breast cancers. AJR Am J Roentgenol 1986;146:661–76.
36. Muller-Schimpfle M, Wersebe A, Xydeas T, et al. Microcalcifications of the breast: how does radiologic classification correlate with histology? Acta Radiol 2005;46(8):774–81.
37. D'Orsi C, Bassett L, Berg W, et al. ACR Breast Imaging Reporting and Data System (BI-RADS Atlas). 4th edition. Reston (VA): American College of Radiology; 2003.
38. D'Orsi CJ, Kopans DB. Mammography interpretation: the BI-RADS method. Am Fam Physician 1997;55:1548–50, 52.

39. Balleyguier C, Ayadi S, Van Nguyen K, et al. BI-RADS classification in mammography. Eur J Radiol 2007;61(2):192–4.
40. Hirunpat S, Tanomkiat W, Khojarern R, et al. Accuracy of the mammographic report category according to BI-RADS. J Med Assoc Thai 2005;88(1):62–5.
41. Lacquement MA, Mitchell D, Hollingsworth AB. Positive predictive value of the Breast Imaging Reporting and Data System. J Am Coll Surg 1999;189(1):34–40.
42. Liberman L, Abramson AF, Squires FB, et al. The breast imaging reporting and data system: positive predictive value of mammographic features and final assessment categories. AJR Am J Roentgenol 1998;171(1):35–40.
43. Mammography teaching files. Available at: http://www.rad.washington.edu/academics/academic-sections/mbi/education/mammoed/teaching-files. Accessed July 17, 2010.
44. Mammography teaching files. Available at: http://www.radiologyeducation.com/#RadiologyTeachingFiles. Accessed July 17, 2010.
45. Ng KH, Muttarak M. Advances in mammography have improved early detection of breast cancer. J HK Coll Radiol 2003;6:126–31.
46. ACR Committee on quality assurance. American College of Radiology (ACR) mammography quality control manual for radiologists, radiologic technologists, and medical physicists. Reston (VA): American College of Radiology; 1999.
47. Hendrick RE, Bassett L, Botsco MA, et al. Mammography quality control manual. Reston (VA): American College of Radiology; 1999.
48. MQSA. Mammography Quality Standards Act. Available at: http://www.fda.gov/cdrh/mammography. Accessed July 17, 2010.
49. Skaane P, Hofvind S, Skjennald A. Randomized trial of screen-film versus full-field digital mammography with soft-copy reading in population-based screening program: follow-up and final results of Oslo II study. Radiology 2007;244(3):708–17.
50. Van Ongeval C, Bosmans H, Van Steen A. Current status of digital mammography for screening and diagnosis of breast cancer. Curr Opin Oncol 2006; 18(6):547–54.
51. Stomper PC, Margolin FR. Ductal carcinoma in situ: the mammographer's perspective. AJR Am J Roentgenol 1994;162:585–91.
52. Feig SA. Ductal carcinoma in situ: implications for screening mammography. Radiol Clin North Am 2000;38:653–68.
53. Breast Cancer Surveillance Consortium. Available at: http://breastscreening.cancer.gov/. Accessed July 17, 2010.
54. Weaver DL, Rosenberg RD, Barlow WE, et al. Pathologic findings from the Breast Cancer Surveillance Consortium: population-based outcomes in women undergoing biopsy after screening mammography. Cancer 2006;106(4):732–42.
55. Tabar L, Tony Chen HH, Amy Yen MF, et al. Mammographic tumor features can predict long-term outcomes reliably in women with 1-14-mm invasive breast carcinoma. Cancer 2004;101(8):1745–59.
56. Tabar L, Dean PB. Thirty years of experience with mammography screening: a new approach to the diagnosis and treatment of breast cancer. Breast Cancer Res 2008;10(Suppl 4):S3.
57. Tabár L, Chen HH, Duffy SW, et al. A novel method for prediction of long-term outcome of women with T1a, T1b, and 10-14 mm invasive breast cancers: a prospective study. Lancet 2000;355(9202):429–33.
58. Zunzunegui RG, Chung MA, Oruwari J, et al. Casting-type calcifications with invasion and high-grade ductal carcinoma in situ: a more aggressive disease? Arch Surg 2003;138(5):537–40.

59. Thompson M, Klimberg VS. Use of ultrasound in breast surgery. Surg Clin North Am 2007;87:469–84.
60. Thompson M, Henry-Tillman R, Margulies A, et al. Hematoma-directed ultrasound-guided (HUG) breast lumpectomy. Ann Surg Oncol 2007;14(1): 148–56.
61. Kopans DB. Breast imaging. 3rd edition. Philadelphia: Lippincott Williams & Wilkins, a Wolters Kluwer Business; 2007. p. 555–606, 691–732, 783–888.
62. Stavros AT. Breast ultrasound. Philadelphia: Lippincott Williams & Wilkins, a Wolters Kluwer Business; 2004. p. 16–41, 276–350, 445–528,528–96, 834–76.
63. Guideline for performance of a breast ultrasound examination. Available at: http://www.acr.org/secondarymainmenucategories/quality_safety/guidelines/breast/us_guided_breast.aspx. Accessed July 17, 2010.
64. American Society of Breast Surgeons position statements. Available at: http://breastsurgeons.org/statements/index.php. Accessed July 17, 2010.
65. NCCN indications for breast US in breast cancer screening and diagnosis guidelines. Available at: http://www.nccn.org/professionals/physician_gls/f_guidelines.asp. Accessed July 17, 2010.
66. American College of Radiology BI-RADS Atlas for US. Available at: http://www.acr.org/SecondaryMainMenuCategories/quality_safety/BI-RADSAtlas/BI-RADSAtlasexcerptedtext/BI-RADSUltrasoundFirstEdition.aspx. Accessed July 17, 2010.
67. American College of Radiology US Lexicon. Available at: http://www.acr.org/SecondaryMainMenuCategories/quality_safety/BI-RADSAtlas/BI-RADSAtlasexcerptedtext/BI-RADSUltrasoundFirstEdition.aspx. Accessed July 17, 2010.
68. Lazarus M, Mainiero MB, Schepps B, et al. BI-RADS lexicon for US and mammography: interobserver variability and positive predictive value. Radiology 2006;239:385–91.
69. Bruening W, Fontanarosa J, Tipton K, et al. Systematic review: comparative effectiveness of core-needle and open surgical biopsy to diagnose breast lesions. Ann Intern Med 2010;1152(4):238–46.
70. Bruening W, Schoelles K, Treadwell J, et al. Comparative effectiveness of core-needle and open surgical biopsy for the diagnosis of breast lesions. Comparative effectiveness review No. 19. (Prepared by ECRI Institute Evidence-based Practice Center under Contract No. 290-02-0019.). Rockville (MD): Agency for Healthcare Research and Quality; 2009. Available at: http://www.effective healthcare.ahrq.gov/reports/final.cfm. Accessed December 15, 2009.
71. Silverstein M. Where's the outrage? J Am Coll Surg 2009;208(1):78–9.
72. Pocock B, Taback B, Klein L, et al. Preoperative needle biopsy as a potential quality measure in breast cancer surgery. Ann Surg Oncol 2009;16(5): 1108–11.
73. American Society of Breast Surgeons Mastery Program for quality measurement. Available at: http://www.breastsurgeons.org. Accessed July 26, 2010.
74. Landercasper J, Tafra L. The relationship between quality and cost during the perioperative breast cancer episode of care. Breast 2010;19(4):289–96.
75. Golub RM, Bennett CL, Stinson T, et al. Cost minimization study of image-guided core biopsy versus surgical excisional biopsy for women with abnormal mammograms. J Clin Oncol 2004;22(12):2430–7.
76. Smith TJ, Landercasper J, Gundrum JD, et al. Perioperative quality metrics for one step breast cancer surgery: a patient-centered approach. J Surg Oncol 2010;102(1):34–8.

77. Kaufman CS, Shockney L, Rabinowitz B, et al. Quality Initiative Committee. National Quality Measures for Breast Centers (NQMBC): a robust quality tool: breast center quality measures. Ann Surg Oncol 2010;17(2):377–85.

78. Landercasper J, Ellis RL, Mathiason MA, et al. A community breast center report card determined by participation in the National Quality Measures for Breast Centers Program™. Breast J 2010;16:472–780.

79. Genta F, Zanon E, Camanni M, et al. Cost/accuracy ratio analysis in breast cancer patients undergoing ultrasound-guided fine-needle aspiration cytology, sentinel node biopsy, and frozen section of node. World J Surg 2007;31(6): 1155–63.

80. Cody HS 3rd. One-step surgery for breast cancer: back to the future? World J Surg 2007;31(6):1153–4.

81. Landercasper J, Gundersen SB Jr, Gundersen AL, et al. Needle localization and biopsy of nonpalpable lesions of the breast. Surg Gynecol Obstet 1987;164(5): 399–403.

82. Ellis RL. Interdisciplinary breast care: essential information for the treatment team. Semin Breast Dis 2005;8(1):10–6.

83. American College of Radiology accreditation for US. Available at: http://www.acr.org/accreditation/breast.aspx. Accessed July 17, 2010.

84. Statement on training of non radiologists in performance and interpretation of imaging and image-guided biopsy. Available at: http://www.sbi-online.org/displaycommon.cfm?an=4. Accessed July 17, 2010.

85. The American Institute of US Medicine (AIUM) breast cancer guidelines. Available at: http://www.aium.org/publications/guidelines.aspx. Accessed July 17, 2010.

86. American Society of Breast Surgeons certification criteria for surgeon sonography. Available at: http://www.breastsurgeons.org/certification/breast_ultrasound_certification.php. Accessed July 17, 2010.

87. NAPBC Program Standards. Available at: http://accreditedbreastcenters.org/standards/standards.html. Accessed July 17, 2010.

88. NCCN. Guidelines for genetic/familial high-risk assessment: breast and ovarian. Available at: www.nccn.org. Accessed July 17, 2010.

89. NCCN. Treatment guidelines for breast cancer. Available at: www.nccn.org. Accessed July 17, 2010.

90. Erkonen WE, Smith WL. Radiology 101: the basics and fundamentals of imaging. 3rd edition. Philadelphia: Lippincott Williams & Wilkins, a Wolters Kluwer Business; 2010. p. 8–10.

91. MRI technology in Wikipedia. Available at: http://en.wikipedia.org/wiki/MRI. Accessed July 17, 2010.

92. Ellis RL. Optimal timing of breast MRI examinations for premenopausal women who do not have a normal menstrual cycle. Am J Roentgenol 2009;193(6): 1738–40.

93. Lee CH, Dershaw DD, Kopans D, et al. Breast cancer screening with imaging: recommendations from the Society of Breast Imaging and the ACR on the use of mammography, breast MRI, breast ultrasound, and other technologies for the detection of clinically occult breast cancer. J Am Coll Radiol 2010;7(1):18–27.

94. Orel S. Who should have breast magnetic resonance imaging evaluation? J Clin Oncol 2008;26(5):703–11.

95. Ciocchetti JM, Joy N, Staller S, et al. The effect of magnetic resonance imaging in the workup of breast cancer. Am J Surg 2009;198(6):824–8.

96. Hollingsworth AB, Stough RG, O'Dell CA, et al. Breast magnetic resonance imaging for preoperative locoregional staging. Am J Surg 2008;196(3):389–97.

97. Houssami N, Hayes DF. Review of preoperative magnetic resonance imaging (MRI) in breast cancer: should MRI be performed on all women with newly diagnosed, early stage breast cancer? CA Cancer J Clin 2009;59(5):290–302.

98. de Bresser J, de Vos B, van der Ent F, et al. Breast MRI in clinically and mammographically occult breast cancer presenting with an axillary metastasis: a systematic review. Eur J Surg Oncol 2010;36(2):114–9.

99. Houssami N, Morrow M. Pre-operative breast MRI in women with recently diagnosed breast cancer—where to next? Breast 2010;19(1):1–2.

100. Katipamula R, Degnim AC, Hoskin T, et al. Trends in mastectomy rates at the Mayo Clinic Rochester: effect of surgical year and preoperative magnetic resonance imaging. J Clin Oncol 2009;27(25):4082–8.

101. Bleicher RJ, Ciocca RM, Egleston BL, et al. Association of routine pretreatment magnetic resonance imaging with time to surgery, mastectomy rate, and margin status. J Am Coll Surg 2009;209(2):180–7 [quiz: 294–5]. Erratum appears in J Am Coll Surg 2009;209(5):679.

102. Siegmann KC, Baur A, Vogel U, et al. Risk-benefit analysis of preoperative breast MRI in patients with primary breast cancer. Clin Radiol 2009;64(4): 403–13.

103. Solin LJ. Counterview: pre-operative breast MRI (magnetic resonance imaging) is not recommended for all patients with newly diagnosed breast cancer. Breast 2010;19(1):7–9.

104. Morrow M. Magnetic resonance imaging for screening, diagnosis, and eligibility for breast-conserving surgery: promises and pitfalls. Surg Oncol Clin N Am 2010;19(3):475–92.

105. Demicheli R, Ardoino I, Boracchi P, et al. Ipsilateral breast tumour recurrence (IBTR) dynamics in breast conserving treatments with or without radiotherapy. Int J Radiat Biol 2010;86(7):542–7.

106. Liau SS, Cariati M, Noble D, et al. Audit of local recurrence following breast conservation surgery with 5-mm target margin and hypofractionated 40-Gray breast radiotherapy for invasive breast cancer. Ann R Coll Surg Engl 2010;92: 562–8.

107. Tuli R, Christodouleas J, Roberts L, et al. Prognostic indicators following ipsilateral tumor recurrence in patients treated with breast-conserving therapy. Am J Surg 2009;198(4):557–61.

108. Clarke M, Collins R, Darby S, et al. Effects of radiotherapy and of differences in the extent of surgery for early breast cancer on local recurrence and 15-year survival: an overview of the randomised trials. Early Breast Cancer Trialists' Collaborative Group (EBCTCG). Lancet 2005;366(9503):2087–106.

109. Tot T. Towards a renaissance of subgross breast morphology. Eur J Cancer 2010;46(11):1946–8.

110. Lagios MD. Multicentricity of breast carcinoma demonstrated by routine correlated serial subgross and radiographic examination. Cancer 1977;40(4): 1726–34.

111. Holland R, Veling SH, Mravunac M, et al. Histologic multifocality of Tis, T1-2 breast carcinomas. Implications for clinical trials of breast-conserving surgery. Cancer 1985;56(5):979–90.

112. Fisher B, Anderson S, Redmond CK, et al. Reanalysis and results after 12 years of follow-up in a randomized clinical trial comparing total mastectomy with

lumpectomy with or without irradiation in the treatment of breast cancer. N Engl J Med 1995;333(22):1456–61.

113. Fischer U, Baum F, Luftner-Nagel S. Preoperative MR imaging in patients with breast cancer: preoperative staging, effects on recurrence rates, and outcome analysis. Magn Reson Imaging Clin N Am 2006;14(3):351–62, vi.

114. Solin LJ, Orel SG, Hwang WT, et al. Relationship of breast magnetic resonance imaging to outcome after breast-conservation treatment with radiation for women with early-stage invasive breast carcinoma or ductal carcinoma in situ. J Clin Oncol 2008;26(3):386–91.

115. Turnbull LW, Brown SR, Olivier C, et al. Multicentre randomised controlled trial examining the cost-effectiveness of contrast-enhanced high field magnetic resonance imaging in women with primary breast cancer scheduled for wide local excision (COMICE). COMICE Trial Group. Health Technol Assess 2010; 14(1):1–182.

116. Landercasper J, Linebarger JH, Ellis RL, et al. A quality review of the timeliness of breast cancer diagnosis and treatment in an integrated breast center. J Am Coll Surg 2010;210(4):449–55.

117. Sorbero ME, Dick AW, Beckjord EB, et al. Diagnostic breast magnetic resonance imaging and contralateral prophylactic mastectomy. Ann Surg Oncol 2009;16(6):1597–605.

118. Newman E, Guest A, Helvie M, et al. Changes in surgical management resulting from case review at a breast cancer multidisciplinary tumor board. Cancer 2006; 107:2346–51.

119. Masood S. Raising the bar: a plea for standardization and quality improvement in the practice of breast pathology. Breast J 2006;12(5):409–12.

120. Kern KA. The delayed diagnosis of breast cancer: medicolegal implications and risk prevention for surgeons. Breast Dis 2001;12:145–58.

121. Tracy TF, Crawford LS, Krizek TJ, et al. When medical error becomes medical malpractice: the victims and the circumstances. Arch Surg 2003;138:447–54.

122. Johnson NB, Collins LC. Update on percutaneous needle biopsy of nonmalignant breast lesions. Adv Anat Pathol 2009;16(4):183–95.

123. Colloquium ASBD. Ensuring optimal interdisciplinary breast care in the United States: gaps, implications, and potential measures to assess optimal care early detection and diagnosis local-regional treatment systemic treatment. Copyright © 2009 American Society of Breast Disease. All rights reserved. Available at: http://www.asbd.org. Accessed July 17, 2010.

Biliary, Pancreatic, and Hepatic Imaging for the General Surgeon

Steven Reitz, MD[a,b], Kristine Slam, MD[c],
Lowell W. Chambers, MD[c],*

KEYWORDS

- Diagnostic imaging • Neoplasm • Biliary system • Pancreas
- Liver • General surgery

Disorders of the hepatobiliary system and pancreas are commonly encountered by the general surgeon. Recent refinements in cross-sectional and other imaging technologies have greatly enhanced the ability to make definitive preoperative diagnoses and help better select patients who will benefit from surgical intervention. It is critical that surgeons treating these patients have a good understanding of the usefulness and limitations of these imaging modalities to deliver optimal and efficient care. This article provides an overview of these imaging modalities within the context of those disorders most commonly seen in general surgical practice.

BILIARY
Cholelithiasis and Cholecystitis

Laparoscopic cholecystectomy is currently the most frequently performed abdominal surgery in the United States.[1,2] Transabdominal ultrasonography (US) is the primary imaging modality used to evaluate for the presence of cholelithiasis, with a sensitivity of 96% to 98% and specificity of 95% for gallstones greater than 2 to 5 mm in size.[2,3] Sonographically, cholelithiasis is characterized by echogenic foci, which cause acoustic shadows and are gravitationally dependent (**Fig. 1**).[3] Stones less than 2 to 3 mm (microlithiasis) are seen inconsistently on transabdominal US but can be seen with greater sensitivity on endoscopic ultrasonography (EUS).[4] This has clinical

The authors have nothing to disclose.
[a] Department of Surgery, Mount Carmel Health System, 793 West State Street, Columbus, OH 43222, USA
[b] Department of Medical Education, Mount Carmel Health System, 750 Mount Carmel Mall, Columbus, OH 43222, USA
[c] Metropolitan Surgery, 750 Mount Carmel Mall, Suite 350, Columbus, OH 43222, USA
* Corresponding author.
E-mail address: lwchambers76@hotmail.com

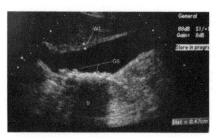

Fig. 1. Transabdominal US with layering, shadowing (S), echogenic foci consistent with gallstones (GS) and thickened gallbladder wall (WT).

applicability in the work-up of idiopathic pancreatitis, which is often associated with microlithiasis.[5,6] The presence of lower-amplitude, nonshadowing echoes layering in the dependent portion of the gallbladder on US constitutes biliary sludge, which represents an intermediate step in gallstone formation. This sludge can cause cholecystitis, cholangitis, and pancreatitis by the same mechanisms as larger stones and warrants similar therapeutic interventions.[3,7–9]

Cholelithiasis has a 1% to 2% likelihood of leading to acute cholecystitis or other complications each year.[1–3] Several signs, seen on US, are suggestive, but not necessarily diagnostic, of acute cholecystitis, including the presence of gallstones or sludge, luminal distension, wall thickening of greater than 3 mm, pericholecystic fluid, sonographic Murphy's sign (ie, the presence of maximal tenderness elicited by direct pressure of the US transducer over the gallbladder), and increased Doppler flow.[1,3,10] The greater the number of findings present, the more likely the diagnosis, in the proper clinical context.[3] Ralls and colleagues[11] showed that the presence of gallstones with concurrently observed wall thickening or sonographic Murphy's sign had a positive predictive value (PPV) of 92% to 95% for acute cholecystitis, whereas the absence of all 3 of these signs had a negative predictive value (NPV) of 95%.

Computed tomography (CT) is less sensitive (75%) than US in the detection of cholelithiasis because of the variable appearance depending on composition; more heavily calcified stones are easier to see than those with high cholesterol content, which are isodense with bile.[3,12] Therefore, CT has a limited role in the initial evaluation of patients with suspected cholelithiasis. It is important to be aware of CT findings of cholelithiasis-related complications, because it is being used increasingly as a screening examination in patients presenting with abdominal pain. CT findings of acute cholecystitis include most of those noted on US, with pericholecystic stranding representing a specific CT sign of acute cholecystitis.[3] However, the primary usefulness of CT in this setting is to assist in evaluation for complications such as emphysematous changes or acute pancreatitis.[3]

Recently, magnetic resonance imaging (MRI) and magnetic resonance cholangiopancreatography (MRCP) have gained widespread use in the secondary evaluation of cholelithiasis-related complications such as choledocholithiasis.[2,3] Gallstones produce little signal because of the restricted motion of water and cholesterol within the crystalline lattice of the stones. They are best seen on T2-weighted images, which produce bright bile against which the signal voids of gallstones can stand out prominently (**Fig. 2**). Gadolinium-enhanced, fat-suppressed, T1-weighted images are sensitive for inflammatory changes within the gallbladder wall, and T2-weighted images will show increased signal intensity with cholecystitis.[2]

Acute acalculous cholecystitis manifests the same clinical and radiologic findings of acute calculous disease but without evidence of gallstones. This diagnosis must be

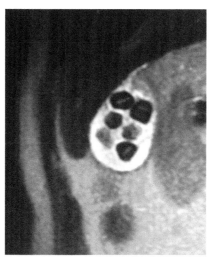

Fig. 2. Gallstones on T2-weighted MRI.

considered in critically or chronically ill hospitalized patients with unexplained abdominal pain or sepsis. Consequently, the general surgeon will often be called on to evaluate such patients who are noted to have gallbladder wall thickening or other findings suggestive of acalculous cholecystitis. To avoid the potential morbidity of nontherapeutic biliary procedures, it is important to recognize that several nonbiliary conditions, including hepatitis, hypoproteinemia, congestive heart failure, and chronic liver failure, can also produce many of these findings on US and CT.[3] Hepatobiliary scintigraphy provides physiologic imaging of the gallbladder and can be helpful in such scenarios.[1,3] Hepatobiliary scintigraphy is performed most commonly with hepatic iminodiacetic acid (HIDA) scanning using technetium-labeled analogues that are taken up by hepatocytes and actively transported through the biliary system. The absence of gallbladder filling 1 hour after intravenous (IV) injection of the isotope is suggestive of cholecystitis, whereas nonfilling after 4 hours is diagnostic provided the isotope has moved through the common bile duct.[1] Alternatively, administration of 0.04 mg/kg of IV morphine induces spasm of the sphincter of Oddi, facilitating filling of the gallbladder. Continued nonfilling 30 minutes after morphine augmentation is equally predictive of the diagnosis of acute cholecystitis[1,13–15] and shortens study duration. A recognized limitation of HIDA scanning is the need for patient transport to nuclear medicine, a move that can be hazardous for critically ill patients.

Chronic acalculous cholecystitis or biliary dyskinesia is also best evaluated with HIDA scanning. Delayed onset of gallbladder filling and slow biliary-to-bowel transit time are associated with chronic gallbladder dysfunction.[14] However, the most reliable criteria for the diagnosis is the gallbladder ejection fraction (EF) observed after administration of synthetic cholecystokinin (CCK) infusion.[16] A gallbladder EF of less than 30% to 40% following 3 to 30 minutes of CCK infusion is predictive of symptom relief after cholecystectomy, provided a supportive clinical setting.[14,16–18] A limitation of HIDA with EF has been inconsistency in diagnostic thresholds and dosing durations. An ongoing Society of Nuclear Medicine multicenter trial is expected to identify and standardize the optimal infusion methodology.[14] Reproduction of pain during the CCK infusion has been regarded as supportive of the diagnosis of chronic cholecystitis, but several investigations have not supported this.[18]

Gallbladder Polyps

Polypoid lesion of the gallbladder (PLG) is a term used to describe a range of elevated mucosal lesions including adenomas, small adenocarcinomas, cholesterol polyps, and adenomyomatosis hyperplasia.[3,19,20] The critical aspect of PLG differentiation is to determine which are at risk for containing, or progressing to, neoplasm. US is the most widely validated imaging modality for these lesions, which typically appear as immobile, nonshadowing echogenic masses (**Fig. 3**). Patients with symptomatic lesions should undergo cholecystectomy. Patients who are asymptomatic with PLGs 1 cm or larger have an 8% to 11% risk of malignancy and should also undergo cholecystectomy.[19,21–23] Lesions that are less than 1 cm have not been associated with neoplasm in the Western population and can therefore be managed nonoperatively, but are recommended to undergo interval US follow-up every 6 months for several years to ensure stability.[19,22] EUS seems to be more sensitive than US in PLG detection but has not been shown to better differentiate malignant from benign lesions.[19,22]

Gallbladder Carcinoma

The most common presentation of gallbladder adenocarcinoma radiographically is a subhepatic mass replacing or obscuring the gallbladder (**Fig. 4**). Less-frequent presentations include focal or diffuse gallbladder wall thickening or an intraluminal mass.[3] On US, malignancies of the gallbladder appear as hypo- or isoechogenic, irregularly shaped lesions. Gallstones are noted in 80% of cases and are occasionally surrounded by the tumor, a finding specific for gallbladder cancer.[23] Overall sensitivity of US in this setting is 85%, with an accuracy of 80%.[23]

CT does not show the mucosal characteristics of gallbladder carcinoma as clearly as US but identifies the presence of liver metastasis or local extension of the tumor. The sensitivity, specificity, PPV, NPV, and accuracy of modern multidetector CT for the primary site of gallbladder cancer are 84%, 71%, 93%, 48%, and 82%, respectively.[24] These tumors show early uptake of contrast within the arterial phase on CT, unlike the delayed uptake typical of cholangiocarcinoma.[23]

MRI is useful in the evaluation of primary gallbladder neoplasms and metastatic sites. Gallbladder adenocarcinoma appears as hypo- or isointense on T1-weighted

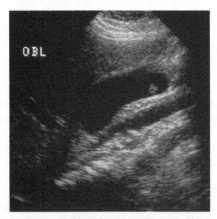

Fig. 3. PLG. US shows an echogenic polypoid mass without shadowing or layering. (*Adapted from* Gore RM, Yaghmai V, Newmark GM, et al. Imaging benign and malignant disease of the gallbladder. Radiol Clin North Am 2002;40:1317; with permission.)

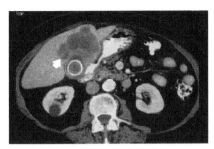

Fig. 4. Gallbladder carcinoma. CT shows a large calcified stone within a gallbladder showing significant mural thickening and invasion into adjacent liver (*arrow*). (*Adapted from* Gore RM, Yaghmai V, Newmark GM, et al. Imaging benign and malignant disease of the gallbladder. Radiol Clin North Am 2002;40:1319; with permission.)

images and is heterogeneously hyperintense on T2-weighted images.[2,23] The primary shows irregular rim early enhancement after gadolinium administration, helping to distinguish neoplastic changes from those of chronic cholecystitis, which is characterized by smooth early enhancement.[2] MRI is accurate for local hepatic invasion, with nearly 100% sensitivity, and also carries a 92% sensitivity in detection of local lymph node involvement.[2] These attributes make MRI the most appropriate secondary imaging modality for evaluation after US in most cases of suspected gallbladder cancer.

Even with concurrent CT scanning, positron emission tomography (PET) does not seem to offer additional benefit to that achieved with US and MRI in regard to primary tumor evaluation, but can be helpful in determination of lymph node involvement (94% PPV) and distant metastasis (95% sensitivity).[24,25]

Choledocholithiasis

Choledocholithiasis complicates 3% to 15% of cases of symptomatic cholelithiasis.[26] Common duct stones may pass harmlessly with time into the duodenum, but severe complications such as cholangitis or pancreatitis can occur. Prevention of such complicated courses, as well as differentiation from other causes of biliary obstruction, makes the diagnosis of choledocholithiasis extremely important.

US is typically the initial imaging modality and can show shadowing echogenic foci within the common bile duct (**Fig. 5**). Obesity and interference from duodenal gas limit

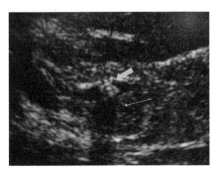

Fig. 5. Choledocholithiasis. US showing shadowing (*small arrow*) echogenic focus (*large arrow*) within the common bile duct.

the usefulness of US for choledocholithiasis, with reported sensitivity ranging between 25% and 63%. The presence of visualized stones on US is highly specific, at 95% to 100%, with PPV of approximately 100%.[4,27–29] It is therefore reasonable to act on positive US findings of choledocholithiasis, but there is no assurance of the reliability of negative findings. US is more sensitive (up to 91%) for indirect findings of choledocholithiasis, such as biliary duct dilatation greater than 6 mm.[26] Such findings are nonspecific and warrant additional radiologic investigation in most instances.

CT does not substantially enhance the imaging of choledocholithiasis beyond that provided by US.[4,27,28,30] CT cholangiography techniques can increase the sensitivity for choledocholithiasis to the 96% range but are limited by a high incidence of nausea and decreased accuracy in the jaundiced patient.[26,31,32] Noncholangiographic CT with coronal reconstruction has been found to be of some increased benefit in other biliary disorders but does not seem to enhance the diagnosis of choledocholithiasis.[33]

MRCP has become the imaging modality of choice in assessment of choledocholithiasis for several authorities.[26,30,34,35] The study is performed with T2-weighted images obtained by rapid acquisition (to minimize breathing artifact), which can be reformatted into three-dimensional, rotatable images. Common duct stones appear as filling defects of variable intensity within the biliary system on MRCP (**Fig. 6**), with a sensitivity of 81% to 100%, specificity of 73% to 100%, PPV of 63% to 97%, NPV of 84% to 100%, and accuracy of 82% to 92%.[4,26,30,34,36–38] Comparisons of MRCP with direct cholangiography via endoscopic retrograde cholangiopancreatography (ERCP) have shown equivalent results with the noted advantages of concurrent hepatic and pancreatic imaging with MRCP, in addition to the noninvasive nature of MRCP.[26,30,39]

The use of MRCP can be limited by patient factors such as claustrophobia, morbid obesity, or indwelling foreign bodies such as pacemakers. In addition, duodenal gas interference causes decreased sensitivity of MRCP for biliary disorders in the periampullary bile duct (**Fig. 7**).[40] The sensitivity of MRCP is also diminished to approximately 70% in the setting of common duct stones less than 5 mm in diameter.[38]

EUS involves the use of a high-frequency US probe on a specialized upper endoscope to facilitate close proximity US imaging of the pancreas, distal bile duct, local lymph nodes, and vessels.[4,41] Placement in the duodenal bulb provides high-resolution US images that can show common duct stones as small as 2 mm (**Fig. 8**). Experience with EUS for choledocholithiasis has shown a sensitivity of 84% to 97%, specificity of 86% to 100%, PPV of 98% to 100%, NPV of 88% to 97%, and accuracy of 91% to 99%.[4,26–30,36,37,42–49]

Limitations of EUS include the inherent risks of upper endoscopy and conscious sedation, poor visualization of the biliary system proximal to the hepatic hilum,

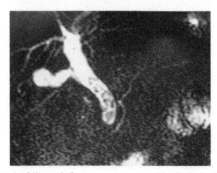

Fig. 6. MRCP with multiple filling defects consistent with choledocholithiasis.

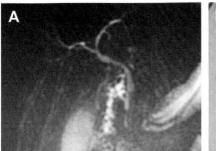
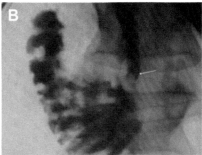

Fig. 7. Periampullary region of decreased sensitivity on MRCP. (*A*) MRCP interpreted as normal. (*B*) A 5-mm distal common bile duct stone (*arrow*) found on intraoperative cholangiography (IOC) after negative MRCP. The stone was removed via transcystic choledochoscopy.

operator dependency, limited availability, and anatomic limitations in some patients having previously undergone upper gastrointestinal operations.[4,26,44] Advantages include the lack of ionizing radiation or contrast exposure and the ability to accurately image small stones and those in the distal common bile duct.[4,30,44,50] These advantages provide an argument to favor EUS as the primary preoperative imaging modality for evaluation of possible choledocholithiasis at institutions where the expertise is available.[4,30,37] For difficult presentations, MRCP and EUS can be complementary, with the former providing good assessment for intrahepatic and proximal biliary causes, whereas the latter can better show smaller stones and the periampullary region.

ERCP has been regarded as the nonoperative gold standard for biliary imaging, with a sensitivity of 84% to 97%, specificity of 87% to 100%, PPV of 79% to 100%, NPV of 93% to 96%, and accuracy of 89% to 97% in the diagnosis of choledocholithiasis.[4,26,29,30,43–45,51] In addition, ERCP has the advantage of allowing for stone removal and biliary drainage (**Fig. 9**). However, the procedure is invasive, with complication rates as high as 15% and mortality ranging between 0.2% and 1.5%.[26,52,53] Acute pancreatitis is the most common notable complication, occurring in approximately 5% of cases. The instrumentation of an obstructed biliary system also poses the risk of cholangitis, particularly if drainage cannot be accomplished. Other substantial morbidities include duodenal and biliary perforation and bleeding.[26,52–54] Because of

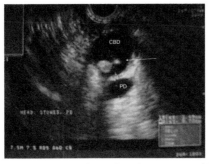

Fig. 8. Choledocholithiasis on EUS. Stone (*arrow*) within common bile duct (CBD) with adjacent pancreatic duct (PD). (*Courtesy of* Sanjay Garuda, MD, Columbus, OH.)

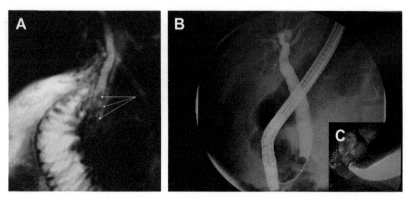

Fig. 9. Common duct clearance with ERCP. (*A*) MRCP obtained for evaluation of acute pancreatitis showing filling defects consistent with choledocholithiasis (*arrows*). (*B, C*) Balloon sweep of duct during ERCP. (*Courtesy of* James Edison, MD, Columbus, OH.)

these risks, ERCP is now reserved for patients with a high likelihood of interventional need based on clinical and/or less-invasive imaging findings.[30,55–58] Intervention via ERCP for choledocholithiasis is successful in 90% to 97% of cases, although 2 or more sessions are required in up to 25% of cases.[30]

Peroral cholangioscopy, as initially described in the 1970s, involved the passage of a small daughter scope through a duodenoscope to directly visualize the bile duct. Early users of the modality were limited by the need for 2 endoscopists and limited resolution.[59–61] More recently, single-operator cholangioscopes with greater resolution and irrigation/operating channels have become available. In experienced hands, choledocholithiasis can be visualized in 90% of cases and the scope permits passage of an electrohydraulic lithotripsy probe or holmium laser for therapeutic purposes.[61] Currently, experience with peroral cholangioscopy is limited but it seems to have great potential for future diagnostic and therapeutic biliary applications.

The first series of direct cholangiography performed intraoperatively was reported in 1932 by Mirizzi.[62] Through the early 1970s, intraoperative cholangiography (IOC) was performed using static images, a time-consuming process that often required repeating.[63] The performance of IOC was greatly aided by the development of c-arm, high-definition fluoroscopy with application as described by Berci and colleagues[64] and others in the late 1970s, allowing for increased resolution and speed of the procedure, the ability to obtain multiple images, and the opportunity to perform fluoroscopically guided biliary interventions.[63,64] Several different instruments and approaches to cannulating the cystic duct laparoscopically have been described, including reusable cholangiograspers, which allow for placement and fixation of 4 to 5 French catheters (**Fig. 10**).[63,65] Laparoscopic IOC can be performed successfully in 92% to 97% of cases,[66–68] typically adding approximately 15 minutes of operating time to cholecystectomy.[26,66,69,70] In addition to providing imaging of the biliary tree, IOC also helps minimize the risk of injury to the common bile duct.[71–73]

In the diagnosis of choledocholithiasis, IOC is 80% to 98% sensitive, 76% to 97% specific, with a PPV of 84% to 100%, NPV of 90% to 98%, and an accuracy of 95% to 100%.[4,26,30,46–49,51] The success rate and diagnostic ability of IOC is equivalent to ERCP but without the risk of acute pancreatitis.[74] As well as an observed rate of common bile duct stones of 8% to 12% on IOC performed after ERCP (because of either false negative ERCP or interval passage of stones),[66] this provides support for an up-front surgical approach for patients presenting with symptomatic biliary

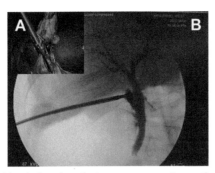

Fig. 10. (*A*) Nondisposable cholangiocatheter passer securing catheter in cystic duct while gallbladder is retracted cephelad. (*B*) Intraoperative cholangiogram with distal filling defect. A single stone was removed transcystically under fluoroscopy.

disease suggestive of choledocholithiasis.[26,30,75] Confirmed choledocholithiasis can then be addressed with laparoscopic common bile duct exploration, with equivalent outcomes to ERCP but with an overall shorter hospital stay and decreased expenses.[30,52,75–84] MRCP, EUS, and/or ERCP can then be limited to use in patients at risk for alternative diagnoses or in the rare instances in which IOC cannot be completed.

A substantial source of false-positive studies in both ERCP and IOC is incidental air-bubble instillation into the biliary system during cannulation and injection of contrast.[4] These can often be simply dealt with by manipulating the operating room (OR) table or flushing them through the system, but they can be persistent (**Fig. 11**A). Definitive assessment of these and other filling defects seen on IOC can be made by direct examination with choledochoscopy (see **Fig. 11**B). Choledochoscopy performance can be simplified by initially passing the scope transcystically into the duodenum under fluoroscopy with flexible wire guidance (**Fig. 12**). Patients with confirmed choledocholithiasis can be managed with basket retrieval of the stones or stone manipulation into the duodenum under choledochoscopic visualization (**Fig. 13**).[26,80,85] The capital outlay costs of purchasing laparoscopic choledochoscopes is problematic for many ORs and can be circumvented by using a flexible ureteroscope for laparoscopic cases and a flexible cystoscope for open cases.

Intraoperative US has been described by several investigators as a study for choledocholithiasis that is equally sensitive as IOC, with the advantage to the patient and operating team of avoiding radiation exposure.[30,86] Intraoperative US can be

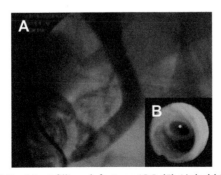

Fig. 11. Air artifact. (*A*) Persistent filling defects on IOC. (*B*) Air bubble on choledochoscopy.

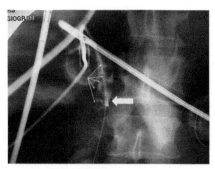

Fig. 12. Fluoroscopic passage of choledochoscope (*large arrow*) past multiple common duct stones (*small arrows*) using flexible guide wire.

performed either laparoscopically or open and, in experienced hands, can be performed within 7 minutes with a sensitivity of 96% to 100% and specificity of 99% to 100%.[26,86] It does not require cystic duct cannulation and can be performed successfully 95% to 99% of the time, which is slightly better than IOC.[67,68] However, it does not delineate ductal abnormalities and anatomic variation as well as IOC, and has a fairly steep learning curve. Perhaps most importantly, intraoperative US does not allow for as expeditious a transition to interventional maneuvers as does IOC.[26]

Cholangiocarcinoma

Cholangiocarcinoma (CC) is classified anatomically as intrahepatic (5%–10% of cases) perihilar (60%–70%), or distal (20%–30%).[87–90] Intrahepatic CC typically

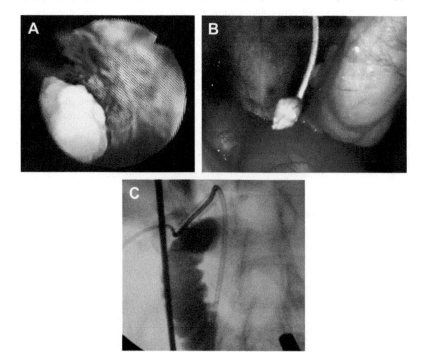

Fig. 13. Choledochoscopy. (*A*) Stone on intraoperative choledochoscopy. (*B*) Basket retrieval of stone. (*C*) Choledochoscope within duodenum.

presents as, and is managed in similar fashion to, hepatocellular carcinoma (HCC), whereas perihilar and distal tumors present most commonly with obstructive jaundice. Surgical resection remains the only potentially curative treatment modality.[87,89,91] A minority of patients seem resectable on presentation, and approximately 25% of these are found to have unresectable disease on exploration.[87,90] Curative surgery requires extensive resections, typically major hepatectomy for intrahepatic and perihilar CC or pancreaticoduodenectomy for distal CC, each of which carries significant risk of morbidity.[87,89,92–94] The preoperative radiographic assessment for resectability is consequently as critical as that for diagnosis. Radiographic criteria for resectability of intrahepatic CC mirror those of HCC, whereas resectability of distal CC is identical to that of other periampullary malignancies. Perihilar CC presents unique challenges in both diagnosis and determination of respectability because CC tends to grow along the biliary tree and frequently invades proximally, resulting in nonresectability.[89]

The most common findings with CC on US is indirect evidence such as proximal biliary ductal dilatation, hepatomegaly, and hepatic atrophy, which are detected with a sensitivity of 80% to 96% and carry a poor specificity of 20% to 40%.[88,95–98] US has poor sensitivity for detecting metastases in the lymph nodes (LN) (37%), liver (66%), and peritoneum (33%).[97] The addition of color flow Doppler enhances the sensitivity of US for portal vein (PV) occlusion (100%) and infiltration (83%), but sensitivity for hepatic arterial involvement remains poor (43%). Consequently, additional imaging modalities are required in essentially all cases for accurate diagnosis and determination of resectability.[87,96]

Both CT and MRI can image the primary site of CC in 70% to 90% of cases as lesions that are hypo- or isoattenuating relative to normal hepatic parenchyma and tend to remain so during arterial and portal venous phases before showing enhancement during delayed phase images.[87,88,99–101] This is reflective of the hypovascular desmoplastic composition typifying CC, and contrasts with the arterial enhancement seen with most cases of gallbladder cancer and HCC.[23,88,99,102,103] MRI additionally allows cholangiographic capability and the opportunity of tissue differentiation based on different pulse sequences with increased signal being noted within most CC primary sites on T2-weighted images. This capability results in near 100% sensitivity in diagnosing biliary obstruction, 98% accuracy in identifying the level of obstruction, and an 88% to 95% accurate assessment of the cause of obstruction; performance equivalent to that of direct cholangiography.[40,87–89,104–108] Given this cholangiographic performance, the ability to concurrently evaluate for intra-abdominal local or distant metastasis and its noninvasive nature, MRCP has become the imaging modality of choice in evaluation of biliary strictures and CC (**Fig. 14**A).[87,91,94,109,110] An accurate assessment of resectability of CC is rendered by MRI/MRCP in 70% to 80% of cases, a rate equivalent to that provided by the combination of CT and direct cholangiography in prospective comparison.[111] From a strategic standpoint, it is important to recognize that stenting and percutaneous drainage procedures cause mild bile duct wall inflammation that is indistinguishable on MRI from CC spread. Consequently, MRCP should be performed before interventional procedures whenever possible.[112]

EUS is a more sensitive modality for the periampullary region, with the ability to show lesions as small as 2 mm, and is therefore a helpful adjunct to MRCP when distal biliary abnormalities are suspected.[4,30,41,44,50] Determination of LN involvement by MRI is 66% to 74% accurate,[87,111,113] whereas the sensitivity and specificity for PV invasion are 78% and 91%, respectively.[87,114] Evaluation of hepatic arterial invasion is more limited, with a 58% to 73% sensitivity and 93% specificity.[87,115] These limitations can also be offset by EUS, which seems to be more accurate at determination of

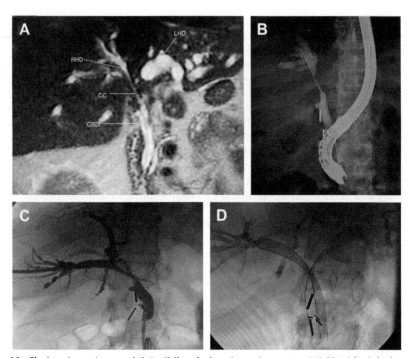

Fig. 14. Cholangiocarcinoma. (*A*) Perihilar cholangiocarcinoma on MRCP with right hepatic duct (RHD), left hepatic duct (LHD), common bile duct (CBD), and tumor site (CC) noted. (*B*) ERCP evaluation. (*C*) Percutaneous transhepatic cholangiogram. (*D*) Palliative and therapeutic stenting with bilateral approach taken to address clinical cholangitis. (*Courtesy of Andrew Verrill, MD, Columbus, OH.*)

regional LN and vascular involvement.[116,117] An additional benefit of EUS is the ability to perform direct-guided, fine-needle aspiration (FNA) on primary tumors as well as local LNs with sensitivity, specificity, and accuracy of 86% to 89%, 100%, and 88% to 91%, respectively.[41,87,118–120] Hypothetically the risk of needle tract seeding should be less than that of percutaneous FNA/biopsy given the shorter needle tract, but data concerning this are limited currently.[87,121]

Evaluation of metastatic disease from several neoplasms has recently been aided with the development of PET scanning, particularly when fused with CT. PET does not currently have a routine role in CC, although it can be helpful when there is a question of possible metastatic disease.[89,122,123]

Direct cholangiography in the setting of CC is typically performed via ERCP or percutaneous transhepatic cholangiography (PTC). The choice between ERCP and PTC is dictated by institutional experience and anatomic characteristics of the tumor. Distal CC tends to be better imaged via ERCP, whereas hilar and intrahepatic lesions typically can be viewed better with PTC (see **Fig. 14**B, C).[87,91] Both modalities carry an overall sensitivity of 75% to 85%, a specificity of 70% to 75%, and an accuracy of 95% in identifying the presence and extent of CC.[87,89,106,107,124] The invasiveness of both procedures is a notable limiting factor, favoring routine use of MRCP with or without EUS during the diagnostic stage of most cases unless the development of cholangitis demands early interventional therapy.[40,87,125,126] The primary role of direct cholangiography in CC is in palliative or preoperative stenting procedures to relieve biliary obstruction (see **Fig. 14**D).[87,89] In addition, direct cholangiography affords the opportunity of obtaining brush cytology and/or biopsy specimens, which can assist with making a definitive diagnosis. Although these sampling methods carry sensitivities ranging from 10% to 80% in the diagnosis of CC, the experience of most authorities has been at the lower end of this range, reflective of the substantial associated desmoplastic reaction and low cellularity seen in many CCs.[87,123,127] This limitation has frequently led to the need to make definitive treatment decisions without the advantage of tissue diagnosis.

Two emerging adjunctive modalities to direct cholangiography have the potential to substantially enhance preoperative diagnosis and staging of CC. Peroneal cholangioscopy, an extension of ERCP techniques, permits direct visualization of the bile duct, with sensitivities and specificities up to 100% and 80%, in patients with CC.[59,61,87] Cholangioscopy also can be performed percutaneously, although published experiences with this technique are more limited.[61]

Intraductal ultrasound (IDUS) uses small-diameter probes that can be inserted over a 9-mm guide wire at the time of direct cholangiography, providing US views that are 89% accurate at determining the benign or malignant nature of biliary strictures and 82% accurate at determining resectability.[41,128] As with any US procedure, the accuracy of IDUS is operator dependent.

PANCREAS
Acute Pancreatitis

More than 300,000 patients are hospitalized each year with acute pancreatitis (AP) and 20,000 ultimately die from the condition.[129,130] The diagnosis of AP is usually made when a patient has 2 of the following 3 criteria: upper abdominal pain, increased pancreatic enzymes, and imaging findings of pancreatic inflammation. In addition to the diagnostic yield, imaging assists with determination of the cause, severity, and prognosis of AP.

AP cannot be definitively diagnosed with plain abdominal films, but abdominal radiography is performed in many cases to rule out other causes of upper abdominal pain, such as gastrointestinal perforation.[131] Inconsistently seen findings suggestive of pancreatitis include localized sentinel loop formation caused by focally dilated small bowel with distal spasm caused by the inflammatory process. Similarly, a colon cutoff sign occurs via the same mechanism and can be seen at the splenic flexure, descending colon, or transverse colon.[132,133] Peripancreatic inflammation can cause widening of the duodenum or produce a generalized ileus with multiple air-fluid levels. Chest films may reveal left-sided pleural effusions, pulmonary infiltrates, or elevation of the left hemidiaphragm.

US is the primary imaging modality in screening for gallstones or ductal abnormalities associated with AP. The inflamed pancreas can be visualized successfully between 62% and 90% of the time.[134] Overlying intestinal gas and large body habitus can severely limit the examination of the pancreatic head and common bile duct.

CT is the most useful modality for making the diagnosis of AP. Patients should receive oral and IV contrast (except if contraindicated for ileus or renal insufficiency) for optimal sensitivity. CT can identify peripancreatic inflammation, nonuniform parenchymal density, acute fluid collections, hematoma, splenic and PV thrombosis, peripancreatic gas, and pancreatic necrosis (**Figs. 15** and **16**). The severity of inflammation and necrosis can be graded according to the Balthazar criteria or CT severity index, which have important prognostic implications.[135] A recent study placed greater emphasis on the presence of extrapancreatic complications, such as

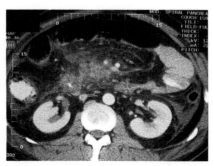

Fig. 15. Pancreatic and peripancreatic inflammatory changes in patient with severe clinical presentation of pancreatitis.

ascites, pleural effusions, or intestinal involvement, which also correlate with patient outcomes.[136]

MRI is a viable alternative to CT for imaging AP and has been shown to possess similar diagnostic ability.[137] T2-weighted images of the pancreas depict the severity of surrounding edema and may be superior in characterizing fluid collections and determination of cause. Arvanitakis and colleagues[138] showed an MRI severity index to be superior in both sensitivity and specificity when characterizing AP compared with CT criteria. MRCP also shows ductal anatomy better than CT.

EUS is primarily useful in cases of idiopathic AP, most of which are caused by microlithiasis. The sensitivity of EUS for stones less than 2 to 3 mm makes the modality the optimal study currently available to select out patients who will benefit from cholecystectomy[4–6] in this setting. EUS also permits more accurate assessment of retained choledocholithiasis compared with MRCP and other noninvasive modalities and is safe to use in pregnant patients and in those with contraindications to MRI. ERCP is of limited use in AP because of the risk of worsening the process. Although performing ERCP is not routinely recommended, patients with AP who benefit from early ERCP are those with cholangitis or severe pancreatitis with evidence of retained stones.[139]

Pancreatic Cysts

Incidental pancreatic cysts are being discovered more frequently as abdominal imaging has increased, and it seems that as many as 1% of inpatients have a detectable pancreatic cyst.[140] Most (85%–90%) pancreatic cystic lesions are pseudocysts related to a prior episode of pancreatitis or trauma resulting in a pancreatic ductal

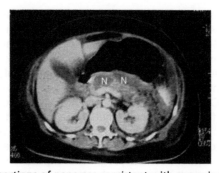

Fig. 16. Nonperfused portions of pancreas consistent with necrosis (N).

disruption.[141] Although these instances can result in free spillage of pancreatic fluid into the free peritoneal cavity (pancreatic ascites) most are walled off and remain localized. Such collections present for less than 4 weeks lack a well-defined wall and are termed acute fluid collections to distinguish them from pseudocysts, which are more mature collections that will typically be encased in a fibrous wall after 4 to 6 weeks.[142,143] Uncomplicated pseudocysts typically appear as simple fluid collections (hypo- or anechoic on US, central low attenuation on CT without septation), which are noted to contain high levels of amylase if aspirated (**Fig. 17**). In the absence of infection, bleeding, mass effect, or other complications, pseudocysts can be observed regardless of size.[143]

Cystic neoplasms represent 10% to 15% of pancreatic cystic masses and are suggested by the presence of internal septa, multiple cysts, or lack of prior history of pancreatitis.[141] The 3 most common cystic neoplasms of the pancreas are serous cystadenomas (also known as microcystic adenomas), mucinous cystic neoplasms (also known as macrocystic adenomas), and intraductal papillary mucinous neoplasms (IPMN).[141] Serous cystadenomas most commonly occur within the pancreatic head of older female patients and are composed of multiple cysts that are hyperintense on T2-weighted MRI and create a honeycomb appearance (**Fig. 18**). Also frequently noted is the presence of a central stellate scar and heterogeneous contrast enhancement. Serous cystadenomas typically have a benign course with operative intervention being reserved for symptomatic or enlarging cases. Mucinous cystic neoplasms of the pancreas tend to occur within the body or tail and radiographically appear as multilocular, enhancing, complex cystic masses, often with a solid component, which contain mucin but do not communicate with the main pancreatic duct.[141] It is difficult to distinguish between a mucinous cystadenoma and cystadenocarcinoma, so resection is favored for most mucin-containing neoplasms.[141] IPMNs encompass a spectrum of mucin-producing cystic neoplasms arising from the pancreatic ductal epithelium. They are classified into main or branch duct types based on their point of origin, with the main duct subtype carrying an increased potential for malignancy (**Fig. 19**). Imaging findings of IPMNs are variable and can mimic mucinous cystic neoplasms, chronic pancreatitis, or adenocarcinoma.[141]

Either CT or MRI is an appropriate initial study for the radiologic evaluation of a cystic pancreatic lesion. However, there is a paucity of data on the accuracy of these imaging techniques in diagnosing pancreatic cysts because of the extensive overlap in early morphology of IPMN and mucinous cystic neoplasm (MCN), and between neoplastic

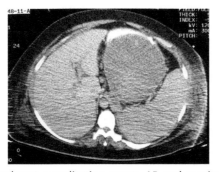

Fig. 17. Pancreatic pseudocyst complicating severe AP and causing displacement of the stomach (S).

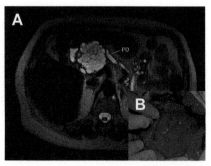

Fig. 18. Large serous cystadenoma. (*A*) T2-weighted MRI with honeycomb appearance of serous cystadenoma (SC) and dilated pancreatic duct (PD). (*B*) Polycystic mass seen on exploration. The patient underwent pancreaticoduodenectomy for 8-cm SC that was increasing in size and obstructing the pancreatic duct.

cysts and reactive cystic lesions.[142] Obstruction of the common bile duct, dilation of the main pancreatic duct, mural nodularity, large size, or multifocal involvement are all ominous findings[142,143] but, because of the inability to effectively diagnose pancreatic cystic lesions, sole reliance on CT or MRI is not recommended.

EUS plays an important role in establishing the diagnosis of pancreatic cysts, not only by allowing further imaging features to be obtained but also by using FNA for sampling cyst contents. Cyst septations, solid components, and mural nodules are more likely to occur in cystic tumors, whereas pseudocysts are likely to show internal echogenic debris with surrounding parenchymal edema.[144,145] EUS features alone are not typically diagnostic because even experienced endosonographers have poor interobserver agreement in the diagnosis of neoplastic versus nonneoplastic cystic lesions.[146] Brugge and colleagues[147] showed low sensitivity (56%), specificity (45%), and diagnostic accuracy (51%) in a large multicenter study on the differentiation between mucinous cystadenoma, cystadenocarcinoma, and nonmucinous lesions with EUS features. More definitive data can be obtained via FNA-obtained cyst fluid analysis, which may differentiate benign lesions from malignant ones. Fluid containing mucin, high levels of carcinoembryonic antigen, or atypical cells is worrying for underlying malignant or premalignant cystic lesions and warrant resection in the appropriate clinical setting.[148–151]

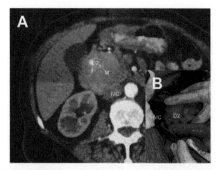

Fig. 19. Large IPMN. (*A*) CT after presentation with gastric outlet obstruction revealing duodenal (D2) obstruction by large pancreatic mass (M) found to be an IPMN. The patient underwent pancreaticoduodenectomy with negative margins. (*B*) Findings in the OR: IPMN invading duodenum (D2) but free from the inferior vena cava and other critical structures.

Pancreatic Cancer

Pancreatic cancer is the fourth leading cancer-related cause of death in the United States.[152] Because of its metastatic tendencies and late presentation, few patients are surgical candidates and those who are typically require extensive operative procedures such as pancreaticoduodenectomy or en-block distal pancreatectomy. In addition to diagnosis, imaging modalities play a vital role in identifying patients in whom surgery will be beneficial, and then helps guide the plan and conduct of operative intervention.

CT remains the most useful imaging modality for diagnosing and staging of pancreatic cancer. Multidetector CT protocols are able to characterize pancreatic parenchyma and surrounding viscera in multiple temporal phases. The pancreas is maximally enhanced after the arterial phase and, because most pancreatic adenocarcinomas are hypovascular, they tend to appear dark at this phase before gradually becoming isointense with normal parenchyma (**Fig. 20A**).[145] The sensitivity of CT is nearly 100% for lesions greater than 2 cm, but is only 70% for smaller lesions.[153,154] For staging purposes, CT has been reported to identify tumor extension and vascular invasion with greater than 90% accuracy.[149,155–157]

MRCP is comparable to CT in evaluating pancreatic masses, with the advantage of providing a more sensitive evaluation for hepatic metastasis and better definition of the ductal anatomy (see **Fig. 20B**; **Fig. 21**).[145,156,158,159] Lopez-Hanninen and colleagues[159] prospectively reported a sensitivity of 95% for MRI in 66 patients with suspected solid pancreatic tumors. Tumor extension and vascular involvement were accurately classified in 89% and 94%, respectively, in those patients undergoing resection.

The sensitivity for EUS is comparable to CT and MRI in detecting pancreatic lesions of more than 2 cm, but the modality provides a more accurate assessment of smaller lesions, with the ability to detect lesions as small as 2 mm.[160] In meta-analysis, EUS was shown to have a higher rate of tumor detection (97% vs 73%), higher sensitivity for vascular invasion (91% vs 64%) (**Fig. 22**), and higher accuracy in determining resectability (91% vs 83%) versus CT.[116] A retrospective comparison of EUS, PET, MRI, and laparoscopy for the detection and staging of potentially malignant pancreatic tumors reported a higher sensitivity with EUS than with PET and MRI (98% vs 88% vs 88%, respectively), although differences did not reach statistical significance.[161] EUS with FNA also allows for tissue diagnosis because pancreatic masses or suspicious LN can be assessed with reported sensitivities of 76% to 90%.[156,162,163] Tumor

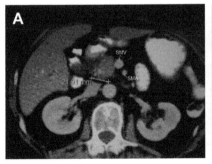
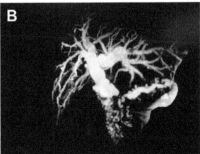

Fig. 20. Pancreatic adenocarcinoma. (*A*) CT findings of hypovascular 2-cm mass in pancreatic head with adjacent superior mesenteric vessels (SMV, SMA). (*B*) MRCP findings of dilated common bile and pancreatic ducts.

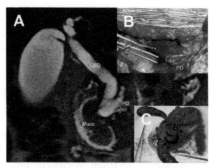

Fig. 21. MRCP delineation of ductal anatomy. (*A*) Dilated common bile duct (CBD) and pancreatic duct (PD) associated with duodenal mass on T2-weighted MRI. (*B*) Dilated PD after resectional portion of pancreaticoduodenectomy. (*C*) Large dysplastic villous adenoma within pancreaticoduodenectomy specimen.

seeding along EUS-FNA tracts, bleeding, and pancreatitis are rare but significant complications that can occur, dampening enthusiasm for routine use on patients with symptomatic, resectable disease.[164,165] Current data do not support the routine use of PET or PET/CT in the setting of pancreatic cancer.[166]

HEPATIC
Benign Masses

Benign conditions of the liver are common; with autopsy series showing that up to 52% of patients display some type of benign liver abnormality.[167] These abnormalities may be difficult to differentiate from malignant processes. The most common benign conditions noted on liver imaging include cysts, abscesses, hemangiomas, focal nodular hyperplasia (FNH), adenomas, and regenerative cirrhotic-associated nodules. It critically important to distinguish these benign pathologies from malignant conditions, and radiographic imaging plays a central role in this.

Benign Cysts

Nonmalignant cysts within the liver occur in up to 5% of the world's population and may be congenital or acquired by infection or trauma.[168] Radiographic studies and patient history can determine the type of cyst and, therefore, its natural history, to

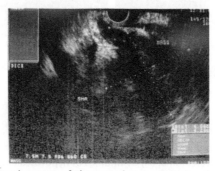

Fig. 22. EUS showing involvement of the superior mesenteric artery (SMA) by pancreatic head mass (M).

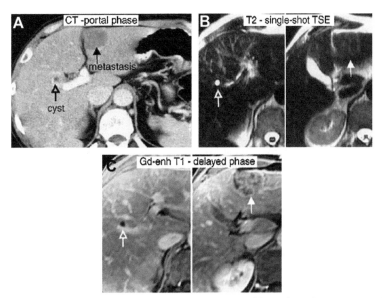

Fig. 23. Hepatic cyst versus neoplasm with illustration of benefits of MRI with different pulse sequences. (*A*) CT with contrast (venous phase) with small cyst (*open arrow*) appearing similar to metastatic lesion (*solid arrow*). (*B*) T2-weighted MRI with the cyst appearing bright because of high fluid content (open arrow), whereas the metastatic lesion is barely visible (*solid arrow*). (*C*) Gadolinium-enhanced T1-weighted MRI images showing no enhancement of the cyst (open arrow) but typical heterogenous enhancement of the metastatic lesion (*solid arrow*). (*Adapted from* Hussain SM, Semelka RC. Hepatic imaging: comparison of modalities. Radiol Clin North Am 2005;43:938; with permission.)

guide management. US is suggested as the first imaging modality for evaluation of liver cysts because of its simplicity, low cost, lack of radiation exposure, and sensitivity and specificity of more than 90%.[169] A simple liver cyst on ultrasound appears uniloc-ular and anechoic, with smooth margins and a thin wall. Posterior wall enhancement is noted, caused by the difference in sound wave reflection between the cyst fluid and the solid liver parenchyma.[170–172] Multiloculation, internal debris, or septation suggest the possibility of a neoplastic cyst, prompting further investigation.

On CT, the wall of a simple hepatic cyst typically will not enhance after IV contrast administration, and the Hounsfield units will be in the water range, from 0 to 10.[171,172] CT is a good modality for cysts larger than 1 cm and can be used to determine the anatomic relationship of the cyst to bile ducts and vasculature. MRI is not commonly used as the primary imaging study for simple hepatic cysts, but knowledge of MRI characteristics of cysts is important if they are noted incidentally while imaging for other conditions. A benign hepatic cyst appears homogeneous and hypointense on T1 images, is bright and hyperintense on T2 images **Fig. 23**, and does not enhance after gadolinium contrast administration.[171,173]

Neoplastic Cysts

Biliary cystadenomas are neoplastic, premalignant cysts, and biliary cystadenocarci-nomas are their malignant counterpart. On US or CT, these lesions are multiloculated, with septae or papillary frond–like projections within the cyst.[174] However, all imaging modalities have limitations in diagnosing these cysts, and the physician must maintain a high index of suspicion. These lesions are more common in middle-aged women and occur more frequently in the right hepatic lobe.[170] Malignant cysts account for only 10% of all neoplastic hepatic cysts, with invasion into surrounding liver and contrast enhancement suggesting malignancy.[170,175] Before surgery, biliary cystadenoma typically cannot be differentiated reliably from biliary cystadenocarcinoma by radiographic or cytologic findings, leading some investigators to recommend an aggressive surgical approach to these lesions.[176]

Hepatic Abscess

Pyogenic liver abscesses may result from biliary, colonic, hematogenous, or cryptogenic sources, and imaging is crucial to quickly diagnose and percutaneously treat the condition. On contrasted CT or MRI, a hepatic abscess appears as a multiloculated, thick-walled lesion that can appear similar to a malignant lesion. There will be peripheral rim enhancement after contrast administration (ie, the double target sign) caused by increased wall permeability (**Fig. 24**).[170,177] Air within a cystic hepatic lesion, with Hounsfield units in the range of -1000 to -100, in a patient who has not undergone some type of intervention is diagnostic for hepatic abscess.[170]

Hemangiomas

The most common benign liver tumors are hemangiomas, occurring in up to 20% of the population.[167] These tumors are usually found in noncirrhotic livers, are more common in women, and typically are less than 5 cm in diameter. These lesions are well defined, hyperintense on T2-weighted MRI, and, on contrasted CT or MRI, display a characteristic peripheral nodular enhancement on early phases, then have progressive centripetal fill in on later phases (**Fig. 25**).[173,178] One study showed that up to 94% of lesions displaying this type of enhancement were hemangiomas, differentiating them from neoplastic lesions.[178,179]

FNH

FNH is the second most common benign liver tumor and has no malignant potential. These lesions are usually singular but may be multiple or associated with other lesions such as adenoma or hemangioma. Focal nodular hyperplasia is usually less than 3 to 5 cm in diameter, typically occurs in a subcapsular location, and is commonly seen in young women.[171,180] CT can diagnose FNH confidently in most cases by the typical

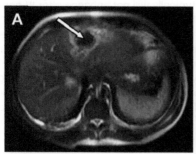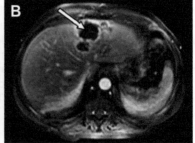

Fig. 24. Hepatic abscess on MRI. (*A*) T2-weighted image with perilesional high signal from edema fluid. (*B*) T1-weighted image with early rim enhancement after gadolinium administration. The lesion center has no enhancement and variable low signal (*arrow*). (*Adapted from* Martin DR, Danrad R, Hussain SM. MR imaging of the liver. Radiol Clin North Am 2005;43:864; with permission.)

A   **B**

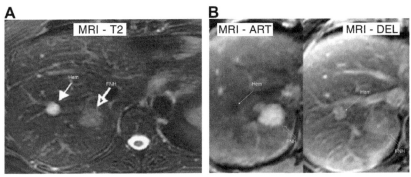

Fig. 25. FNH versus hemangioma. (*A*) T2-weighted image shows 2 lesions: one much brighter than the liver (*solid arrow*) and a larger lesion that is only slightly brighter (*open arrow*). (*B*) Gadolinium-enhanced T1-weighted images show intense homogeneous enhancement of FNH during the arterial phase, with subsequent washout to near isointensity except for ongoing enhancement of a central scar during delayed phase imaging (open arrows). The hemangioma shows peripheral nodular enhancement during the arterial phase but then retains contrast during delayed phases (*solid arrows*). (*Adopted from* Hussain SM, Semelka RC. Hepatic imaging: comparison of modalities. Radiol Clin North Am 2005;43:937; with permission.)

early and bright enhancement with subsequent washout (see **Fig. 25**B).[171,173,180] On delayed scans, most of these lesions are isoattenuating to the liver. A central scar is more common in larger lesions and, when present, results in the lesion remaining centrally bright because of delayed washout.[180] Up to 20% of FNH have a nonclassic appearance, including presence of a pseudocapsule, dilated sinusoids, or vessels surrounding the lesion.[181] MRI has been suggested to be the most sensitive (70%) and specific (98%) imaging modality for FNH[182] because of the additional information available from differing pulse sequences. FNH is iso- or hypointense on T1 imaging and is isointense or minimally hyperintense on T2 imaging (see **Fig. 25**A).[173] If present, the central scar is of high intensity on T2 imaging and low intensity on T1 imaging.[173,183]

Hepatic Adenoma

Hepatic adenomas are almost exclusively diagnosed in young women taking oral contraceptives, so clinical history is useful when coupled to radiographic imaging. There is a risk of hemorrhage or rupture, and a small risk of malignant transformation. Adenoma, the fibrolamellar variant of hepatocellular carcinoma (HCC), and FNH are all typically hypervascular lesions. Because of management being significantly different, accurate radiographic diagnosis is critical. Hepatic adenomas are well defined without lobulation or calcification, and central hemorrhage may be noted in up to 40% of symptomatic patients.[184] Smaller adenomas are hyperattenuated lesions relative to the surrounding liver, with up to 80% of lesions having nearly homogeneous enhancement, unless there has been recent hemorrhage. Larger adenomas may be more heterogeneous on CT imaging and can have less-specific features. Adenoma characteristics on MRI vary within the literature, ranging from hypo- to hyperintense compared with the liver. Fat, necrosis, and hemorrhage within the adenoma contribute to its heterogeneous and varied appearance on MRI. Most adenomas are hyperintense on T1 images but heterogeneous on T2 images.[173,184] Because of the variable radiographic findings, adenoma may be diagnosed more accurately by what is not noted on imaging. Typically, the fibrolamellar variant of HCC has calcifications and lobulations, possible surrounding tissue invasion, and is also associated with lymph-adenopathy in most cases.[185] FNH can have central scarring and is typically more homogeneous on imaging.

HCC

HCC is the most common primary liver malignancy, and its incidence has tripled in the United States in the past 30 years. Currently, the age-adjusted incidence is 4.9 cases per 100,000 individuals.[186] Most cases of HCC arise in the setting of cirrhosis or hepa-titis C or B infection. A meta-analysis on the usefulness of US in detecting HCC found that the sensitivity for detecting early HCC in cirrhotic patients was 63%, but this increased to 94% with routine biennial screening.[187]

If a lesion is noted on screening US, or if a patient has an increased α-fetoprotein level, additional imaging is necessary to evaluate for a dysplastic nodule or HCC. The main diagnostic criteria of HCC is depiction of changes of vascular supply, which is typically reflected by inhomogeneous enhancement in the arterial phase that then washes out to iso- or hypodensity in the portal venous phase (**Fig. 26**).[173] This vari-ability of enhancement across the different phases of contrast administration can be shown on CT, MRI, or, with the recent development of US contrast agents (most involving the use of coated microbubbles to function as an acoustic reflector), by specialized US studies.[102,103,110] However, a significant minority of HCC tumors are hypovascular without significant arterial enhancement (**Fig. 27**).[102,173] In this regard, MRI is advantageous in allowing further tissue differentiation based on different pulse sequences, with increased signal being noted on T2-weighted images in more than 90% of HCC cases in contrast with the eqo- or hypointensity seen with regenerative or dysplastic nodules (**Fig. 28**).[102,103,173,177] The sensitivity of MRI is 100% for HCC larger than 2 cm and 89% for those 1 to 2 cm, but decreases to 34% sensitivity for tumors of less than 1 cm, as documented on explant studies.[103,188]

Smaller HCCs, less than 3 cm in diameter, tend to present as a solid mass or possible multifocal tumor, whereas larger HCCs tend to behave more as an infiltrative process.[189] HCC has a tendency to invade vasculature such as the portal and hepatic veins in up to 40%.[190] Less commonly, HCC will invade the biliary system and result in obstructive jaundice.

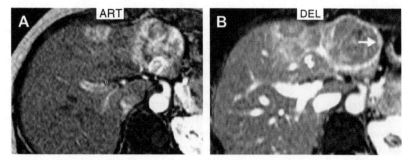

Fig. 26. HCC on MRI. (*A*) Intense heterogenous uptake of contrast during arterial phase. (*B*) Washout and capsular enhancement (*arrow*) on delayed images. (*Adapted from* Hussain SM, Semelka RC. Hepatic imaging: comparison of modalities. Radiol Clin North Am 2005;43:940; with permission.)

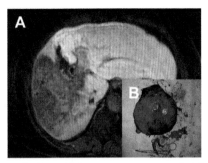

Fig. 27. Large HCC. (*A*) MR findings. Subsequent contrast administration did not result in enhancement. (*B*) HCC in right hepatic resection specimen.

Several advanced MRI techniques, such as diffusion-weighted imaging and specialized contrast agents like superparamagnetic iron oxide, are being investigated and used in some centers and may offer benefits in the future.

Hepatic Metastases

Although HCC is the most common primary liver tumor in the US, the most common hepatic malignancy overall is metastatic disease. The imaging appearance of hepatic metastases varies depending on the primary, with neuroendocrine tumors tending to

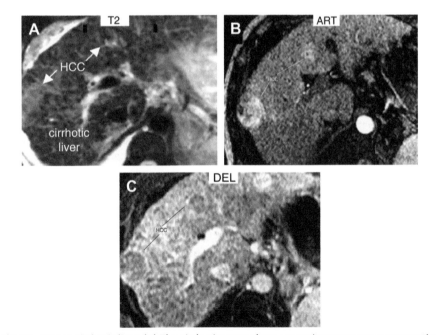

Fig. 28. HCC in cirrhotic liver. (*A*) The cirrhotic parenchyma contains numerous regenerative dark nodules adjacent to 2 brighter lesions consistent with HCC on nonenhanced T2 images. (*B*) These 2 lesions (HCC) enhance during the arterial phase of contrast administration. (*C*) Washout and delayed capsule enhancement (HCC) consistent with HCC is noted on delayed images. (*Adapted from* Hussain SM, Semelka RC. Hepatic imaging: comparison of modalities. Radiol Clin North Am 2005;43:940; with permission.)

be hypervascular and most solid organ metastasis (breast, colon, lung, pancreatic) being hypovascular with ring enhancement only. Particular attention will be directed to evaluation of colorectal metastasis because this is the most common scenario within which general surgeons will be asked to consider resectional intervention in patients with metastatic disease.

Multiple studies and meta-analyses have attempted to delineate the best imaging modality for detection of colorectal cancer liver metastasis. Bipat and colleagues[191] reviewed studies published between January 1990 and December 2003 comparing helical and nonhelical CT, MRI, and PET. On a per-patient analysis, this group concluded that PET was the most accurate imaging modality for detecting hepatic metastasis at 94.6% sensitivity, compared with 60.2% for nonhelical CT, 64.7% for helical CT, and 75.8% for MRI. However, they noted no significant difference between MRI and PET for detection of hepatic metastasis on a per-lesion basis.[191] In a second meta-analysis of literature from 1994 to 2003, and specifically comparing CT with PET, Wiering and colleagues[192] found that PET had a pooled sensitivity of 96% for hepatic lesions and 95.4% for extrahepatic lesions, superior to CT at 84.1% and 91.1%, respectively. The conclusion of this meta-analysis was that PET can have an influence on the preoperative work-up of patients with potentially resectable colorectal hepatic metastasis, particularly in the detection of extrahepatic disease. A third meta-analysis of literature from 2000 to 2008 compared US, multidetector and helical CT, MRI, and PET. This group found that MRI outperformed the other imaging modalities on a per-patient basis, with 74.8% sensitivity and 97.2% specificity, and also showed better sensitivity than CT on a per-lesion basis, especially when liver-specific contrast was administered.[193] The most recent meta-analysis reviewing studies from 2004 to 2009 concluded that, on a per-lesion basis, MRI had the highest sensitivity at 87.3%, which was statistically significant compared with CT, PET, and PET/CT. On a per-patient basis, all 4 modalities had comparable sensitivity estimates, ranging from 88.7% for CT to 96.2% for PET/CT.

It is clear from these separate meta-analyses that MRI and PET are superior to CT for the evaluation of patients with colorectal liver metastasis. It is also clear that there is a distinct gap in prospective, randomized data in all of these reviews, which probably contributes to the differing conclusions and sensitivity estimates. Although additional study is needed, current data therefore support obtaining either MRI or PET/CT, or both, before operating on patients with metastatic colon cancer.

SUMMARY

Multiple imaging modalities including US, CT, MRI/MRCP, direct cholangiography, and PET are now available to assist surgeons with preoperative assessment of hepatobiliary and pancreatic disorders. Having a thorough understanding of the benefits and limitations of each is necessary to guide optimal management of these cases.

ACKNOWLEDGMENTS

The authors wish to thank Paul Buehrer, MD, Mansfield, OH, for editorial supervision.

REFERENCES

1. Strasberg SM. Clinical practice. Acute calculus cholecystitis. N Engl J Med 2008;358:2804–11.

2. Catalano OA, Sahani DV, Kalva SP, et al. MR imaging of the gallbladder: a pictorial essay. Radiographics 2008;28:135–55.
3. Gore RM, Yaghmai V, Newmark GM, et al. Imaging benign and malignant disease of the gallbladder. Radiol Clin North Am 2002;40:1307–23.
4. Sgouros SN, Bergele C. Endoscopic ultrasonography versus other diagnostic modalities in the diagnosis of choledocholithiasis. Dig Dis Sci 2006;51:2280–6.
5. Petrone MC, Arcidiacono PG, Testoni PA. Endoscopic ultrasonography for evaluating patients with recurrent pancreatitis. World J Gastroenterol 2008;14:1016–22.
6. Ardengh JC, Malheiros CA, Rahal F, et al. Microlithiasis of the gallbladder: role of endoscopic ultrasonography in patients with idiopathic acute pancreatitis. Rev Assoc Med Bras 2010;56:27–31.
7. Jüngst C, Kullak-Ublick GA, Jüngst D. Gallstone disease: microlithiasis and sludge. Best Pract Res Clin Gastroenterol 2006;20:1053–62.
8. Shaffer EA. Gallbladder sludge: what is its clinical significance? Curr Gastroenterol Rep 2001;3:166–73.
9. Lee SP, Nicholls JF, Park HZ. Biliary sludge as a cause of acute pancreatitis. N Engl J Med 1992;326:589–93.
10. Draghi F, Ferrozzi G, Calliada F, et al. Power Doppler ultrasound of gallbladder wall vascularization in inflammation: clinical implications. Eur Radiol 2000;10:1587–90.
11. Ralls PW, Colletti PM, Lapin SA, et al. Real-time sonography in suspected acute cholecystitis: prospective evaluation of primary and secondary signs. Radiology 1985;155:767–71.
12. Van Beers BE, Pringot JH. Imaging of cholelithiasis: helical CT. Abdom Imaging 2001;26:15–20.
13. Hicks RJ, Kelly MJ, Kalff V. Association between false negative hepatobiliary scans and initial gallbladder visualization after 30 min. Eur J Nucl Med 1990;16:747–53.
14. Chamarthy M, Freeman LM. Hepatobiliary scan findings in chronic cholecystitis. Clin Nucl Med 2010;35:244–51.
15. Chen CC, Holder LE, Maunoury C, et al. Morphine augmentation increases gallbladder visualization patients pretreated with cholecystokinin. J Nucl Med 1997;38:644–7.
16. Al-Muqbel KM. Diagnostic value of gallbladder emptying variables in chronic acalculous cholecystitis as assessed by fatty meal cholescintigraphy. Nucl Med Commun 2009;30:669–74.
17. Krishnamurthy S, Krishnamurthy GT. Cholecystokinin and morphine pharmacological intervention during 99m Tc-HIDA cholescintigraphy: a rational approach. Semin Nucl Med 1996;26:16–24.
18. Riyad K, Chalmers CP, Aldouri A, et al. The role of (99m) technetium-labeled hepatoiminodiacetic acid (HIDA) scan in the management of biliary pain. HPB (Oxford) 2007;9:219–24.
19. Ito H, Hann LE, D'Angelica M, et al. Polypoid lesions of the gallbladder: diagnosis and follow up. J Am Coll Surg 2009;208:570–5.
20. Elsayes KM, Oliveira EP, Narra VR, et al. Magnetic resonance imaging of the gallbladder: spectrum of abnormalities. Acta Radiol 2007;48:476–82.
21. Kubota K, Bandai Y, Noli T, et al. How should polypoid lesions of the gallbladder be treated in the era of laparoscopic cholecystectomy? Surgery 1995;17:481–7.
22. Cheon YK, Cho WY, Lee TH, et al. Endoscopic ultrasonography does not differentiate neoplastic from non-neoplastic small gallbladder polyps. World J Gastroenterol 2009;15:2361–6.

23. Gourgiotis S, Kocher HM, Solaini L, et al. Gallbladder cancer. Am J Surg 2008; 196:252–64.
24. Lee SW, Kim HJ, Park JH, et al. Clinical usefulness of 18F-FDG PET-CT for patients with gallbladder cancer and cholangiocarcinoma. J Gastroenterol 2010;45:560–6.
25. Shukla PJ, Barreto SG, Arya S, et al. Does PET-CT scan have a role prior to radical re-resection for incidental gallbladder cancer? HPB (Oxford) 2008;10: 439–45.
26. Freitas ML, Bell RL, Duffy AJ. Choledocholithiasis: evolving standards for diagnosis and management. World J Gastroenterol 2006;12:3162–7.
27. Amouyal P, Amouyal G, Lévy P, et al. Diagnosis of choledocholithiasis by endoscopic ultrasonography. Gastroenterology 1994;106:1061–7.
28. Sugiyama M, Atomi Y. Endoscopic ultrasonography for diagnosing choledocholithiasis: a prospective comparative study with ultrasonography and computed tomography. Gastrointest Endosc 1997;45:143–6.
29. Chak A, Hawes RH, Cooper GS, et al. Prospective assessment of the utility of EUS in the evaluation of gallstone pancreatitis. Gastrointest Endosc 1999;49:599–604.
30. Williams EJ, Green J, Beckingham I, et al. Guidelines on the management of common bile duct stones (CBDS). Gut 2008;57:1004–21.
31. Cabada Giádas T, Sarría Octavio de Toledo L, Martínez-Berganza Asensio MT, et al. Helical CT cholangiography in the evaluation of the biliary tract: application for the diagnosis of choledocholithiasis. Abdom Imaging 2002;27:61–70.
32. Maniatis P, Triantopoulous C, Sofianou E, et al. Virtual CT cholangiography in patients with choledocholithiasis. Abdom Imaging 2003;28:536–44.
33. Tseng CW, Chen CC, Chen TS, et al. Can computed tomography with coronal reconstruction improve the diagnosis of choledocholithiasis? J Gastroenterol Hepatol 2008;23:1586–9.
34. Hallal AH, Amortegui JD, Jeroukhimov IM, et al. Magnetic resonance cholangiopancreatography accurately detects common bile duct stones in resolving gallstone pancreatitis. J Am Coll Surg 2005;200:869–75.
35. Shanmugam V, Beattie GC, Yule SR, et al. Is magnetic resonance cholangiopancreatography the new gold standard in biliary imaging? Br J Radiol 2005;78: 888–93.
36. Materne R, Van Beers BE, Gigot JF, et al. Extrahepatic biliary obstruction: magnetic resonance imaging compared with endoscopic ultrasonography. Endoscopy 2000;32:3–9.
37. de Lédinghen V, Lecesne R, Raymond JM, et al. Diagnosis of choledocholithiasis: EUS or magnetic resonance cholangiopancreatography? A prospective controlled study. Gastrointest Endosc 1999;49:26–31.
38. Sugiyama M, Atomi Y, Hachiya J. Magnetic resonance cholangiography using half-Fournier acquisition for diagnosing choledocholithiasis. Am J Gastroenterol 1998;93:1886–90.
39. Varghese JC, Liddell RP, Farrell MA, et al. Diagnostic accuracy of magnetic resonance cholangiopancreatography and ultrasound compared with direct cholangiography in the detection of choledocholithiasis. Clin Radiol 2000;55: 25–35.
40. Romagnuolo J, Bardou M, Rahme E, et al. Magnetic resonance cholangiopancreatography: a meta-analysis of test performance in suspected biliary disease. Ann Intern Med 2003;139:547–57.
41. Varadarajulu S, Eloubeidi M. The role of endoscopic ultrasonography in the evaluation of pancreatico-biliary cancer. Surg Clin North Am 2010;90:251–63.

42. Polkowski M, Palucki J, Regulu J, et al. Helical computed tomographic cholangiography versus endosonography for suspected bile duct stones: a prospective blinded study in non-jaundiced patients. Gut 1999;45:744–9.
43. Palazzo L, Girollet PP, Salmeron M, et al. Value of endoscopic ultrasonography in the diagnosis of common bile duct stones: comparison with surgical exploration and ERCP. Gastrointest Endosc 1995;42:225–31.
44. Prat F, Amouyal G, Amouyal P, et al. Prospective controlled study of endoscopic ultrasonography and endoscopic retrograde cholangiopancreatography in patients with suspected common bile duct lithiasis. Lancet 1996; 347:75–9.
45. Canto MI, Chak A, Stellato T, et al. Endoscopic ultrasonography versus cholangiography for the diagnosis of choledocholithiasis. Gastrointest Endosc 1998; 47:439–48.
46. Aubertin JM, Levoir D, Bouillot JL, et al. Endoscopic ultrasonography immediately prior to laparoscopic cholecystectomy: a prospective evaluation. Endoscopy 1996;28:667–73.
47. Ohtani T, Kawai C, Shirai Y, et al. Intraoperative ultrasonography versus cholangiography during laparoscopic cholecystectomy: a prospective comparative study. J Am Coll Surg 1997;185:274–82.
48. Birth M, Ehlers KU, Delinikolas R, et al. Prospective randomized comparison of laparoscopic ultrasonography using a flexible-tip ultrasound probe and intraoperative dynamic cholangiography during laparoscopic cholecystectomy. Surg Endosc 1998;12:30–6.
49. Sahai AV, Mauldin PD, Marsi V, et al. Bile duct stones and laparoscopic cholecystectomy: a decision analysis to assess the roles of intraoperative cholangiography, EUS, and ERCP. Gastrointest Endosc 1999;49:334–43.
50. Aubé C, Delorme B, Yzet T. MR cholangiopancreatography versus endoscopic sonography in suspected common bile duct lithiasis: a prospective, comparative study. AJR Am J Roentgenol 2005;184:55–62.
51. Griniatsos J, Karvounis E, Isla AM. Limitations of fluoroscopic intraoperative cholangiography in cases suggestive of choledocholithiasis. J Laparoendosc Adv Surg Tech A 2005;15:312–7.
52. Rhodes M, Sussman L, Cohen L, et al. Randomised trial of laparoscopic exploration of common bile duct versus postoperative endoscopic retrograde cholangiopancreatography for common bile duct stones. Lancet 1998;351: 159–61.
53. Stapfer M, Selby RR, Stain SC, et al. Management of duodenal perforation after endoscopic retrograde cholangiopancreatography and sphincterotomy. Ann Surg 2000;23:191–8.
54. Ong TZ, Khor JL, Selamat DS, et al. Complications of endoscopic retrograde cholangiopancreatography in the post-MRCP era: a tertiary center experience. World J Gastroenterol 2005;11:5209–12.
55. Nathan T, Kjeldsen J, Schaffalitzky de Muckadell OB. Prediction of therapy in primary endoscopic retrograde cholangiopancreatography. Endoscopy 2004; 36:527–34.
56. Onken JE, Brazer SR, Elsen GM, et al. Predicting the presence of choledocholithiasis in patients with symptomatic cholelithiasis. Am J Gastroenterol 1996;91: 762–7.
57. Trondsen E, Edwin B, Reiertsen O, et al. Prediction of common duct stones prior to cholecystectomy: a prospective validation of a discriminant analysis function. Arch Surg 1998;133:162–6.

58. Petrov MS, Savides TJ. Systematic review of endoscopic ultrasonography versus endoscopic retrograde cholangiopancreatography for suspected chole-docholithiasis. Br J Surg 2009;96:967–74.

59. Fukuda Y, Tsuyuguchi T, Sakai Y, et al. Diagnostic utility of peroral cholangio-scopy for various bile-duct lesions. Gastrointest Endosc 2005;62:374–82.

60. Chen YK, Pleskow DK. SpyGlass single-operator peroral cholangiopancreato-scopy system for the diagnosis and therapy of bile-duct disorders: a clinical feasibility study (with video). Gastrointest Endosc 2007;65:832–41.

61. Fishman DS, Tarnasky PR, Patel SN, et al. Management of pancreaticobiliary disease using a new intra-ductal endoscope: the Texas experience. World J Gastroenterol 2009;15:1353–8.

62. Mirizzi PL. [La cholangiografia durante las operaciones de las vias biliares]. Bol Soc Cir Buenos Aires 1932;16:1133 [in Spanish].

63. MacFadyen BV. Intraoperative cholangiography: past, present, and future. Surg Endosc 2006;20:S436–40.

64. Berci G, Shore JM, Hamlin JA, et al. Operative fluoroscopy and cholangiog-raphy. Ann Surg 1978;135:32.

65. Berci G. Laparoscopic cholecystectomy: cholangiography. In: Scott-Conner CEH, editor. The SAGES manual: fundamentals of laparoscopy and GI endoscopy. 1st edition. New York: Springer; 1999. p. 143–66.

66. Pierce RA, Jonnalagadda S, Spitler JA, et al. Incidence of residual choledocho-lithiasis detected by intraoperative cholangiography at the time of laparoscopic cholecystectomy in patients having undergone preoperative ERCP. Surg En-dosc 2008;22:2365–72.

67. Hublet A, Dili A, Lemaire J, et al. Laparoscopic ultrasonography as a good alter-native to intraoperative cholangiography during laparoscopic cholecystectomy: results of a prospective study. Acta Chir Belg 2009;109:312–6.

68. Tateishi MJ, Oishi AJ, Furumoto NL, et al. Laparoscopic US versus operative cholangiography during laparoscopic cholecystectomy: review of the literature and a comparison with open intraoperative cholangiography. J Am Coll Surg 1999;188:360–7.

69. Bresadola V, Intini S, Terrosu G, et al. Intraoperative cholangiography in laparo-scopic cholecystectomy during residency in general surgery. Surg Endosc 2001;15:812–5.

70. Amott D, Webb A, Tulloh B. Prospective comparison of routine and selective operative cholangiography. ANZ J Surg 2005;75:378–82.

71. Flum DR, Koepsell T, Heagerty P, et al. Common bile duct injury during laparo-scopic cholecystectomy and the use of intraoperative cholangiography: adverse outcome or preventable error? Arch Surg 2001;136:1287–92.

72. Traverso LW. Intraoperative cholangiography lowers the risk of bile duct injury during cholecystectomy. Surg Endosc 2006;20:1659–61.

73. Flum DR, Dellinger EP, Cheadle A, et al. Intraoperative cholangiography and risk of common bile duct injury during cholecystectomy. JAMA 2003;289:1639–44.

74. Morgan S, Traverso LW. Intraoperative cholangiography and postoperative pancreatitis. Surg Endosc 2000;14:264–6.

75. Horwood J, Akbar F, Davis K, et al. Prospective evaluation of a selective approach to cholangiography for suspected common bile duct stones. Ann R Coll Surg Engl 2010;92:206–10.

76. Cuschieri A, Lezocke E, Morino M, et al. EAES multicenter prospective random-ized trial comparing two-stage vs. single-stage management of patients with gallstone disease and ductal calculi. Surg Endosc 1999;13:952–7.

77. Martin DJ, Vernon DL, Tooul J. Surgical versus endoscopic treatment of bile duct stones. Cochrane Database Syst Rev 2006;2:CD003327.
78. Franklin ME Jr, Pharand D, Rosenthal D. Laparoscopic common bile duct exploration. Surg Laparosc Endosc 1994;4:119–24.
79. Berci G, Morgenstern L. Laparoscopic management of common bile duct stones. A multi-institutional SAGES study. Society of the American Gastrointestinal Endoscopic Surgeons. Surg Endosc 1994;8:1168–74.
80. Petelin JB. Laparoscopic common bile duct exploration. Surg Endosc 2003;17: 1705–15.
81. DePaula AL, Hashiba K, Bafutto M. Laparoscopic management of choledocholithiasis. Surg Endosc 1994;8:1399–403.
82. Waage A, Strömberg C, Leijonmarck CE, et al. Long-term results from laparoscopic common bile duct exploration. Surg Endosc 2003;17:1181–5.
83. Riciardi R, Islam S, Canete JJ, et al. Effectiveness and long-term results of laparoscopic common bile duct exploration. Surg Endosc 2003;17:19–22.
84. Kharbutli B, Velanovich V. Management of preoperatively suspected choledocholithiasis: a decision analysis. J Gastrointest Surg 2008;12:1973–80.
85. Topal B, Aerts R, Penninckx F. Laparoscopic common bile duct stone clearance with flexible choledochoscopy. Surg Endosc 2007;21:2317–21.
86. Tranter SE, Thompson MN. A prospective single-blinded controlled study comparing laparoscopic ultrasonography of the common bile duct with operative cholangiography. Surg Endosc 2003;17:216–9.
87. Aljiffry M, Walsh MJ, Molinari M. Advances in diagnosis, treatment and palliation of cholangiocarcinoma 1990–2009. World J Gastroenterol 2009;15(34): 4240–62.
88. Sainani NI, Catalano OA, Holalkere NS, et al. Cholangiocarcinoma: current and novel imaging techniques. Radiographics 2008;28:1263–87.
89. Aljiffry M, Abdulelah A, Walsh M, et al. Evidenced-based approach to cholangiocarcinoma: a systematic review of the current literature. J Am Coll Surg 2009;208:134–47.
90. Nakeeb A, Pitt KA, Sohn TA, et al. Cholangiocarcinoma. A spectrum of intrahepatic, perihilar, and distal tumors. Ann Surg 1996;224:463–73.
91. Khan SA, Davidson BR, Goldin R, et al. Guidelines for the diagnosis and treatment of cholangiocarcinoma: consensus document. Gut 2002;51(Suppl V1): Vi1–9.
92. Jarnagin WR, Shoup M. Surgical management of cholangiocarcinoma. Semin Liver Dis 2004;24:189–99.
93. Jonas S, Benckert C, Thelen A, et al. Radical surgical for hilar cholangiocarcinoma. Eur J Surg Oncol 2008;34:263–71.
94. Khan SA, Thomas HE, Davidson BR, et al. Cholangiocarcinoma. Lancet 2005; 366:1303–14.
95. Honickman SP, Mueller PR, Wittenberg J, et al. Ultrasonography in obstructive jaundice: prospective evaluation of site and cause. Radiology 1983;147:511–5.
96. Robledo R, Muro A, Prieto ML. Extrahepatic bile duct carcinoma: US characteristics and accuracy in demonstration of tumors. Radiology 1996;198:869–73.
97. Neumaier CE, Bertolotto M, Perrone R, et al. Staging of hilar cholangiocarcinoma with ultrasound. J Clin Ultrasound 1995;23:173–8.
98. Choi BI, Lee JH, Han MC, et al. Hilar cholangiocarcinoma: comparative study with sonography and CT. Radiology 1989;172:689–92.
99. Kim TK, Choi BI, Han JK, et al. Peripheral cholangiocarcinoma of the liver: two-phase spiral CT findings. Radiology 1997;204:539–43.

100. Watadani T, Akahane M, Yoshikawa T, et al. Preoperative assessment of hilar cholangiocarcinoma using multidetector-row CT: correlation with histopathological findings. Radiat Med 2008;26:402–7.
101. Choi BI, Lee SJ, Han JK. Imaging of intrahepatic and hilar cholangiocarcinoma. Abdom Imaging 2004;29:548–57.
102. Ariff B, Lloyd CR, Khan S, et al. Imaging of liver cancer. World J Gastroenterol 2009;15:1289–300.
103. Zech C, Reiser MF, Herrmann KA. Imaging of hepatocellular carcinoma by CT and MRI: state of the Art. Dig Dis 2009;27:114–24.
104. Sodickson A, Mortele KJ, Barish MA, et al. Three-dimensional fast-recovery fast spin-echo MRCP: comparison with two-dimensional single-shot fast spin-echo techniques. Radiology 2006;238:549–59.
105. Manfredi R, Brizi MG, Maselli G, et al. Malignant biliary hilar stenosis: MR cholangiography compared with direct cholangiography. Radiol Med 2001;102:48–54.
106. Rösch T, Meining A, Frühmorgen S, et al. A prospective comparison of the diagnostic accuracy of ERCP, MRCP, CT, and EUS in biliary strictures. Gastrointest Endosc 2002;55:870–6.
107. Park MS, Kim TK, Kim KW, et al. Differentiation of extrahepatic bile duct cholangiocarcinoma from benign structure: findings at MRCP versus ERCP. Radiology 2004;233:234–40.
108. Varghese JC, Farrell MA, Courtney G, et al. A prospective comparison of magnetic resonance cholangiopancreatography with endoscopic retrograde cholangiopancreatography in the evaluation of patients with suspected biliary tract disease. Clin Radiol 1999;54:513–20.
109. Manfredi R, Barbaro B, Masselli G, et al. Magnetic resonance imaging of cholangiocarcinomas. Semin Liver Dis 2004;24:155–64.
110. Outwater EK. Imaging of the liver for hepatocellular cancer. Cancer Control 2009;17:72–82.
111. Park HS, Lee JM, Choi JY, et al. Preoperative evaluation of bile duct cancer: MRI combined with MR cholangiopancreatography versus MDCT with direct cholangiography. AJR Am J Roentgenol 2008;90:396–405.
112. Masselli G, Gualdi G. Hilar cholangiocarcinoma: MRI/MRCP in staging and treatment planning. Abdom Imaging 2008;33:444–51.
113. Hänninen EL, Pech M, Jonas S, et al. Magnetic resonance imaging including magnetic resonance cholangiopancreatography for tumor localization and therapy planning in malignant hilar obstructions. Acta Radiol 2005;46:462–70.
114. Masselli G, Manfredi R, Vecchioli A, et al. MR imaging and magnetic resonance cholangiopancreatography in the preoperative evaluation of hilar cholangiocarcinoma: correlation with surgical and pathologic findings. Eur Radiol 2008;18:2213–21.
115. Lee MG, Park KB, Shin YM, et al. Preoperative evaluation of hilar cholangiocarcinoma with contrast-enhanced three-dimensional fast imaging with steady-state precession magnetic resonance angiography: comparison with intra-arterial digital subtraction angiography. World J Surg 2003;27:278–83.
116. Hunt GC, Faigel DO. Assessment of EUS for diagnosing, staging, and determining resectability of pancreatic cancer: a review. Gastrointest Endosc 2002;55:232–7.
117. Garrow D, Miller S, Sinha D, et al. Endoscopic ultrasound: a meta-analysis of test performance in suspected biliary obstruction. Clin Gastroenterol Hepatol 2007;5:616–23.

118. Lee JH, Salem R, Aslanian H, et al. Endoscopic ultrasonography and fine-needle aspiration of unexplained bile duct strictures. Am J Gastroenterol 2004;99: 1069–73.

119. Fritscher-Ravens A, Broering DC, Sriram PV, et al. EUS-guided fine-needle aspiration cytodiagnosis of hilar cholangiocarcinoma: a case series. Gastrointest Endosc 2000;52:534–40.

120. Eloubeidi MA, Chen VK, Jhala HC, et al. Endoscopic ultrasound-guided FNA biopsy of suspected cholangiocarcinoma. Clin Gastroenterol Hepatol 2004;2: 209–13.

121. Malhi H, Gores G. Review article: the modern diagnosis and therapy of cholangiocarcinoma. Aliment Pharmacol Ther 2006;23:1287–96.

122. Wakabayashi H, Akamoto S, Yachida S, et al. Significance of fluorodeoxyglucose PET imaging in the diagnosis of malignancies in patients with biliary stricture. Eur J Surg Oncol 2005;31:1175–9.

123. Weber A, Schmid R, Prinz C. Diagnostic approaches for cholangiocarcinoma. World J Gastroenterol 2008;14:4131–6.

124. Kumar M, Prashad R, Kumar A, et al. Relative merits of ultrasonography, computed tomography, and cholangiography in patients of surgical obstructive jaundice. Hepatogastroenterology 1998;45:2027–32.

125. Loperfido S, Angelina G, Benedetti G, et al. Major early complications from diagnostic and therapeutic ERCP: a prospective multicenter study. Gastrointest Endosc 1998;48:1–10.

126. Hochwald SN, Burke EC, Jarnagin WR, et al. Association of preoperative biliary stenting with increased postoperative infectious complications in proximal cholangiocarcinoma. Arch Surg 1999;134:261–6.

127. Lazaridis KN, Gores GJ. Cholangiocarcinoma. Gastroenterology 2005;128: 16555–67.

128. Menzel J, Poremba C, Dietl KJ. Preoperative diagnosis of bile duct strictures – comparison of intraductal ultrasonography with conventional endosonography. Scand J Gastroenterol 2000;35:77–82.

129. Cavallini G, Frulloni L, Bassi C, et al. Prospective multicentre survey on acute pancreatitis in Italy (ProInf-AISP): results on 1005 patients. Dig Liver Dis 2004; 36(3):205–11.

130. Sandler RS, Everhart JE, Donowitz M, et al. The burden of selective digestive diseases in the United States. Gastroenterology 2002;122(5):1500–11.

131. Stein GN, Kalser MH, Sarian NN, et al. An evaluation of the roentgen changes in acute pancreatitis: correlation with clinical findings. Gastroenterology 1959;36: 354–61.

132. Davis S, Parbhoo SP, Gibson MJ. The plain abdominal radiograph in acute pancreatitis. Clin Radiol 1980;31(1):87–93.

133. Negro P, D'Amore L, Saputelli A, et al. Colonic lesions in pancreatitis. Ann Ital Chir 1995;66(2):223–31.

134. Jeffrey RB Jr, Laing FC, Wing VW. Extrapancreatic spread of acute pancreatitis: new observations with real-time US. Radiology 1986;159:707–11.

135. Balthazar EJ, Robinson DL, Megibow AJ, et al. Acute pancreatitis: value of CT in establishing diagnosis. Radiology 1990;174:331–6.

136. Mortele KJ, Wiesner W, Intriere L, et al. A modified CT severity index for evaluating acute pancreatitis: improved correlation with patient outcome. AJR Am J Roentgenol 2004;183(5):1261–5.

137. Miller FH, Keppke AI, Dalal K, et al. MRI of pancreatitis and its complications: part 1. Acute pancreatitis. AJR Am J Roentgenol 2004;183:1637–44.

138. Arvanitakis M, Delhaye M, De Maertelaere V, et al. Computed tomography and magnetic resonance imaging in the assessment of acute pancreatitis. Gastroenterology 2004;126(3):715–23.

139. Banks PA, Freeman ML. Practice guidelines in acute pancreatitis. Am J Gastroenterol 2006;101:2379–400.

140. Khalid AK, Brugge W. ACG practice guidelines for the diagnosis and management of neoplastic pancreatic cysts. Am J Gastroenterol 2007;102:2339–49.

141. Hammond N, Miller FH, Sica GT, et al. Imaging of cystic diseases of the pancreas. Radiol Clin North Am 2002;40:1243–62.

142. Baille J. Technical review: pancreatic pseudocysts (Part 1). Gastrointest Endosc 2004;59:873–9.

143. Baille J. Technical review: pancreatic pseudocysts (Part 2). Gastrointest Endosc 2005;43:929–47.

144. Song MH, Lee SK, Kim MH, et al. EUS in the evaluation of pancreatic cystic lesions. Gastrointest Endosc 2003;57:891–6.

145. Kinney T. Evidence-based imaging of pancreatic malignancies. Surg Clin North Am 2010;90:235–49.

146. Ahmad NA, Kochman ML, Brensinger C, et al. Interobserver agreement among endosonographers for the diagnosis of neoplastic versus non-neoplastic pancreatic cystic lesions. Gastrointest Endosc 2003;58(1):59–64.

147. Brugge WR, Lewandrowski K, Lee-Lewandrowski E, et al. Diagnosis of pancreatic cystic neoplasms: a report of the cooperative pancreatic cyst study. Gastroenterology 2004;126:1330–6.

148. Maire F, Couvelard A, Hammel P, et al. Intraductal papillary mucinous tumors of the pancreas: the preoperative value of cytologic and histopathologic diagnosis. Gastrointest Endosc 2003;58:701–6.

149. Uehara H, Nakaizumi A, Iishi H, et al. Cytologic examination of pancreatic juice for differential diagnosis of benign and malignant mucin-producing tumors of the pancreas. Cancer 1994;74:826–33.

150. Frossard JL, Amouyal P, Amouyal G, et al. Performance of endosonography-guided fine needle aspiration and biopsy in the diagnosis of pancreatic cystic lesions. Am J Gastroenterol 2003;98:1516–24.

151. Hutchins G, Draganov PV. Diagnostic evaluation of pancreatic cyst malignancies. Surg Clin North Am 2010;90:399–410.

152. Ries LA, Ksary CL, Hankey BF, et al. SEER cancer statistics review, 1973–1996. Bethesda (MD): National Cancer Institute; 1999.

153. Legman P, Vignaux O, Dousset B, et al. Pancreatic tumors: comparison of dual-phase helical CT and endoscopic sonography. AJR Am J Roentgenol 1998;170:1315–22.

154. Bronstein YL, Loyer EM, Kaur H, et al. Detection of small pancreatic tumors with multiphasic helical CT. AJR Am J Roentgenol 2004;182:619–23.

155. Karmazanovsky G, Federov V, Kubyshkin V, et al. Pancreatic head cancer: accuracy of CT in determination of resectability. Abdom Imaging 2005;30:488–500.

156. Bipat S, Phoa SS, van Delden OM, et al. Ultrasonography, computed tomography and magnetic resonance imaging for diagnosis and determining resectability of pancreatic adenocarcinoma: a meta-analysis. J Comput Assist Tomogr 2005;29:438–45.

157. Ellsmere J, Mortele K, Sahani D, et al. Does multidetector-row CT eliminate the role of diagnostic laparoscopy in assessing the respectability of pancreatic head carcinoma? Surg Endosc 2005;19:369–73.

158. Adamek HE, Albert J, Breer H, et al. Pancreatic cancer detection with magnetic resonance cholangiopancreatography and endoscopic retrograde cholangio-pancreatography: a prospective controlled study. Lancet 2000;365(9225):190–3.
159. Lopez-Hanninen E, Amthauer H, Hosten N, et al. Prospective evaluation of pancreatic tumors: accuracy of MR imaging with MR cholangiopancreatography and MR angiography. Radiology 2002;224(1):34–41.
160. Rosch T, Lightdale CJ, Botet JF, et al. Localization of pancreatic endocrine tumors by endoscopic ultrasonography. N Engl J Med 1992;326:1721–6.
161. Borbath I, Van Ceers BE, Lonneux M, et al. Preoperative assessment of pancreatic tumors using magnetic resonance imaging, endoscopic ultrasonography, positron emission tomography, and laparoscopy. Pancreatology 2005;5(6):553–61.
162. Gress F, Gotltlieb K, Sherman S, et al. Endoscopic ultrasonography-guided fine-needle aspiration biopsy of suspected pancreatic cancer. Ann Intern Med 2001;134:459–64.
163. Harewood GC, Wiersma MJ. Endosonography-guided fine-needle aspiration biopsy in the evaluation of pancreatic masses. Am J Gastroenterol 2002;97:1386–91.
164. Paquin SC, Gariepy G, Lepanto L, et al. A first report of tumor seeding because of EUS-guided FNA of a pancreatic adenocarcinoma. Gastrointest Endosc 2005;61(4):610–1.
165. Shah JN, Fraker D, Guerry D, et al. Melanoma seeding of an EUS-guided fine needle track. Gastrointest Endosc 2004;59(7):923–4.
166. Orlando LA, Kulasingam SL, Matchar DB. Meta-analysis: the detection of pancreatic malignancy with positron emission tomography. Aliment Pharmacol Ther 2004;20:1063–70.
167. Karhunen PJ. Benign hepatic tumours and tumour-like conditions in men. J Clin Pathol 1986;39:183–8.
168. Caremani M, Vincenti A, Benci A, et al. Echographic epidemiology of non-parasitic hepatic cysts. J Clin Ultrasound 1993;21:115–8.
169. Cowles RA, Mulholland MW. Solitary hepatic cysts. J Am Coll Surg 2000;191(3):311–21.
170. Mortele KJ, Ros PR. Cystic focal liver lesions in the adult: differential CT and MR imaging features. Radiographics 2001;21:895–910.
171. Horton KM, Bluemke DA, Hruban RRH, et al. CT and MR imaging of benign hepatic and biliary tumors. Radiographics 1999;19(2):431–51.
172. Gaines PA, Sampson MA. The prevalence and characterization of simple hepatic cysts by ultrasound examination. Br J Radiol 1989;62(736):335–7.
173. Hussain SM, Semelka RC. Hepatic imaging: comparison modalties. Radiol Clin North Am 2005;43:929–47.
174. Korobkin M, Stephens DH, Lee JK, et al. Biliary cystadenoma and cystadenocarcinoma: CT and sonographic findings. AJR Am J Roentgenol 1989;153(3):507–11.
175. Lewin M, Mourra N, Honigman I, et al. Assessment of MRI and MRCP in diagnosis of biliary cystadenoma and cystadenocarcinoma. Eur Radiol 2006;16:407–13.
176. Hai S, Hirohashi K, Uenishi T, et al. Surgical management of cystic hepatic neoplasms. J Gastroenterol 2003;38:759–64.
177. Martin DR, Danrad R, Hussain SM. MR imaging of the liver. Radiol Clin North Am 2005;43:861–6.

178. Heiken JP. Distinguishing benign from malignant liver tumors. Cancer Imaging 2007;7:S1–14.
179. Leslie DF, Johnson CD, Johnson CM, et al. Distinction between cavernous hemangiomas of the liver and hepatic metastases on CT: value of contrast enhancement patterns. AJR Am J Roentgenol 1995;164:625–9.
180. Brancatelli G, Federle MP, Grazioli L, et al. Focal nodular hyperplasia: CT findings with emphasis on multiphasic helical CT in 78 patients. Radiology 2001; 219:61–8.
181. Choi CS, Freeny PC. Triphasic helical CT of focal nodular hyperplasia: incidence of atypical findings. AJR Am J Roentgenol 1998;170:391–5.
182. Mortele KJ, Praet M, Van Vlierberghe H, et al. CT and MR imaging findings in focal nodular hyperplasia of the liver: radiologic-pathologic correlation. AJR Am J Roentgenol 2000;175:687–92.
183. Hussain SM, Terkivatan T, Zondervan PE, et al. Focal nodular hyperplasia: findings at state-of-the art MR imaging US, CT and pathologic analysis. Radiographics 2004;24:3–17.
184. Grazioli L, Federle MP, Brancatelli G, et al. Hepatic adenomas: imaging and pathologic findings. Radiographics 2001;21:877–92.
185. Ichikawa T, Federle MP, Grazioli L, et al. Fibrolamellar hepatocellular carcinoma: imaging and pathologic findings in 31 recent cases. Radiology 1999;213: 352–61.
186. Altekruse SF, McGlynn KA, Reichman ME. Hepatocellular carcinoma incidence, mortality, and survival trends in the United States from 1975 to 2005. J Clin Oncol 2009;27(9):1485–91.
187. Singal A, Volk ML, Waljee A, et al. Meta-analysis: surveillance with ultrasound for early-stage hepatocellular carcinoma in patients with cirrhosis. Aliment Pharmacol Ther 2009;30(1):37–47.
188. Burrel M, Llovet JM, Ayuso C, et al. MRI angiography is superior to helical CT for detection of HCC prior to liver transplantation: an explant correlation. Hepatology 2003;38:1034–42.
189. Digumarthy SR, Sahani DV, Saini S. MRI for the detection of hepatocellular carcinoma (HCC). Cancer Imaging 2005;5:20–4.
190. Fong Y, Sun RL, Jarnagin W, et al. An analysis of 412 cases of hepatocellular carcinoma at a Western center. Ann Surg 1999;229(6):790–9.
191. Bipat S, van Leeuwen MS, Comans EF, et al. Colorectal liver metastases: CT, MR imaging, and PET for diagnosis. Radiology 2005;237(1):123–31.
192. Wiering B, Krabbe PF, Jager GJ, et al. The impact of fluor-18-deoxyglucose-positron emission tomography in the management of colorectal liver metastases: a systematic review and meta-analysis. Cancer 2005;104(12):2658–70.
193. Floriani I, Torri V, Rulli E, et al. Performance of imaging modalities in diagnosis of liver metastasis from colorectal cancer: a systematic review and meta-analysis. J Magn Reson 2010;31:19–31.

Imaging of Gastrointestinal Bleeding

John D. Mellinger, MD[a],*, James G. Bittner IV, MD[b],
Michael A. Edwards, MD[b], William Bates, MD[b],
Hadyn T. Williams, MD[b]

KEYWORDS

- Gastrointestinal bleeding • Tagged erythrocyte scanning
- Mesenteric angiography • Meckel • CT angiography

Radiological imaging has played an increasingly important role in the diagnosis and management of gastrointestinal bleeding over the past 30 years. The initial description of selective mesenteric angiography in 1965[1] and radiolabeled sulfur colloid scintigraphy in 1977,[2] along with subsequent refinements in these techniques, have had a significant effect in this regard. Current computed tomographic (CT) techniques, including multidetector CT, CT enterography (CTE), and CT angiography, as well as magnetic resonance enterography (MRE) are capable of playing a role in the evaluation of the patient with gastrointestinal bleeding. Mesenteric angiography in particular has allowed therapeutic intervention, and the evolution of selective coaxial catheter systems has improved the safety and efficacy of this modality in the therapeutic armamentarium. Given the fact that gastrointestinal bleeding results in up to 500,000 hospital admissions per year in the United States[3] and that mortality rates as high as 23% may be associated with such presentations when bleeding is massive or recurrent,[4,5] it is incumbent on the surgical provider to understand the utility and efficacy of these radiological techniques in the spectrum of patient evaluation and management. This review summarizes the current literature with regard to radiological imaging and its role in the care of the patient with gastrointestinal bleeding. Scintigraphy, angiography, and solid organ imaging techniques are discussed, including a review of their relative roles in comparison with those of nonradiological management tools such as endoscopy and surgical therapy.

[a] Department of Surgery, Southern Illinois University, 701 North First Street, Springfield, IL 62794, USA
[b] Departments of Surgery and Radiology Medical College of Georgia, 1120 15th Street, Augusta, GA 30912, USA
* Corresponding author. 701 North First Street, PO Box 19638, Springfield, IL 62794-9638.
E-mail address: jmellinger@siumed.edu

Surg Clin N Am 91 (2011) 93–108
doi:10.1016/j.suc.2010.10.014   **surgical.theclinics.com**
0039-6109/11/$ – see front matter © 2011 Elsevier Inc. All rights reserved.

SCINTIGRAPHIC EVALUATION

Technetium Tc 99m sulfur colloid scintigraphy is based on the principle of early phase vascular imaging with rapid clearance of the radiotracer by reticuloendothelial elements in the liver, spleen, and bone marrow. Radionuclide extravasated from the vascular space accordingly can be recognized as an area of concentrated and slower clearing activity against the background. Thus, a positive scan result is dependent on active bleeding occurring within a few minutes after administration of the agent. Limitations of the study other than the need for active bleeding within a short time interval after administration include the fact that extravasation over areas of high background activity, such as the liver or spleen, may be obscured by the same. Oblique views may help in reducing missed bleeding overlying these areas. False-positive results secondary to accessory spleens and retroperitoneal varices have been described.[1] Standardized techniques for gastrointestinal bleeding include the administration of 10 millicurie (mCi; 370 megabecquerel [MBq]) of technetium Tc 99m sulfur colloid intravenously, followed by large-field scanning of the abdomen and pelvis in the supine position with an initial dynamic flow sequence for the first minute followed by continuous static images for up to 30 minutes.[6]

Several variations in scintigraphic technique have been developed to attempt to improve diagnostic yield. Technetium Tc 99m–labeled autologous erythrocyte or tagged red blood cell scanning (**Fig. 1**) allows imaging to occur in both the dynamic early phase captured by sulfur colloid scanning and also during an expanded equilibrium or blood pool phase. This imaging allows the potential for detection of bleeding that is intermittent and not active during the dynamic phase or that occurs at such a slow rate as to not be captured during that phase of imaging. The period of imaging is limited only by the half-life of the radiotracer used and access to the scanner. The labeling itself is accomplished by adding 5 mL of anticoagulated blood to a vial containing stannous pyrophosphate, which reduces the erythrocyte membrane valence, trapping the added 25 mCi (925 MBq) Technetium Tc 99m pertechnetate intracellularly, and typically allows a labeling efficiency of 98% or greater. Bleeding rates of 0.3 mL/min are detectable with this technique,[7] and experimental models have suggested that rates even in the range of 0.1 mL/min may be detected with this modality, depending on the volume of the bleed.[8] Bleeding volumes from a minimum of 3 to 5 mL to as high as 50 to 70 mL are reported as necessary for scintigraphic detection in adults.[8–10] Potential sources of false-positive results with this technique may be expanded from those seen with sulfur colloid studies and include horseshoe kidney, hepatic hemangiomata, ischemic bowel, uterine leiomyomata, and aneurysmal disease.[1] Nonhemorrhagic gallbladder visualization, particularly in patients with renal failure, and labeling of the porphyrin group of degraded erythrocyte hemoglobin have also been described after erythrocyte-labeled scintigraphy.[11] Spontaneous elution of free technetium Tc 99m pertechnetate from erythrocytes can occur at a variable rate and lead to gastric, thyroid, and urinary secretion, which can confound image interpretation, especially on delayed images.[12,13]

Despite the theoretical benefit of tagged erythrocyte scanning, some studies have questioned its effect when assessed in light of the realities of prolonged scanning. In a retrospective review of 359 consecutive scans, there was no statistical difference in bleeding detection rates between sulfur colloid and tagged red cell techniques.[14] Furthermore, in patients who had sulfur colloid scans followed by tagged red cell studies, only 14% showed positive findings on tagged red cell study after initial negative findings on sulfur colloid scan. The investigators found that the likelihood of positive study results with either scan method was higher during daytime hours, which the

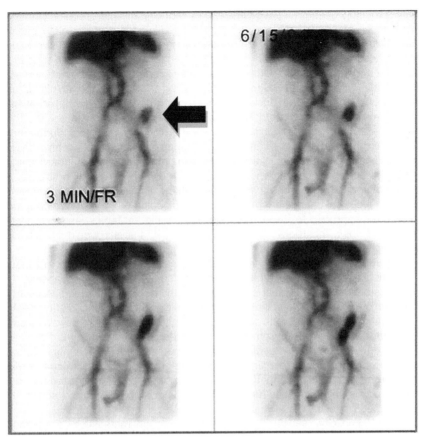

Fig. 1. Technetium Tc 99m–tagged autologous erythrocyte scan demonstrating active bleeding from a sigmoid diverticular source after a negative colonoscopic result. The arrow highlights the bleeding site.

investigators attributed to longer delays between test ordering and execution when the study was ordered during off hours. This study highlights the importance of scan timing, and given the propensity of lower gastrointestinal bleeds to spontaneously cease, prolonged scanning after significant delays may not be a cost-effective strategy.

Several other techniques have been studied for scintigraphic assessment of bleeding. Technetium Tc 99m–labeled albumin was one of the first agents studied,[10] but subsequent techniques, including those described earlier, have proved more reliable. Technetium Tc 99m–labeled heat-damaged erythrocytes have also been evaluated in the hope that accelerated clearance of the heat-damaged cells by the spleen would improve target to background ratios in the setting of an acute bleed.[15] Indium 111 has also been evaluated as a longer half-life labeling agent that could allow prolonged imaging in settings of intermittent bleeding.[16,17] Higher cost and radiation exposure have prevented this technique from being clinically useful.[18]

Standard technetium Tc 99m–labeled erythrocyte scanning has also been evaluated regarding optimal duration of scanning and technique. Some studies have suggested that scanning for periods longer than the standard 1 to 2 hours[19,20] or with a second injection of radiotracer[21] could improve diagnostic yield by increasing sensitivity for slow or intermittent bleeds and by reducing misinterpretation stemming from previously extravasated blood noted on delayed images. A study of 137 patients in which 24 underwent imaging beyond 3 hours suggested that nearly half the patients with prolonged scan intervals had positive scans that would have been missed on a scan of standard duration.[22] Other series have reported similar rates of increased positive results with scanning beyond 90 minutes and associated this with higher rates of surgery and increased transfusion requirements in patients with delayed positive scans.[23] Nevertheless, most studies that are initially negative remain so, and there is a resource cost obviously associated with prolonged scanning. Furthermore, some studies have suggested that delayed scanning, even when positive, fails to impact patient management or clinical outcome in comparison with standard imaging duration protocols.[24] The retrospective nature of all these studies precludes the formation of strong conclusions or recommendations. Repeat imaging on a selective basis when a clinical change suggests recurrent bleeding might prove to be a more cost-effective approach to the use of delayed imaging strategies, and prospective multicenter studies incorporating outcome and cost analysis would be useful in addressing this issue in the future.

Other studies have highlighted the potential for subtraction techniques to enhance the detection and localization rates of standard tagged erythrocyte scanning. This method has been used in nuclear studies for parathyroid imaging and in assessment for infection of prosthetic joints. In this technique, either the initial image after injection or a summation of all images with normalization for count density are used as a background image and subtracted from each subsequent image, providing a mechanism to capture only accumulated bleeding on the delayed images. Proponents have highlighted the potential of this technique to offer the high-contrast advantage of sulfur colloid scanning with the prolonged time capacity of tagged erythrocyte techniques.[25] Studies exploring this technique have suggested its potential to improve sensitivity[23] and cost-effectiveness.[26]

Given its simplicity, sensitivity, and noninvasive characteristics, scintigraphic screening has been assessed as an important early diagnostic tool in gastrointestinal bleeding. The potential of the screening to risk-stratify patients and to guide decisions regarding surgical or angiographic intervention has clear appeal in the setting of a disease process characterized by spontaneous cessation in 75% to 89% of cases[27,28] and potential high mortality in those who continue to bleed. Negative study results have been shown to correlate with a good clinical outcome,[29] and positive study results have been predictive of heightened hospital morbidity and mortality.[30,31] Positive scan results have also been used to calculate estimated bleeding rates in patients with anemia, transfusion requirement, and heme-positive stool.[29] Optimal timing of the study within 24 hours of a 500-mL blood transfusion has been demonstrated in such studies.[29,32] Specifically, patients transfused with more than 2 units of packed red blood cells within 24 hours preceding the study were found to be twice as likely to have a positive scan result compared with those transfused with 2 units or less.[32] Retrospective studies attempting to correlate scan results with surgical indication and outcome have documented that most patients requiring surgery have positive scan results (70%); conversely, nearly a third of patients coming to surgery may have negative study results.[33] Perhaps of greater interest to surgeons in operative planning is not the positivity of the study but its accuracy as a localization tool. Studies in which positive scan results have been correlated with other localizations via endoscopy, angiography, and/or surgical intervention have reported accuracy for scintigraphy as low as 40% and as high as 100%.[1,34–41] Despite the variability in published reports, positive study results have a mean likelihood of accurate localization in the range of 75%, and inaccurate localization may be expected in approximately 25% of cases.[34,41,42] Of these 25% cases, many can be seen in settings of relatively slow rates of hemorrhage in which bowel peristalsis in response to the cathartic effect of intraluminal blood may result in confusing imaging. For these reasons, most surgeons operate on positive scan results alone (ie, as the only localization study) only in settings in which clinical deterioration dictates or other more precise localization studies, such as endoscopy and angiography, have been unsuccessful in confirming the location of the bleed.

Because of its potential to identify bleeding at rates less than those required for a positive angiogram, which typically requires bleeding approaching the range of 1.0 mL/min for detection,[43] scintigraphy has been investigated as a tool to guide decisions regarding mesenteric angiography as well. Studies evaluating this strategy are mixed, with some suggesting a benefit of scintigraphy before angiography[44] and others showing no advantage of such a strategy.[38,41,45] Perhaps the greatest correlation would be expected when the scintigraphic study is rapidly positive and angiography can follow immediately because this pattern would be most predictive of active bleeding at more significant volumes. Some studies have suggested accordingly that the presence or absence of positive scintigraphic findings in the first 2 minutes of a study provides a meaningful positive and negative predictive value with regard to the utility of angiography in patients with clinically significant bleeding.[46] Scintigraphy in such settings may also provide the angiographer with a strategy for localization priorities at the time of catheter placement and injection. Based on this feature, many angiographers request that scintigraphy be performed before committing a patient to angiography. It is important to remember that in the patient with ongoing bleeding and hemodynamic changes, prioritization toward urgent therapeutic intervention may make the potential delay involved in scintigraphy unwise, both from the standpoint of patient safety and because of the opportune timing issue on which angiography depends.

Before leaving the subject of radionuclide scanning, the role of scintigraphy in assessing for Meckel's diverticula is worthy of mention. Meckel's diverticula are a commonly encountered anomaly of the small intestine, occurring in 2% of the general population, and may contain heterotopic mucosa of various types, including gastric mucosa in 50% of cases.[47] Although most of these diverticula are clinically silent and found incidentally during autopsy, during laparotomy, or on contrast studies, there is a lifetime risk of a complicating illness related to the diverticulum in 4% of cases.[48] Furthermore, 25% of those with complicating illness may present with lower gastrointestinal bleeding.[49] Hemorrhage is in fact the most common presenting symptom of Meckel's diverticula in patients in the first decade of life, although it has been described even in a nonagenarian.[50] In children, the single most useful diagnostic test is scintigraphy using sodium technetium Tc 99m pertechnetate (**Fig. 2**). The success of this imaging modality relies on preferential uptake of technetium Tc 99m pertechnetate by the mucous-secreting cells of the ectopic gastric mucosa within the diverticulum.[47,51] In adults, scintigraphy is less accurate because of the lower prevalence of heterotopic gastric mucosa in the base of the diverticulum in the older population. To improve the diagnostic yield of technetium Tc 99m pertechnetate scintigraphy in adults, pentagastrin, histamine2 (H_2) receptor antagonists (cimetidine, ranitidine), and glucagon have all been used. Pentagastrin is a potent metabolic stimulator of the ectopic gastric mucosa within the diverticulum and can enhance radionuclide uptake. When administered subcutaneously (6 μg/kg), approximately 15 to 20 minutes before injection of technetium Tc 99m pertechnetate, pentagastrin may increase the sensitivity of scintigraphy. H_2 receptor antagonists limit

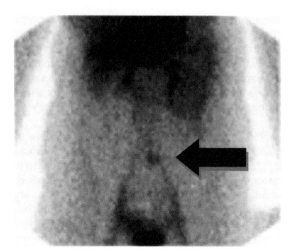

Fig. 2. Technetium Tc 99m pertechnetate scan in a 17-year-old adolescent girl with gastro-intestinal bleeding, demonstrating focal increased activity overlying the area of the aortic bifurcation (*arrow*) consistent with Meckel diverticulum.

gastric acid secretion and slow the rate of radionuclide washout from the diverticular lumen. Glucagon (50 μg/kg), given intravenously 10 minutes after technetium Tc 99m pertechnetate, can further inhibit gastrointestinal motility and delay emptying of radionuclide from the lumen of the diverticulum.[52,53] Although these methods may serve to improve the diagnostic yield of scintigraphy for Meckel's diverticula, the utility of pharmacologic manipulation is controversial and is not required to achieve diagnostic results in appropriate clinical settings. Other technical details of the scanning protocol have been well described.[53] Overall, the sensitivity and specificity of scintigraphy for children with Meckel's diverticula approaches 85% and 95%, respectively. The sensitivity and specificity for adults is much lower (63% and 9%, respectively) and is again related to the lower prevalence of ectopic gastric mucosa in the older population.[47]

Scintigraphy for Meckel's diverticula is limited by certain physiologic, pharmacologic, and technical parameters. The most frequent causes of false-positive Meckel scintigraphy results include intussusception, inflammation of the bowel caused by underlying disease or previous endoscopy, uterine bleeding, retention of radionuclide tracer within the urine collecting system, hemangiomas, and arteriovenous malformations. Alternatively, false-negative imaging results, which can delay timely diagnosis and appropriate therapy, can be a consequence of diminutive volumes (<1 cm^2) or absence of heterotopic gastric mucosa within the diverticulum or excreted radionuclide tracer throughout the urine collecting system, obscuring a small focus of heterotopic gastric mucosa.[51–54]

MESENTERIC ANGIOGRAPHY

As outlined earlier, angiography is often performed in settings of urgent lower gastrointestinal bleeding or in the setting of a positive radionuclide scan and can be useful both as a localization tool (**Figs. 3** and **4**) and as a means of therapy. Digital subtraction techniques may enhance diagnostic yield compared with standard imaging, which generally requires a bleeding rate in the range of 0.5 to 1.0 mL/min for a positive study result.[43,55] For suspected upper gastrointestinal hemorrhage, the celiac artery is first evaluated, followed by the superior mesenteric artery, which supplies the duodenum

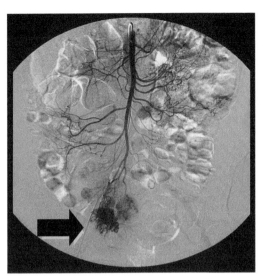

Fig. 3. Angiogram demonstrating active bleeding and tumor blush (*arrow*) on superior mesenteric artery injection from what proved to be a small intestinal neurofibroma.

via the inferior pancreaticoduodenal arteries. Inferior mesenteric artery injections are required for bleeding sites at or beyond the splenic flexure. The internal iliac arteries supply the rectosigmoid junction area and rectum and are studied to assess for bleeding from these sites. Variations related to occlusive disease of one or more of the main mesenteric vessels or congenital variations, such as anomalous vessels arising directly from the aorta, are important considerations when standard injections fail to demonstrate a source. Magnification and projection techniques are critical in the performance of angiographic assessment of gastrointestinal bleeding.

Several sources of false-positive examination results have been described, including hypervascular bowel mucosa, adrenal gland blush, and digital artifact

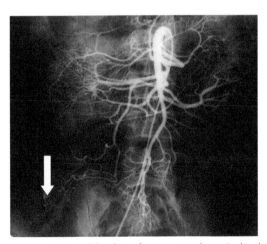

Fig. 4. Angiogram demonstrating bleeding from a cecal angiodysplastic lesion (*white arrow*).

related to peristalsis or respiratory motion.[46] Extravasation of contrast into the bowel lumen is the classic sign of true bleeding. Additional suggestive stigmata can include the presence of pseudoaneurysmal changes in an area of suspicion or the presence of a "pseudovein" sign caused by the linear pooling of extravasated blood along a rugal or haustral fold. When bleeding is caused by angiodysplastic or arteriovenous malformation, early and prolonged opacification of a draining vein or near-simultaneous filling of the feeding artery and draining vein may be noted.

A variety of tools are available to the angiographer in treating gastrointestinal bleeding. A detailed discussion of these is beyond the scope of this review.[56] Superselective microcatheter access to feeding vessels is accomplished typically with 3F coaxial catheters manipulated over 0.018-in or smaller hydrophilic wires. Vasospasm can occur during catheter manipulation and may be treated with vasodilating agents, such as verapamil or nitroglycerin, to preserve luminal access. Absorbable gelatin pledgets, particles including polyvinyl alcohol, microspheres, cyanoacrylate, and microcoils, alone or in combinations, have been used in achieving successful embolization (**Figs. 5** and **6**). Particulate agents allow occlusion of more distal vessels but accordingly may also reflux into nontarget arteries. These agents can also be associated with higher ischemia rates because of their potential to reach more distal vessels without collateral circulation.[56] So-called sandwich techniques, involving occlusion of potential feeding points on either side of a lesion such as an ulcer, are sometimes required if there is a potential tangential or dual blood supply. Stents that allow exclusion of pseudoaneurysmal sources of hemorrhage may also be required in appropriate settings.

Initial reports of angiographic therapy for gastrointestinal bleeding were associated with relatively high rebleeding and complication rates.[57] In these early experiences, proximal occlusion of major mesenteric vessels was being performed. Refinements in technique and experience, including the development of microcatheters capable of providing superselective cannulation of feeding vessels, have resulted in success rates approaching 100% when an active bleeding site can be seen, with mortality and complication rates of less than 5%.[58–60] Rebleeding rates seem higher in some colonic series with right-sided pathology,[60] which may correlate with more massive

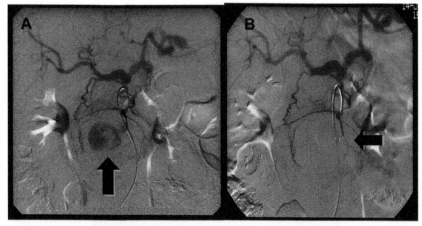

Fig. 5. (A) Active extravasation (arrow) on selective injection of the superior mesenteric artery from a source in the third portion of the duodenum. (B) Control after selective embolization. The coils are highlighted by the arrow.

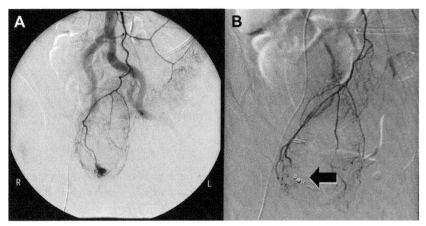

Fig. 6. Angiogram of inferior mesenteric artery demonstrating active bleeding in rectum (*A*) and cessation (*B*) after selective coil embolization (*arrow*).

hemorrhage associated with right-sided diverticular hemorrhage in particular.[61,62] A combined series of 144 patients with lower gastrointestinal bleeding treated angiographically has reported major complication rates of 0% and minor complication rates of 9%.[63] In the direct experience of the investigators (n = 22), an initial embolization success rate of 86% was reported and all cases of rebleeding were successfully treated by colonoscopy. Studies focusing on the upper gastrointestinal tract have reported technical success in 94% of procedures but with lower success rates of 51% after initial procedure and 56% if repeat embolization was included.[64] Recent failed duodenal ulcer suture ligation and blood transfusion of more than 6 units before angiography were independent predictors of poor outcome in this study, and major ischemic complications of embolization were noted in 7%, with previous foregut surgery being a predisposing factor. Clinical failure of angiographic therapy has been associated with coagulopathy and multiple organ system failure in other series of upper gastrointestinal hemorrhage, although successful embolization improved survival from 4% to 69%, suggesting that the technique was still a worthy modality in a highly morbid population.[65] Other combined series of more than 400 patients with significant hemorrhage from peptic ulcers have reported success rates of 75% for arterial embolization, with 25% rebleeding, 18% surgery, 4% major complication, and 25% thirty-day mortality rates.[66] There is ample experience to support the role of angiographic therapy in patients failing or unsuitable for endoscopic therapy, and success is best attested in the lower gastrointestinal tract, perhaps as a function of disease processes more likely to spontaneously improve in that anatomic setting.

One of the greatest challenges encountered in the management of patients with gastrointestinal bleeding, and especially that of the lower gastrointestinal tract with its particular propensity for spontaneous resolution and subsequent recurrence, is the nonlocalization of episodes in patients after careful endoscopic and radiological evaluation. In this setting, provocative radionuclide scanning has been reported.[67] Greater interest has been shown in provocative angiographic assessment because of the potential for immediate therapy via embolization if a bleeding site is identified. Methods used have included the administration of intravenous heparin[68] and intra-arterial administration of fibrinolytics and vasodilators,[69,70] alone and in combination.[71] Some series have reported significant improvement in diagnostic yield from 33% to 67% with such approaches,[68] and small series have reported successful inducement of hemorrhage in even higher ranges of nearly 90%.[71] Conversely, others have reported continued unsuccessful localization in most patients, with positive study results in the range of 30%.[72,73] Given the variability in the protocols used and results achieved in these studies, appropriate use of such approaches requires further investigation with standardized protocols and multicenter designs. In the meantime, appropriate use dictates that these strategies can be used in settings of recurring and otherwise occult hemorrhage, with appropriate preparation and therapeutic options immediately available.

CT AND MAGNETIC RESONANCE IMAGING

Traditionally, solid organ imaging studies have not had meaningful utility in the evaluation of the patient with acute gastrointestinal hemorrhage. However, with the advent of newer modalities, including CTA, CTE, MRE, and single-photon emission CT (SPECT), this is changing. There are now several studies documenting the utility of these techniques in the patient with gastrointestinal bleeding, and even some comparative studies that are now being published.

CTA has been evaluated in several studies and relies on contrast extravasation into the bowel lumen along with subtler signs, such as abnormal dynamic enhancement of the bowel wall including bowel wall thickening and high density of the peribowel adipose tissue, as signs of bleeding and underlying pathologic condition contributory to the same.[74] Combined reviews have suggested a sensitivity of 86% and a specificity of 95% with CTA.[74] Single-slice scanners have been able to detect bleeding at rates as low as 0.3 mL/min in animal model studies,[75] and in human studies, there has been documentation of positive CTA findings in patients with negative mesenteric angiography findings.[76] As with other modalities, CT is the most sensitive in the setting of massive bleeding and may be unrevealing if bleeding is intermittent or of limited rate.[77] CTA has been touted as being less invasive and perhaps more sensitive than angiography, while providing a much higher resolution degree of localization than scintigraphic methods.[74] Challenges include the issue of artifact with metallic objects, such as joint or spinal prostheses; the unavailability of therapeutic option; and the occurrence of contrast allergy or toxicity, given the required contrast load.

CTE and MRE, like traditional small bowel follow through or enteroclysis studies, are more appropriate for the evaluation of the patient with occult bleeding and possible small bowel pathology beyond the reach of standard endoscopic tools than for the evaluation of the patient with acute bleeding. CTE and MRE have proven useful in identifying pathologic conditions in patients with slow or occult bleeding and negative traditional and capsule endoscopic evaluations.[78] Such experiences highlight the utility of these techniques in the evaluation of the patient with slower gastrointestinal bleeding and also highlight the fact that with current reconstructive techniques, CT- and magnetic resonance imaging (MRI)-based studies can potentially combine the benefits of angiography, evaluating for active bleeding, and the imaging qualities of enterographic techniques, exploring for underlying bowel pathology. Thus, these modalities have the potential to delineate a cause and localization of a bleeding site in the presence or absence of active hemorrhage.[79,80] Reformatted imaging techniques using current generation multidetector CT (MDCT) scans also have the potential to clarify pathology and guide subsequent intervention via angiographic or surgical approaches, including the demonstration of underlying vascular lesions such as angiodysplasia.[80]

Early studies are exploring the utility of CT techniques, including CTA and triphasic CT scanning, in comparison with, or in concert with, other tools to assess the patient with gastrointestinal bleeding. Triphasic scanning involves multiple phases of scanning, including arterial, enteric, and delayed, in the hopes of delineating active bleeding as well as bowel wall lesions or vascular anomalies, which might predispose to hemorrhage in the absence of active bleeding (**Fig. 7**). Developing experience suggests a complimentary role for such techniques alongside tools such as endoscopy and capsule studies and highlights the importance of experience in image interpretation.[81] Other studies have suggested that MDCT imaging techniques do not meaningfully add to the results of capsule endoscopy in patients with obscure bleeding.[82] Conversely, in patients with acute gastrointestinal bleeding as defined by transfusion of at least 4 units of packed red cells in 24 hours or overt bleeding and a decrease in hemoglobin level to less than 9 g/dl, MDCT has been shown in a prospective study of 29 patients to compare favorably to endoscopy for the determination of both cause and location of bleeding.[83] In this study, MDCT had superior sensitivity in identifying the site of bleeding in comparison with endoscopy for both upper (100% vs 73%) and lower (100% vs 53%) acute gastrointestinal hemorrhage. Several patients diagnosed by CT and missed on endoscopy had extraluminal, small intestinal, or vascular pathology that could not be recognized endoscopically. MDCT has also been compared with tagged erythrocyte scintigraphy.[84] The investigators found scintigraphy to be more sensitive but felt that MDCT offered advantages in anatomic detail and elucidation of ancillary findings that proved helpful in therapeutic planning, with recognized disadvantages, including relative radiation exposure and intravenous contrast requirement. MDCT has also, like scintigraphy, been evaluated as a less-invasive tool to select patients for angiographic or surgical intervention.[85] Similar to reports mentioned earlier for scintigraphic screening, a negative CTA was associated with spontaneous cessation of bleeding. Furthermore, a positive study facilitated decisions regarding surgical versus angiographic intervention based on localization and characterization of pathology. Hemodynamically stable patients were found to have a low likelihood of significant findings on CTA. SPECT scanning in combination with CT has been found to offer the sensitivity advantages of scintigraphy with the localization benefits of CT when an active bleeding site is demonstrated on radionuclide examination.[86] Early investigations of the cost and other advantages

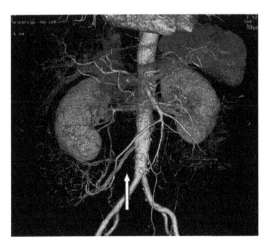

Fig. 7. Reconstructive images from CT scan demonstrating prominent and early filling vein (*white arrow*) draining ileocecal region in a patient with cecal angiodysplasia.

and disadvantages of MDCT in comparison to other investigative strategies for acute gastrointestinal bleeding have been performed.[87] The investigators felt that MDCT compared favorably with radionuclide studies, angiography, and endoscopy from the standpoint of time, sensitivity, and accuracy.

The increasingly widespread availability of MDCT and advanced-generation CT and MRI reformatting techniques, with the attendant potential for simultaneous evaluation of active bleeding and localization of predisposing luminal, extraluminal, and underlying vascular pathology even in the absence of active hemorrhage, make these techniques of growing interest in the evaluation of both acute and obscure gastrointestinal bleeding. It is likely that they will play an expanding future role in the evaluation of the patient with gastrointestinal bleeding.

SUMMARY

Radiological techniques play a critical role in the evaluation and treatment of the patient with gastrointestinal bleeding. Scintigraphic and CT-based techniques have demonstrated the capability to be useful in patient triage based on their sensitivity and potential to stratify and select patients for therapeutic intervention. Solid organ imaging techniques have now demonstrated the potential to couple relatively high sensitivity for active bleeding with tissue imaging capable of detecting underlying pathology even in the absence of vascular extravasation. With the development of microcatheter technology and selective embolization techniques, angiography has attested safety as a therapeutic modality for acute bleeding. As technologic advances and experience continue to develop, radiological methods will be increasingly prominent components of patient evaluation and management strategies, occupying defined and critical roles alongside endoscopic and surgical approaches to diagnosis and therapy.

REFERENCES

1. Howarth D. The role of nuclear medicine in the detection of acute gastrointestinal bleeding. Semin Nucl Med 2006;36:133–46.
2. Alavi A, Dann RW, Baum S, et al. Scintigraphic detection of acute gastrointestinal bleeding. Radiology 1977;124:753–6.
3. Terdiman JP. Colonoscopic management of lower gastrointestinal hemorrhage. Curr Gastroenterol Rep 2001;3:425–32.
4. Longstreth GF, Longstreth GF. Epidemiology and outcome of patients with acute lower gastrointestinal hemorrhage: a population-based study. Am J Gastroenterol 1997;92:419–24.
5. Leitman IM, Paull DE, Shires GT 3rd. Evaluation and management of massive lower gastrointestinal hemorrhage. Ann Surg 1989;209:175–80.
6. Alavi A, Ring EJ. Localization of gastrointestinal bleeding: superiority of Tc-99m sulfur colloid compared with angiography. Am J Roentgenol 1981;137:741–8.
7. Winzelberg GG, MCKusick KA, Strauss HW, et al. Evaluation of gastrointestinal bleeding by red blood cells labeled in vivo with technetium-99m. J Nucl Med 1979;20:1080–6.
8. Thorne DA, Datz FL, Remley K, et al. Bleeding rates necessary for detecting acute gastrointestinal bleeding with technetium-99m-labelled red blood cells in an experimental model. J Nucl Med 1987;28:514–20.
9. Smith RK, Arterburn G. Detection and localization of gastrointestinal bleeding using Tc-99m-pyrophosphate in vivo labeled red blood cells. Clin Nucl Med 1980;5:57–60.

10. Miskowiak J, Nielsen SL, Munck O, et al. Abdominal scintiphotography with Tc99m technetium labeled albumin in acute gastrointestinal bleeding. Lancet 1977;2:852–4.
11. Brill DR. Gallbladder visualization during technetium-99m labeled red cell scintigraphy for gastrointestinal bleeding. J Nucl Med 1985;26:1408–11.
12. Srivastava S, Rao CL. Radionuclide-labeled red blood cells: current status and future prospects. Semin Nucl Med 1984;14:68–82.
13. Ferrant A, Lewis SM, Szur L. The elution of 99m Tc from red cells and its effect on red cell volume measurement. J Clin Pathol 1974;27:983–5.
14. Ponzo F, Zhuang H, Liu FM, et al. Tc-99m sulfur colloid and Tc-99m tagged red blood cell methods are comparable for detecting lower gastrointestinal bleeding in clinical practice. Clin Nucl Med 2002;27:405–9.
15. Som P, Oster ZH, Atkins HL, et al. Detection of gastrointestinal blood loss with Tc-99m-labeled heat-treated red blood cells. Radiology 1981;138:207–9.
16. Winzelburg GG. Detection of intermittent gastrointestinal bleeding with indium 111 labeled erythrocytes. J Nucl Med 1981;22:96–7.
17. Mole DJ, Hughes SJ, Khosraviani K. 111-indium-labeled red-cell scintigraphy to detect intermittent gastrointestinal bleeding from synchronous small and large bowel adenocarcinomas. Eur J Gastroenterol Hepatol 2004;16:795–9.
18. Ferrant A, Dehasque N, Leners N, et al. Scintigraphy with In-111-labeled red cells in intermittent gastrointestinal bleeding. J Nucl Med 1980;21:844–5.
19. Markisz JA, Front D, Royal HD, et al. An evaluation of Tc-99m-labeled red blood cell scintigraphy for the detection and localization of gastrointestinal bleeding sites. Gastroenterology 1982;83:394–8.
20. Zettinig G, Staudenherz A, Leitha T. The importance of delayed images in gastrointestinal bleeding scintigraphy. Nucl Med Commun 2002;23:803–8.
21. Jacobson AF. Delayed positive gastrointestinal bleeding studies with technetium-99m red blood cells: utility of a second injection. J Nucl Med 1991;32:330–2.
22. Howarth DM, Tang K, Lees W. The clinical utility of nuclear medicine imaging for the detection of occult gastrointestinal haemorrhage. Nucl Med Commun 2002;23:591–4.
23. Jacobson AF, Cerqueira MD. Prognostic significance of late imaging results in technetium-99m-labeled red blood cell gastrointestinal bleeding studies with early negative images. J Nucl Med 1992;33:202–7.
24. Kan JH, Funaki B, O'Rourke BD, et al. Delayed 99m Tc-labeled erythrocyte scintigraphy in patients with lower gastrointestinal tract hemorrhage. Acad Radiol 2003;10:497–501.
25. Currie GM, Towers PA, Wheat JM. Improved detection and localization of lower gastrointestinal tract hemorrhage by subtraction scintigraphy: phantom analysis. J Nucl Med Technol 2006;34:160–8.
26. Currie GM. Cost-effectiveness analysis of subtraction scintigraphy in patients with acute lower gastrointestinal tract hemorrhage. J Nucl Med Technol 2007;35:140–7.
27. Gayer C, Chino A, Lucas C, et al. Acute lower gastrointestinal bleeding in 1112 patients admitted to an urban emergency medical center. Surgery 2009;146:600–6.
28. Schmulewitz N, Fisher DA, Rockey DC. Early colonoscopy for acute lower GI bleeding predicts shorter hospital stay; a retrospective study of experience in a single center. Gastrointest Endosc 2003;6:841–6.
29. Smith R, Copely DJ, Bolen FH. 99m-Tc RBC scintigraphy: correlation of gastrointestinal bleeding with scintigraphic findings. Am J Roentgenol 1987;148:869–74.

30. O'Neill BB, Gosnell JE, Lull RJ, et al. Cinematic nuclear scintigraphy reliably directs surgical intervention for patients with gastrointestinal bleeding. Arch Surg 2000;135:1076–82.
31. Kourakis G, Misiakos E, Koratzas G, et al. Diagnostic approach and management of active lower gastrointestinal hemorrhage. Int Surg 1995;80:138–40.
32. Olds GD, Cooper GS, Chak A, et al. The yield of bleeding scans in acute lower gastrointestinal hemorrhage. J Clin Gastroenterol 2005;39:273–7.
33. Levy R, Barto W, Gani J. Retrospective study of the utility of nuclear scintigraphic-labeled red cell scanning for lower gastrointestinal bleeding. ANZ J Surg 2003; 73:205–9.
34. Hunter JM, Pizim ME. Limited value of technetium 99m-labeled red cell scintigraphy in localization of lower gastrointestinal bleeding. Am J Surg 1990;159:504–6.
35. Suzman MS, Talmor M, Jennis R, et al. Accurate localization and surgical management of active lower gastrointestinal hemorrhage with technetium-labeled erythrocyte scintigraphy. Ann Surg 1996;224:29–36.
36. Nicholson ML, Neoptolemos JP, Sharp JF, et al. Localization of lower gastrointestinal bleeding using in vivo technetium-99m-labeled red blood cell scintigraphy. Br J Surg 1989;76:358–61.
37. Ryan P, Styles CB, Chmiel R. Identification of the site of severe colonic bleeding by technetium-labeled red cell scan. Dis Colon Rectum 1992;35:219–22.
38. Bentley DE, Richardson JD. The role of tagged red blood cell imaging in the localization of gastrointestinal bleeding. Arch Surg 1991;126:821–4.
39. Dusold R, Burke K, Carpentier W, et al. The accuracy of technetium-99m-labeled red cell scintigraphy in localizing gastrointestinal bleeding. Am J Gastroenterol 1994;89:345–8.
40. Guiterrez C, Mariano M, Vander Laan T, et al. The use of technetium-labeled erythrocyte scintigraphy in the evaluation and treatment of lower gastrointestinal bleeding. Am Surg 1998;64:989–92.
41. Pennoyer WP, Vignati PV, Cohen JL. Mesenteric angiography for lower gastrointestinal hemorrhage. Are there predictors for a positive study? Dis Colon Rectum 1997;40:1014–8.
42. Orrechia PM, Hensley EK, McDonald PT, et al. Localization of lower gastrointestinal hemorrhage: experiences with red blood cells labeled in vitro with technetium Tc-99m. Arch Surg 1985;120:621–4.
43. Athanasoulis CA, Waltman AC, Novelline RA, et al. Angiography: its contribution to the emergency management of gastrointestinal hemorrhage. Radiol Clin North Am 1976;14:265–80.
44. Gunderman R, Leef J, Ong K, et al. Scintigraphic screening prior to visceral areteriography in acute lower gastrointestinal bleeding. J Nucl Med 1998;39:1081–3.
45. Voeller GR, Bunch G, Britt LG. Use of technetium-labeled red blood cell scintigraphy in the detection and management of gastrointestinal hemorrhage. Surgery 1991;110:799–804.
46. Ng DA, Opelka FG, Beck DE. Predictive value of technetium-99m labeled red blood cell scintigraphy for positive angiogram in massive lower gastrointestinal hemorrhage. Dis Colon Rectum 1997;40:471–7.
47. Tavakkolizadeh A, Goldberg JE, Ashley SW. Acute gastrointestinal hemorrhage. In: Towsend CM, Beauchamp RD, Evers BM, et al, editors. Sabiston textbook of surgery: the biological basis of modern surgical practice. 18th edition. Philadelphia: WB Saunders; 2008. p. 1199–222.
48. Yahchouchy EK, Marano AF, Etienne JC, et al. Meckel's diverticulum. J Am Coll Surg 2001;192:658–62.

49. Mackey WC, Dineen P. A fifty year experience with Meckel's diverticulum. Surg Gynecol Obstet 1983;156:56–64.
50. Lichenstein DM, Herskowitz B. Massive gastrointestinal bleeding from Meckel's diverticulum in a 91-year old man. South Med J 1998;91:753–4.
51. Sfakianakis CN, Conway JJ. Detection of ectopic gastric mucosa in Meckel's diverticulum and in other aberrations by scintigraphy: pathophysiology and 10 year clinical experience. J Nucl Med 1981;22:647–54.
52. Ford PV, Bartold SB, Fink-Bennett DM, et al. Society of Nuclear Medicine procedure guideline for gastrointestinal bleeding and Meckel's diverticulum scintigraphy. J Nucl Med 1999;40:1226–32.
53. Sfakianakis GN, Conway JJ. Detection of ectopic gastric mucosa in Meckel's diverticulum and in other aberrations by scintigraphy: indications and methods—a 10 year experience. J Nucl Med 1981;22:732–8.
54. Kiratli PO, Aksoy T, Bozkurt MF, et al. Detection of ectopic gastric mucosa using 99mTc pertechnetate: review of the literature. Ann Nucl Med 2009;23:97–105.
55. Kruger K, Heindel W, Dolken W, et al. Angiographic detection of gastrointestinal bleeding: an experimental comparison of conventional screen-film angiography and digital subtraction angiography. Invest Radiol 1996;31:451–7.
56. Walker TG. Acute gastrointestinal hemorrhage. Tech Vasc Interv Radiol 2009;12: 80–91.
57. Funaki B, Kostelic JK, Lorenz J, et al. Superselective microcoil embolization of colonic hemorrhage. Am J Roentgenol 2001;177:829–36.
58. Silver A, Bendick P, Wasvary H. Safety and efficacy of superselective angioembolization in control of lower gastrointestinal hemorrhage. Am J Surg 2005;189: 361–3.
59. Tan KK, Wong D, Sim R. Superselective embolization for lower gastrointestinal hemorrhage: an institutional review over 7 years. World J Surg 2008;32:2707–15.
60. Tan KK, Nallathamby V, Wong D, et al. Can superselective embolization be definitive for colonic diverticular hemorrhage? An institution's experience over 9 years. J Gastrointest Surg 2010;14:112–8.
61. Wong SK, Ho YH, Leong AP, et al. Clinical behavior of complicated right-sided and left sided diverticulosis. Dis Colon Rectum 1997;40:344–8.
62. Luchtefeld MA, Senagore AJ, Szomstein M, et al. Evaluation of transarterial embolization for lower gastrointestinal bleeding. Dis Colon Rectum 2000;43: 532–4.
63. Kuo WT, Lee DE, Saad WE, et al. Superselective microcoil embolization for the treatment of gastrointestinal hemorrhage. J Vasc Interv Radiol 2003;14:1503–9.
64. Poultsides GA, Kim CJ, Orlando R, et al. Angiographic embolization for gastroduodenal hemorrhage. Arch Surg 2008;143:457–61.
65. Schneker MP, Duxzak R Jr, Soulen MC, et al. Upper gastrointestinal hemorrhage and transcatheter embolotherapy: clinical and technical factors impacting success and survival. J Vasc Interv Radiol 2001;12:1263–71.
66. Loffroy R, Guiu B. Role transcatheter arterial embolization for massive bleeding from gastroduodenal ulcers. World J Gastroenterol 2009;15:5889–97.
67. Bakalar RS, Tourigny PR, Silverman ED, et al. Provocative red blood cell scintiscan in occult gastrointestinal hemorrhage. Clin Nucl Med 1994;19:945–8.
68. Merragh JR, O'Donovan N, Somers S, et al. Use of heparin in the investigation of obscure gastrointestinal bleeding. Can Assoc Radiol J 2001;52:232–5.
69. Sandstede J, Wittneberg G, Schmitt S, et al. [The diagnostic localization of acute gastrointestinal bleeding in a primarily negative angiographic finding]. Rofo 1997; 166:258–9 [in German].

70. Ryan MJ, Key SM, Dumbleton SA, et al. Nonlocalized lower gastrointestinal bleeding: provocative bleeding studies with intra-arterial tPA, heparin, and tolazoline. J Vasc Interv Radiol 2001;12:1273–7.
71. Willus DM, Salis AI. Reteplase provocative visceral angiography. J Clin Gastroenterol 2007;41:830–3.
72. Kim CY, Suhocki PV, Miller MJ, et al. Provocative mesenteric angiography for lower gastrointestinal hemorrhage: results from a single institution study. J Vasc Interv Radiol 2010;21:477–83.
73. Bloomifield RS, Smith TP, Schneider AM, et al. Provocative angiography in patients with gastrointestinal hemorrhage of obscure origin. Am J Gastroenterol 2000;95:2807–12.
74. Chua AE, Ridley LJ. Diagnostic accuracy of CT angiography in acute gastrointestinal bleeding. J Med Imaging Radiat Oncol 2008;52:333–8.
75. Kuhle WG, Sheiman RG. Detection of active colonic hemorrhage with use of CT angiography: findings in a swine model. Radiology 2003;228:743–52.
76. Sabharwal R, Vladica P, Chou R, et al. CT angiography in the diagnosis of acute gastrointestinal hemorrhage. Eur J Radiol 2006;58:273–9.
77. Miller FH, Hwang CM. An initial experience using CT angiography imaging to detect obscure gastrointestinal bleeding. Clin Imaging 2004;28:245–51.
78. Postgate A, Despott E, Burling D, et al. Significant small bowel lesions detected by alternative diagnostic modalities after negative capsule endoscopy. Gastrointest Endosc 2008;68:1209–14.
79. Yoon W, Jeong YY, Shin SS, et al. Acute massive gastrointestinal bleeding: detection and localization with arterial phase multi-detector row helical CT. Radiology 2006;239:160–7.
80. Duchat F, Soyer P, Boudiaf M, et al. Multi-detector row CT of patients with acute intestinal bleeding: a new perspective using multiplanar and MIP reformations from submillimeter isotropic voxels. Abdom Imaging 2010;35:296–305.
81. Hara AK, Walker FB, Silva AC, et al. Preliminary estimate of triphasic CT enterography performance in hemodynamically stable patients with suspected gastrointestinal bleeding. AJR 2009;193:1252–60.
82. Zhang BL, Ling-Ling J, Chun-Xiao C, et al. Diagnosis of obscure gastrointestinal hemorrhage with capsule endoscopy in combination with multiple-detector computed tomography. J Gastroenterol Hepatol 2010;25:75–9.
83. Frattaroli FM, Casciani E, Spoletini D, et al. Prospective study comparing multidetector row CT and endoscopy in acute gastrointestinal bleeding. World J Surg 2009;33:2209–17.
84. Zink SI, Ohki SK, Stein B, et al. Noninvasive evaluation of active lower gastrointestinal bleeding: comparison between contrast-enhanced MDCT and 99mTc-labeled RBC scintigraphy. AJR 2008;191:1107–14.
85. Foley PT, Ganeshan A, Anthony S, et al. Multi-detector CT angiography for lower gastrointestinal bleeding: can it select for endovascular intervention? J Med Imaging Radiat Oncol 2010;54:9–16.
86. Schillaci O, Spanu A, Tagliabue L, et al. SPECT/CT with a hybrid imaging system in the study of lower gastrointestinal bleeding with technetium-99m red blood cells. Q J Nucl Med Mol Imaging 2009;53:281–9.
87. Laing CF, Tobias T, Rosenblum DI, et al. Acute gastrointestinal bleeding: emerging role of multidetector CT angiography and review of current imaging techniques. Radiographics 2007;27:1055–70.

Small Bowel Imaging

Benjamin T. Jarman, MD

KEYWORDS
- CT enterography • Meckel diverticulum • Small bowel imaging
- Small bowel obstruction • Small bowel tumor

Imaging of the small intestine and determining accurate diagnoses that parallel the clinical presentations represent a challenge for general surgery practitioners. There is often discordance between the radiologic interpretation of small bowel findings and the clinical symptoms and examination of the patient. The small bowel is the most difficult part of the gastrointestinal tract to image because of its length, diameter, and overlap of loops within the abdomen. Advances have occurred over the past several years with more sophisticated computed tomographic (CT) examination and the refinement of nonradiologic tools such as push enteroscopy and capsule enteroscopy. These techniques certainly have limitations, and optimal small bowel imaging remains elusive. Cope's assertion in 1957 that "overreliance on laboratory tests and radiological evaluation will very often mislead the clinician, especially if the history and physical examination are less than diligent and complete" remains true.[1] This article reviews standard small bowel imaging (plain films, contrast studies, CT, CT enteroclysis), provides information on more advanced tools (CT and magnetic resonance enterography [MRE], ultrasonography [US]), and reviews small bowel pathologic conditions that are common to the practice of general surgery.

ANATOMY

The small bowel consists of the duodenum, jejunum, and ileum and starts at the pylorus and extends to the ileocecal valve. The small bowel normally measures 5.4 to 6.3 m (18–21 ft) in length, and each section has subtle features that are appreciable on gross and radiologic evaluations. The duodenum is divided into 4 anatomic sections. The first (superior) and fourth (ascending) sections are intra-abdominal, and the second (descending) and third (horizontal) sections are retroperitoneal. It terminates at the ligament of Treitz, where the jejunum begins. When compared with the ileum, the jejunum is characterized by prominent valvulae conniventes, larger

Department of General and Vascular Surgery, Gundersen Lutheran Health System, 1900 South Avenue, C05-001, La Crosse, WI 54601, USA
E-mail address: BTJarman@gundluth.org

Surg Clin N Am 91 (2011) 109–125
doi:10.1016/j.suc.2010.10.011   **surgical.theclinics.com**
0039-6109/11/$ – see front matter © 2011 Elsevier Inc. All rights reserved.

diameter, thicker wall, and its position in the left upper abdomen. A precise point of transition to the ileum is difficult to delineate, but the ileum is characterized by less prominent valvulae conniventes and its termination at the ileocecal valve. The terminal ileum represents the last 10 to 20 cm of ileum and is a more common location of small bowel pathologic conditions. The normal intraluminal diameter of the small bowel is 2.5 to 3.0 cm and decreases through its length. The wall is normally 1 to 2 mm thick (**Fig. 1**).

PLAIN FILMS

Plain radiography does not require any patient preparation and usually includes chest, supine abdominal, and upright abdominal radiography to aid in the evaluation of patients with abdominal pain. Radiation exposure is minimal, and the studies are immediately available for review.

CONTRAST STUDIES
Barium Follow Through

Barium follow through (BFT) is performed after nothing-by-mouth status of 8 hours with or without the ingestion of a laxative the day before the procedure. A prokinetic agent is often administered 30 minutes before the examination, and a low-density barium solution is administered orally. An effervescent agent is also often administered to produce a double-contrast effect. Spot films are accomplished until the agent reaches the cecum, and then, compression films are used to define overlapping bowel loops and visualize mucosal variances. The study is radiologist dependent and limited by the lack of bowel distensibility and fixation. In addition, partially obstructing lesions may be overlooked because of intermittent fluoroscopy missing the transient prestenotic dilations. The examination is becoming infrequently used at the author's institution because of the availability of other more sensitive studies.

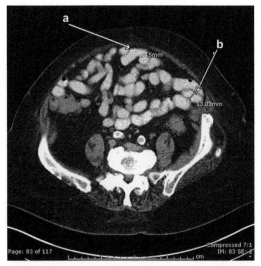

Fig. 1. CT scan demonstrating the normal appearance of small bowel: (a) wall thickness, (b) diameter.

Enteroclysis

Preparation for enteroclysis is similar to that for the BFT. In addition, placement of a nasojejunal tube for controlled infusion of enteric contrast at 75 mL/min is required. Spot and compression films are obtained for analysis. The advantage of controlled infusion of contrast aids in the diagnosis of partial small bowel obstructions (SBOs) and helps clarify mucosal abnormalities. The study depends on intermittent fluoroscopy, with similar drawbacks as noted for BFTs.

US

US is preferably accomplished after nothing-by-mouth status of 6 hours. This status reduces motility and limits gas in the small bowel. Small bowel wall thickness, stratification of layers, and luminal patency with estimations of the degree of luminal narrowing can be evaluated. The addition of duplex scanning provides valuable evaluation of the mesenteric vasculature and small bowel perfusion. Improvements in diagnostic accuracy can be accomplished with hydrosonography. This technique involves the oral or nasojejunal tube administration of polyethylene glycol to aid in bowel distension. Use of US to assess small bowel pathologic conditions is infrequently accomplished. Although US has clear benefits that include cost, portability, flexibility, and lack of radiation exposure, the examination highly depends on user skill, which may vary at any given hour. It is also challenging in obese patients and compromised when intestinal gas is present. These limitations, in addition to the increased volume of information available through other modalities, make the widespread use of US for small bowel assessment unlikely.

CT SCAN

CT was introduced in 1973 and has become a mainstay of small bowel imaging over the ensuing 4 decades. Advancements with helical CT technology and the development of multichannel CT have further refined this modality, permitting quicker allocation of a large volume of data with thinner collimation. This modality makes multiplanar reformatting possible to better evaluate the small bowel.[2] When interpreting CT, it is important to view more than the standard axial sections. Sandrasegaran and colleagues[3] reviewed 50 CTs with additional reconstructions and noted significant findings on sagittal and coronal sections in 23% and 17% of patients, respectively. These findings included all intra-abdominal pathologic conditions in addition to small bowel processes.

CT ENTEROCLYSIS

CT enteroclysis combines traditional enteroclysis with CT to accurately demonstrate small bowel pathologic conditions. The examination requires the placement of a nasojejunal tube that permits controlled infusion (100–150 mL/min) of negative or positive contrast media. Intravenous (IV) contrast is recommended when negative contrast media are used. When fluoroscopic (positive agents) or US (negative agents) evidence of contrast is present in the ascending colon, the patient is transferred to CT and the infusion continues until scanning is complete.[4] Limitations include radiation exposure, cost, failure to delineate mild inflammation, and the need for a radiologist to be present. In addition, some centers routinely use conscious sedation for patient comfort, which further increases cost.[5]

CT ENTEROGRAPHY

CT enterography (CTE) is an adjunct technique that involves the combination of a high-volume (1500–2000 mL) oral negative contrast agent with IV contrast to create small bowel distension. CT slices measuring 3 mm or less in thickness are obtained to provide an accurate image of the bowel lumen, bowel wall, and extraenteric anatomy (**Fig. 2**). Benefits of CTE when compared with contrast studies are the demonstration of extraenteric findings and avoidance of nasojejunal tube placement. One limitation of CTE is the combined need for large-volume ingestion with the timing of IV contrast administration and imaging. Inadequate distension of the small bowel can limit the detection of abnormalities. Relative contraindications for the examination include bowel obstruction, IV contrast allergy, pregnancy, and renal insufficiency.[6]

MRE

MRE is performed in fasting patients without bowel preparation. An oral cathartic agent is ingested before the examination, and images are obtained 20 minutes after ingestion until the contrast medium reaches the colon. Benefits of MRE are the absence of ionizing radiation exposure, pseudodynamic bowel investigation, good temporal and contrast resolution, and lack of nasojejunal intubation to complete the study. Limitations include lower resolution and greater motion artifact than CT.

CLINICAL SCENARIOS
Meckel Diverticulum

Meckel diverticulum (MD) results from the failure of the omphalomesenteric duct to regress and is present in 2% of the population. Although most patients are asymptomatic, complications are reported to occur in 4% to 40% of patients and may include bleeding, obstruction, inflammation, perforation, stone formation, or neoplasm.[7] MD may also be discovered as an incidental radiologic finding. Plain radiographs are not often helpful; however, enteroliths and evidence of bowel obstruction may be identified. BFT studies can demonstrate a blind-ending pouch arising from the antimesenteric side of the small bowel, but this may be difficult to visualize if the ostium is small or if peristalsis is active, which can promptly empty the diverticulum. US may

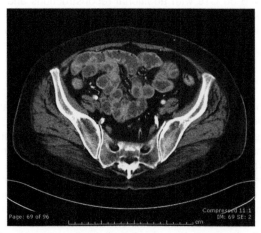

Fig. 2. CTE (negative contrast medium) showing normal appearance of the small bowel.

demonstrate a fluid-filled structure in the right lower abdomen appearing as a blind-ended loop of bowel connected to a peristaltic loop of the small bowel. Enteroliths may also be visualized with US.[8] MD can be identified on CT when complications (obstruction, inflammation) are present, but a normal diverticulum is more difficult to identify. A blind-ending segment of small bowel with associated gas or fluid level may be evident (**Fig. 3**). CTE can more readily identify a normal MD.[9] Scintigraphy with sodium pertechnetate Tc 99m has diagnostic value for some patients with MD. Pertechnetate is absorbed by ectopic gastric tissue, which is present in 60% of MD, and this can aid in diagnosis when ectopic mucosa is present.[10]

Small Bowel Diverticulosis

Small bowel diverticuli are fairly common; however, they are rarely symptomatic, and the incidence is hard to determine. Small bowel diverticuli are readily visualized on contrast studies (**Fig. 4**). Duodenal diverticuli have been incidentally diagnosed on BFT studies in up to 14.5% of patients and have been reported in 22% of cadavers.[11] A duodenal diverticulum typically extends from the medial wall of the junction of the second and third portions of the duodenum and has a thin wall and a collection of gas or oral contrast present. These diverticuli have been confused with cystic neoplasms of the pancreas, and contrast studies can help differentiate these entities.[11] Jejunal and ileal diverticuli are less common, visible on 1% of barium examinations.[11] CT scan is helpful in the diagnosis of small bowel diverticuli and associated inflammatory complications (**Fig. 5**).

Small Bowel Tumors

Small bowel tumors are uncommon and account for 2% of primary gastrointestinal tumors. Most tumors (75%) are benign; however, individuals with malignant tumors are often asymptomatic or present with nonspecific symptoms. Diagnosis is often delayed.[12] Benign tumors include leiomyomas, adenomas, angiomas, hamartomas, hyperplastic polyps, and lipomas. Malignant tumors include carcinoids (44.3%), adenocarcinoma (32.6%), lymphomas (14.8%), and sarcomas (8.3%).[13] Plain films have a limited role in the evaluation of small bowel tumors unless they reveal secondary complications such as perforation or obstruction. BFT can demonstrate

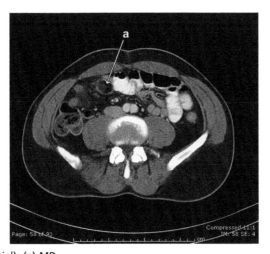

Fig. 3. CT scan (axial): (a) MD.

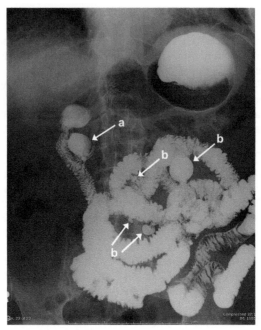

Fig. 4. BFT of small bowel diverticulosis: (a) duodenal, (b) jejunal.

small bowel tumors but is being replaced by more sensitive studies that yield informa-tion about the extraluminal characteristics of these lesions. CT can demonstrate small bowel tumors (**Fig. 6**) but may miss small lesions even if they have caused complica-tions (**Fig. 7**). CTE has 84.7% sensitivity and 90.9% specificity for the detection of small bowel tumors. The positive and negative predictive values were 90.9% and 94.5%, respectively.[14]

Magnetic resonance imaging (MRI) has the advantage of differentiating tumors based on T1- and T2-weighted image characteristics.[15] Carcinoid tumors cause asymmetric mural thickening or a smooth submucosal mass and are markedly enhanced with contrast. Adenocarcinomas are usually focal, with intra- and extralumi-nal growth that is sometimes circumferential. Lymphomas are of variable appearance, ranging from polypoid masses to fungating tumors and diffusely infiltrating full-thick-ness lesions. Gastrointestinal stromal tumors are characterized by large exophytic masses with areas of necrosis. This differentiation may aid in operative planning.

SBO

SBO remains a common problem faced by general surgeons and constitutes 15% of admissions to hospitals in the United States.[16] Clinical history and examination are clearly most important in the evaluation of SBO, with radiology and laboratory testing being important adjuncts. Plain films demonstrating more than 2 fluid levels in dilated small bowels (>2.5 cm) indicate ileus or obstruction. They are diagnostic in 50% to 60% of cases and may obviate further imaging.[17] Dilated small bowels can be distin-guished from large bowels by the presence of valvulae conniventes, the absence of haustra, a central distribution of bowel loops, a small radius of curvature of bowel loops, a paucity of gas in the colon, and the absence of solid feces. With complete SBO, plain films may be diagnostic (**Fig. 8**), but with partial or early complete SBO,

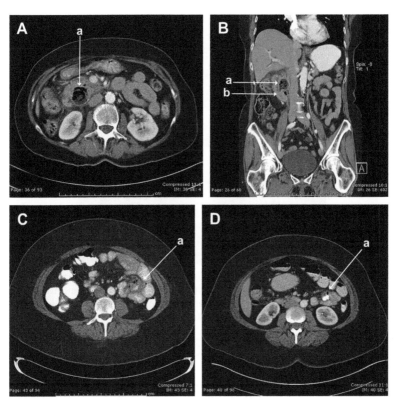

Fig. 5. (*A*) CT scan (axial): (a) perforated duodenal diverticulum. (*B*) CT scan (coronal): (a) duodenal diverticulum, (b) duodenum. (*C*) CT scan (axial) of a 51-year-old woman with jejunal diverticulitis: (a) mesenteric thickening with contained perforation. (*D*) CT scan (axial) of a 51-year-old woman with jejunal diverticulitis: (a) improvement was observed with nonoperative management (6 days after **Fig 5**C).

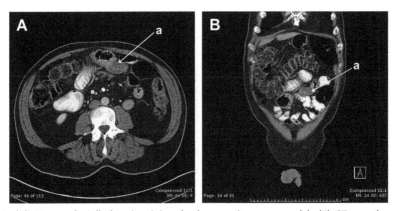

Fig. 6. (*A*) CT scan (axial) showing jejunal adenocarcinoma mass (a). (*B*) CT scan (coronal) showing jejunal adenocarcinoma mass (a).

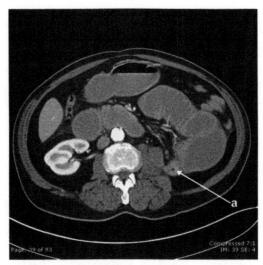

Fig. 7. CT scan (axial) of a 69-year-old man after left nephrectomy for renal cell cancer who presented with SBO and recovered with nonoperative management. He returned 2 weeks later with similar radiologic evaluation, underwent exploration, and was diagnosed with a jejunal adenocarcinoma: (a) high-grade obstruction with transition point.

they may be nonspecific (**Fig. 9**). In the latter case, further imaging with immediate CT or follow-up abdominal films in 2 to 3 hours may be helpful. Differentiating ileus from mechanical SBO is difficult with plain films but may be clear if distension occurs throughout the small bowel and colon (**Fig. 10**). Despite limitations, plain films remain an important initial diagnostic tool because of high sensitivity with high-grade SBO, low cost, and widespread availability.

Schmutz and colleagues[18] demonstrated that US was effective in demonstrating the diagnosis and cause of obstruction in a prospectively designed trial of patients with SBO. The sensitivity and specificity of US for diagnosis of SBO were 95.3% and 84.3%, respectively. The cause of obstruction was confirmed in 80.5% of cases. There was clear benefit over nondiagnostic plain films (gasless abdomen or no evidence of obstruction) when dilated fluid-filled loops could be easily visualized

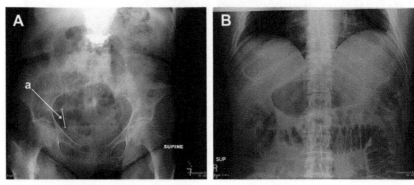

Fig. 8. (A) Plain supine abdominal film of an SBO: (a) dilated small bowel measuring 3.5 cm. (B) Plain upright abdominal film of an SBO.

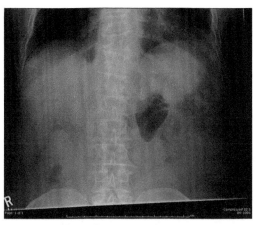

Fig. 9. Plain upright abdominal film of a high-grade SBO in a 69-year-old patient.

with US.[18] A retrospective study by Ko and colleagues[19] demonstrated that US was 89% and 76% accurate in the diagnosis of SBO and determining the level of obstruction, respectively. A prospective trial of US performed by surgeons in the diagnosis of SBO yielded an accuracy of 98%.[20] Although there is mounting evidence that US is a cost-effective adjunct to imaging for SBO, there seem to be significant barriers to incorporating US routinely because CT scan is readily available, whereas US remains dependent on the sonographer.

At present, CT is the examination of choice when acute SBO is suspected. Retained intraluminal fluid serves as a negative contrast agent, obviating oral contrast. CT is readily available in most institutions and is quickly obtainable. In addition, extraenteric evaluation can be accomplished. CT findings of dilated small bowel loops measuring more than 2.5 cm in diameter are diagnostic, and an associated transition point increases diagnostic sensitivity (**Fig. 11**). Transition zones on CT scan are predictive of the obstruction site, with a positive predictive value of 71% as reported by Colon

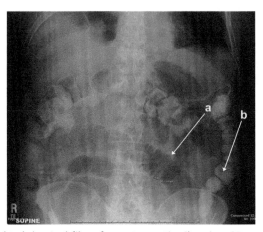

Fig. 10. Plain upright abdominal film of a postoperative ileus in a 98-year-old man on postoperative day 3 after laparoscopic appendectomy with abdominal distension: (a) small bowel dilation, (b) contrast within colon from CT taken 3 days earlier.

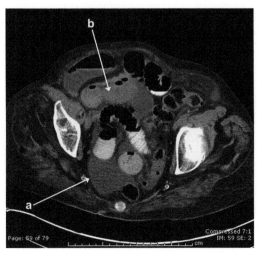

Fig. 11. CT scan (axial) of an SBO: (a) free fluid, (b) dilated small bowel.

and colleagues[21]; however, these zones do not predict the need for surgical intervention. Rocha and colleagues[16] documented successful nonoperative management in 45% of their patients with high-grade obstructions but demonstrated a shorter interval to recurrent SBO and a higher recurrence rate of SBO when this finding was present on the CT scan. CT is 81% to 94% sensitive and 96% specific for the diagnosis of high-grade SBO but is not as favorable for low-grade obstructions (64% and 79%, respectively).[22]

CT enteroclysis has been demonstrated to be more accurate in the diagnosis of low-grade obstructions (sensitivity and specificity of 89% and 100%, respectively).[23,24] Maglinte and colleagues[25] reported the correct prediction of the presence of obstruction in 100% of cases, the correct level of obstruction in 89% of cases, and the correct cause of obstruction in 86% of cases. Small bowel distensibility and fixation are more easily recognized, and the severity of obstruction can be visualized. The role of CT enteroclysis in delineating partial SBOs and excluding complete SBOs constitute it as a valid clinical tool. It also affords characterization of adhesions (parietal vs visceral), which may be of benefit when considering an operative approach.[4] CTE has provided similar results without the requirement for nasoenteric intubation. Diaz and colleagues[26] proposed a well-supported algorithm for the radiologic evaluation and clinical management of patients with SBO.

MRI can be helpful in the evaluation of SBO but is infrequently used because of the availability of CT, inferior resolution, and longer scanning times. However, MRI is not compromised by the presence of barium and avoids exposure of the patients to ionizing radiation. Recent advances with rapid-sequence scans have improved diagnostic accuracy, and MRI may be used more in the future.[22] Recently, MRE has been reported to provide improved diagnostic yield and may become more integral to the evaluation of SBO in the future.[27]

Crohn Disease

Crohn disease (CD) is a chronic inflammatory disease with complex pathophysiology. It frequently involves the terminal ileum and cecum but can involve any segment of the alimentary tract from the mouth to the anus. More than 70% of patients who have CD have small bowel involvement.[28] BFT examinations have traditionally been used to assess patients with CD. Findings consistent with CD on BFT include acute or chronic strictures (**Fig. 12**A), cecal contraction, prestenotic dilation, ulceration with edema yielding a "cobblestone" appearance (**Fig. 13**A), thickening of mucosal folds, bowel loop separation secondary to mesenteric thickening or mass, fistula, and signs of malabsorption.[29] Patients with CD who present with acute abdominal pain may undergo CT scan, which can demonstrate acute disease and complications well (see **Figs. 12**B, C and **13**B; **Fig. 14**). Enteroclysis, cross-sectional imaging (MRI or CT) with or without enteroclysis, and CTE have proven to be more accurate in detecting early inflammatory changes, extraenteric findings, and complications (abscess, stenosis, and fistula) (see **Fig. 12**D; **Fig. 15**).[28,30] CT enteroclysis has been studied extensively and offers the classification of CD, which can have a direct effect on treatment. Differentiation of active inflammatory, fibrostenotic, fistulizing or perforating, and reparative disease can provide a basis for medical or surgical treatment. The enteric volume challenge of enteroclysis is sensitive for fibrostenotic strictures, which may not respond to medical therapy. In addition, CT enteroclysis may be used to ensure that there is no obstruction before considering capsule endoscopy in patients with CD.[25]

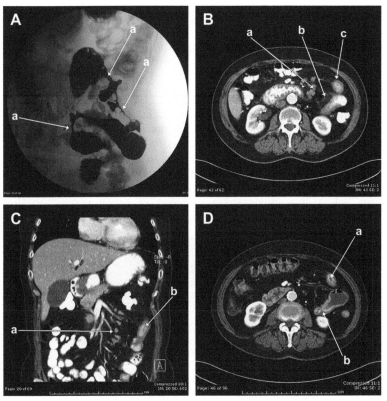

Fig. 12. (*A*) BFT of a 65-year-old woman with acute CD: (a) multiple inflammatory strictures of the proximal jejunum with mucosal edema. (*B*) CT scan (axial): (a) lymphadenopathy, (b) mesenteric stranding, (c) mucosal edema. (*C*) CT scan (coronal): (a) lymphadenopathy, (b) mucosal edema. (*D*) CTE (axial) on follow-up study 2 months after **Fig. 12**A–C: (a) mucosal edema, (b) luminal stenosis.

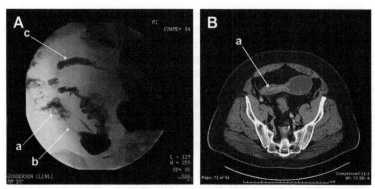

Fig. 13. (A) BFT of a 44-year-old man with acute Crohn ileitis: (a) cecum, (b) terminal ileum with string sign, (c) cobblestoning in ileum. (B) CT scan (axial): (a) ileum with mucosal edema or narrowing.

MRE is more sensitive than conventional enteroclysis in the detection of active CD (89% vs 72%) and is equivalent to CT enteroclysis. Messaris and colleagues[28] demonstrated concordance of MRE interpretation and intraoperative findings. In addition, MRE was able to differentiate fibrostenotic from acute inflammatory lesions that affected patient management. The obvious benefit of no ionizing radiation combined with the chronicity of CD and potential for serial imaging constitute MRE as a critical tool in the evaluation of patients with CD.

Small Bowel Ischemia

Patients diagnosed with small bowel ischemia account for 1% of those who present with acute abdominal pain and 0.1% of hospital admissions.[31] Ischemia may be secondary to SBO, volvulus, arterial embolus, arterial insufficiency (nonocclusive mesenteric ischemia or chronic atherosclerosis), infectious or inflammatory causes, and mesenteric vein thrombosis. Timely clinical and radiologic diagnoses have been documented to reduce both morbidity and mortality.[31] Plain films are typically misleading unless they demonstrate evidence of bowel obstruction, free air,

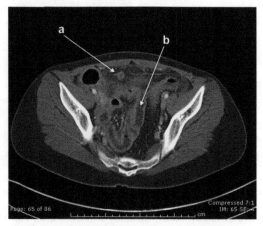

Fig. 14. CT scan (axial) of an acute CD: (a) appendicitis, (b) ileitis.

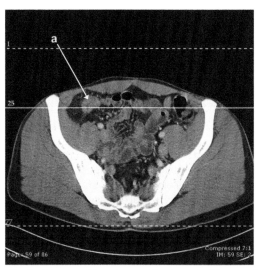

Fig. 15. CT scan (axial) of a 22-year-old patient with CD and a history of ileocolic resection: (a) fibrostenotic anastomotic stricture without evidence of obstruction.

pneumatosis intestinalis, or portal venous gas (**Fig. 16**A). Nonspecific findings include intestinal dilation or a gasless abdomen. The projection of round, smooth, soft tissue densities into the bowel lumen, known as thumbprinting, indicate mucosal and submucosal edema and hemorrhage. CT provides more definitive information with regard to SBI but may appear normal in early stages. Thickening of the bowel, presence of ascites, a target sign (trilaminar appearance of the bowel wall from submucosal edema and contrast enhancement of the mucosa and muscularis layers), pneumatosis intestinalis (see **Fig. 16**B), a whirl sign (twisting of mesentery), engorged mesenteric vessels, and increased bowel wall attenuation on noncontrast studies are all signs that suggest ischemia, especially when several of these findings are present on the same examination.[22]

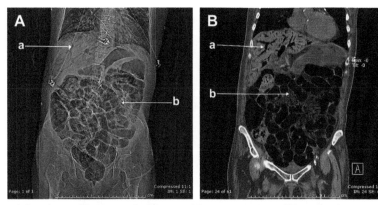

Fig. 16. (*A*) CT (scout film) scan of a 58-year-old woman with small bowel ischemia: (a) portal venous gas, (b) pneumatosis intestinalis. (*B*) CT scan (coronal): (a) portal venous gas, (b) pneumatosis intestinalis.

Malrotation

Failure of normal rotation of the small bowel during intrauterine life may result in the small bowel lying in the right side of the abdomen. This condition predisposes to intestinal volvulus. Plain films are not particularly helpful in the asymptomatic individual but may demonstrate a high-grade proximal obstruction in the case of acute volvulus. Contrast studies are diagnostic and demonstrate the displacement of the duodenal-jejunal junction inferiorly and to the right of the expected location (**Fig. 17**).

Acute Abdominal Pain

Acute abdominal pain is one of the most common complaints of patients presenting to the emergency room. Although multiple causes must be considered, those related to the small bowel include duodenal ulcer disease, small bowel diverticulitis, SBO, SBI, bowel perforation, and inflammatory bowel disease. Plain films continue to be integral to the evaluation of these patients. Valuable information can be obtained, and additional radiologic examination time, radiation exposure, and cost can be reduced.[32] However, plain films often reveal nonspecific findings when acute processes are present, and further imaging may be indicated. As a result, there is a nationwide trend of foregoing plain radiographs and relying on CT as a primary imaging modality.[33,34]

An acute abdominal series typically consists of an upright chest and flat and upright abdominal films. A lateral decubitus film may be needed when patients cannot stand or be placed in an upright position. In this situation, it is important that the patient be in this position for 10 minutes before the film to permit free gas to rise to the highest point.[35] Chest radiographs may demonstrate free intra-abdominal air (**Fig. 18A**), cardiopulmonary causes of abdominal pain (such as congestive heart failure, pneumonia, pneumothorax; see **Fig. 18B**), or secondary cardiothoracic findings (such as aspiration pneumonia, pleural effusions) and serve as a valuable baseline study.[35] Flat and upright abdominal films can demonstrate gastric or small bowel distension, free intra-abdominal air, or paucity of small bowel gas. The loss of normal anatomic landmarks, such as the psoas outline, may indicate soft tissue edema or mass effect.

CT has an important role in the evaluation of the patient with acute abdominal pain when plain films are nondiagnostic and the patient's history and examination suggest an ongoing acute process. CT is more sensitive than plain films in detecting pneumoperitoneum (95% vs 50%–70%) and is 86% accurate in detecting the site of

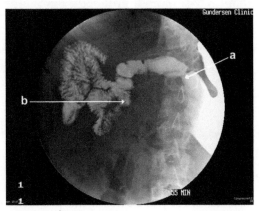

Fig. 17. CT scan of a 20-year-old woman who presented with epigastric pain: (a) duodenal-jejunal junction.

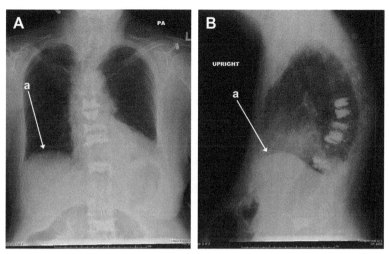

Fig. 18. (*A*) Chest radiograph (anteroposterior) of a perforated duodenal ulcer: (a) pneumo-peritoneum. (*B*) Chest radiograph (lateral) of patient with a perforated duodenal ulcer: (a) pneumoperitoneum.

perforation.[36] CT is also extremely helpful to exclude other nonsmall bowel causes of acute abdominal pain, such as ruptured aneurysms, acute pancreatitis, colonic diverticulitis, renal stones, appendicitis, and abscesses.

SUMMARY

The variety of small bowel imaging studies available to the clinician has undergone significant expansion over the past several decades. Plain films and contrast studies continue to have a role, and more invasive testing, such as enteroclysis, add significant information. Although well supported in the literature, US may not have a significant role in the near future. CT remains the standard for acute processes related to the small bowel and, combined with enteroclysis or enterography, is robust in its diagnostic ability. MRE may be increasingly used as it becomes more accessible and improvements evolve.

REFERENCES

1. Silen W, Cope Z. Cope's early diagnosis of the acute abdomen. 19th edition. New York: Oxford University Press Inc; 1996. p. 57.
2. Maglinte DD. Small bowel imaging–a rapidly changing field and a challenge to radiology. Eur Radiol 2006;16(5):967–71.
3. Sandrasegaran K, Maglinte DD, Rajesh A, et al. CT findings for post-surgical blind pouch of small bowel. AJR Am J Roentgenol 2006;186(1):110–3.
4. Engin G. Computed tomography enteroclysis in the diagnosis of intestinal diseases. J Comput Assist Tomogr 2008;32(1):9–16.
5. Maglinte DD, Sandrasegaran K, Lappas JC, et al. CT enteroclysis. Radiology 2007;245(3):661–71.
6. Fletcher JG, Huprich J, Loftus EV Jr, et al. Computerized tomography enterography and its role in small-bowel imaging. Clin Gastroenterol Hepatol 2008;6(3): 283–9.

7. Elsayes KM, Menias CO, Harvin HJ, et al. Imaging manifestations of Meckel's diverticulum. AJR Am J Roentgenol 2007;189(1):81–8.

8. Elsayes KM, Menias CO, Smullen TL, et al. Closed-loop small-bowel obstruction: diagnostic patterns by multidetector computed tomography. J Comput Assist Tomogr 2007;31(5):697–701.

9. Paulsen SR, Huprich JE, Fletcher JG, et al. CT enterography as a diagnostic tool in evaluating small bowel disorders: review of clinical experience with over 700 cases. Radiographics 2006;26(3):641–57 [discussion: 657–62].

10. Poulsen KA, Qvist N. Sodium pertechnetate scintigraphy in detection of Meckel's diverticulum: is it usable? Eur J Pediatr Surg 2000;10(4):228–31.

11. Macari M, Lazarus D, Israel G, et al. Duodenal diverticula mimicking cystic neoplasms of the pancreas: CT and MR imaging findings in seven patients. AJR Am J Roentgenol 2003;180(1):195–9.

12. Paski SC, Semrad CE. Small bowel tumors. Gastrointest Endosc Clin N Am 2009; 19(3):461–79.

13. Bilimoria KY, Bentrem DJ, Wayne JD, et al. Small bowel cancer in the United States: changes in epidemiology, treatment, and survival over the last 20 years. Ann Surg 2009;249(1):63–71.

14. Pilleul F, Penigaud M, Milot L, et al. Possible small-bowel neoplasms: contrast-enhanced and water-enhanced multidetector CT enteroclysis. Radiology 2006; 241(3):796–801.

15. Masselli G, Polettini E, Casciani E, et al. Small-bowel neoplasms: prospective evaluation of MR enteroclysis. Radiology 2009;251(3):743–50.

16. Rocha FG, Theman TA, Matros E, et al. Nonoperative management of patients with a diagnosis of high-grade small bowel obstruction by computed tomography. Arch Surg 2009;144(11):1000–4.

17. Maglinte DD, Balthazar EJ, Kelvin FM, et al. The role of radiology in the diagnosis of small-bowel obstruction. AJR Am J Roentgenol 1997;168(5):1171–80.

18. Schmutz GR, Benko A, Fournier L, et al. Small bowel obstruction: role and contribution of sonography. Eur Radiol 1997;7(7):1054–8.

19. Ko YT, Lim JH, Lee DH, et al. Small bowel obstruction: sonographic evaluation. Radiology 1993;188(3):649–53.

20. Mucha P Jr. Small intestinal obstruction. Surg Clin North Am 1987;67(3):597–620.

21. Colon MJ, Telem DA, Wong D, et al. The relevance of transition zones on computed tomography in the management of small bowel obstruction. Surgery 2010;147(3):373–7.

22. Nicolaou S, Kai B, Ho S, et al. Imaging of acute small-bowel obstruction. AJR Am J Roentgenol 2005;185(4):1036–44.

23. Walsh DW, Bender GN, Timmons H. Comparison of computed tomography-enteroclysis and traditional computed tomography in the setting of suspected partial small bowel obstruction. Emerg Radiol 1998;5(1):29–37.

24. Kohli MD, Maglinte DD. CT enteroclysis in incomplete small bowel obstruction. Abdom Imaging 2009;34(3):321–7.

25. Maglinte DD, Kohli MD, Romano S, et al. Air (CO2) double-contrast barium enteroclysis. Radiology 2009;252(3):633–41.

26. Diaz JJ Jr, Bokhari F, Mowery NT, et al. Guidelines for management of small bowel obstruction. J Trauma 2008;64(6):1651–64.

27. Cronin CG, Lohan DG, Browne AM, et al. MR enterography in the evaluation of small bowel dilation. Clin Radiol 2009;64(10):1026–34.

28. Messaris E, Chandolias N, Grand D, et al. Role of magnetic resonance enterography in the management of Crohn disease. Arch Surg 2010;145(5):471–5.

29. Armstrong P, Wastie ML, Rockall A. Small intestine. In: Diagnostic imaging. 6th edition. Hoboken (NJ): Wiley Blackwell; 2009. p. 150–9.

30. Hara AK, Swartz PG. CT enterography of Crohn's disease. Abdom Imaging 2009; 34(3):289–95.

31. Gore RM, Thakrar KH, Mehta UK, et al. Imaging in intestinal ischemic disorders. Clin Gastroenterol Hepatol 2008;6(8):849–58.

32. Paslawski M, Gwizdak J, Zlomaniec J. The diagnostic value of different imaging modalities in evaluation of bowel obstruction. Ann Univ Mariae Curie Sklodowska Med 2004;59(2):268–74.

33. Broder J, Warshauer DM. Increasing utilization of computed tomography in the adult emergency department, 2000–2005. Emerg Radiol 2006;13(1):25–30.

34. Pines JM. Trends in the rates of radiography use and important diagnoses in emergency department patients with abdominal pain. Med Care 2009;47(7): 782–6.

35. Field S, Morrison I. The acute abdomen. In: Sutton D, editor. Textbook of radiology and imaging. 7th edition. New York: Churchill Livingstone; 2003. p. 663–89.

36. Singh JP, Steward MJ, Booth TC, et al. Evolution of imaging for abdominal perforation. Ann R Coll Surg Engl 2010;92(3):182–8.

Computed Tomographic Colonography

Ancil K. Philip, MD[a], Meghan G. Lubner, MD[b], Bruce Harms, MD[c],*

KEYWORDS

- Colonography • Colography • Colonoscopy • Colon cancer
- Screening • CT

Initially described in 1994, computed tomographic colonography (CTC; also called CT colonoscopy, virtual colography, and virtual colonoscopy) uses a traditional computed tomography (CT) scanner to reconstruct endoluminal images of the colon. The principal clinical use of CT colonography has been the detection of colon cancer and the surveillance of colorectal polyps. Its use has been growing in popularity among physicians and patients for cancer screening. As opposed to optical (conventional) colonoscopy, CTC does not require conscious sedation or endoscopy, making it less invasive and less time-consuming. However, CT colonography is image based, so some abnormalities require subsequent colonoscopy and tissue sampling for diagnosis and management.

In addition to gains in patient popularity, CTC is diagnostically accurate. The complimentary nature of both two-dimensional (2D) and three-dimensional (3D) imaging in CTC enhances detection of colonic abnormalities. Improved study methods and technology make CTC sensitivity comparable with other screening tests. Because of this, CTC is emerging as a valuable screening tool, as both an adjunct and an alternative to the current gold standard of optical colonoscopy.

HISTORY

CTC was first popularized by Vining and colleagues[1] at the Bowman Gray School of Medicine in 1994, where they used helical CT data to provide 3D images, simulating

This work was not supported by grant money.
The authors have nothing to disclose.
[a] Department of General Surgery, University of Wisconsin-Madison, 600 Highland Avenue, Madison, WI 53792-7375, USA
[b] Department of Radiology, University of Wisconsin-Madison, 600 Highland Avenue, Madison, WI 53792-7375, USA
[c] Section of Colorectal Surgery, Department of General Surgery, University of Wisconsin-Madison, 600 Highland Avenue, Madison, WI 53792-7375, USA
* Corresponding author.
E-mail address: harms@surgery.wisc.edu

the endoluminal view of traditional optical colonoscopy. They called the technique virtual colonoscopy.[2] The term CT colonography (CTC) was later adopted by the American College of Radiology because of its more accurate description of the test.[3]

Early studies of CTC were performed in the supine position, using single- or dual-row CT scanners and 2D imaging. Incorporation of supine and prone positions, multi-detector scanners, and both 2D and 3D imaging has allowed for steady improvement in resolution and detection.[3,4] The use of the supine and prone positions in a single CTC test allows for better displacement of fluid and stool to reduce areas of the colon that may be obscured by retained fluid or poorly distended.

The addition of multidetector scanners and protocols involving decreased CT slice thickness permits more accurate reconstruction of the endoluminal topography. The combination of 2D and 3D imaging has increased sensitivity and specificity of polyp/cancer detection (**Figs. 1–3**).[5] CTC interpretation can start with the 3D endoluminal views; modes can be static or fly-through, allowing both anterograde and retrograde examination of the colon. Abnormalities can be further characterized and verified using 2D axial, coronal, and sagittal images, in which special polyp windows

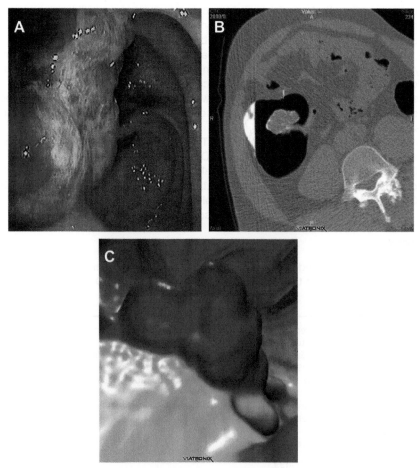

Fig. 1. Tubulovillous adenoma. Cecum as seen by conventional colonoscopy (*A*), 2D CTC (*B*), and 3D CTC (*C*).

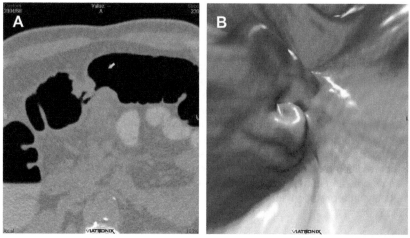

Fig. 2. Annular transverse colon adenocarcinoma. 2D CTC (*A*), and 3D CTC (*B*).

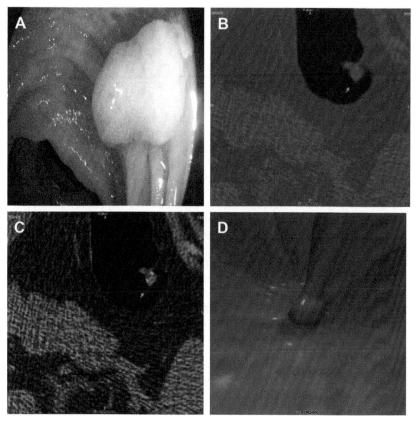

Fig. 3. Tubulovillous adenoma measuring 8 mm in splenic flexure as seen by conventional colonoscopy (*A*), 2D CTC (*B*, *C*), and 3D CTC (*D*).

depict the homogeneous nature and distinct borders of soft tissue lesions, compared with the heterogeneous appearance of irregular fecal matter.[6]

Other advances include reduced radiation exposure, advanced CTC hardware, software, and expanded programs for CTC technologist and radiologist education.[5] Radiation doses for CT imaging have decreased because of improved speed and resolution of CT technology as well as dose reduction techniques such as automatic exposure control. In CTC specifically, given the nature of the soft tissue–air interface, the radiation dose is lower than the traditional CT diagnostic level.[7,8] Dedicated CTC software programs are available that have imaging capabilities specific to the colon. Currently, there are 3 rendering modes available: surface, volume, or perspective. These options allow for more views of the same subject matter, providing the ability to compare different views of the same abnormality.[6,9] In addition to advances in software, an increasing number of radiologists are being trained and tested to ensure the high-quality interpretation that is advocated in 2009 by the American College of Radiology.[6,9,10]

STUDY DETAILS

Four aspects of CTC are essential to produce a successful CTC study: colon preparation, colon distention, CT equipment and operation, and study interpretation.[11] Each of these components is dependent on the others for successful results. As with optical colonoscopy, a radiologist may be skilled at CTC analysis, but in the absence of an adequate colonic preparation, polyp detection may be difficult. The usefulness of CTC results for surgeons is based on multiple factors including patient compliance, technician and technology interfacing, and the 4 components of CTC as noted earlier. Each of these is discussed later.

COLONIC PREPARATION

The goal of colon preparation is to cleanse the colon and to provide contrast for fecal and fluid tagging. This preparation increases the specificity of CTC by tagging residual or adherent fecal material. The fecal material is mixed with high-attenuation contrast that can be well seen on 2D images, which helps with differentiation of a soft tissue polyp from high-attenuation tagged adherent stool. By mixing high-attenuation contrast with retained fluid, this allows for visualization of soft tissue polyps that may be submerged in the fluid pool. The day before CTC, the patient drinks a liquid diet to limit stool formation. The preparation and number of agents required depend on the patient's comorbidities, the referring physician's preference, and the CTC protocols accepted by the CTC facility.[10] In the Department of Defense (DoD) screening trial, patients used 45-mL and 90-mL doses of oral sodium phosphate for bowel preparation.[12] Additional studies have used alternative combinations of cathartics including magnesium citrate, polyethylene glycol, and sodium phosphate.[13,14] However, more recent studies have reported mixed results with non–laxative-based preparations.[15] The correlation between a limited preparation and increased patient satisfaction must be balanced against increased diagnostic capability with a more thorough CTC preparation.

An analysis of bowel preparation regimens compared sodium phosphate versus magnesium citrate and compared thick (40%) barium at 60 mL versus thin (4.6%) barium at 600 mL. A significant improvement in tagging efficacy and compliance with comparable diagnostic performance was reported in the group using magnesium citrate and high-concentration barium.[13] At our institution, the University of Wisconsin-Madison, the standard bowel preparation used for CTC is 2 bottles of magnesium citrate. This preparation is followed by 250 mL of 2% barium sulfate and 1 bottle (60 mL) of diatrizoate used to tag retained stool and fluid respectively. Unlike a sodium phosphate regimen that has a risk of acute phosphate nephropathy, the magnesium citrate regimen can be used for elderly patients with renal insufficiency or hypertension, especially those taking angiotensin-converting enzyme inhibitors.[16] For the 1% of patients who cannot tolerate mild fluid or electrolyte shifts, a polyethylene glycol 4-L solution is recommended.[6]

An additional consideration with CTC includes choosing a preparation with enough contrast to label fecal remnants and polyps, but without impairing visual clarity if same-day colonoscopy is required for pathologic findings. Future advancements in colon preparation for CTC may include incorporation of non–laxative-based solutions and the possibility of same-day contrast and colon preparation.[17] Both of these options show increased patient satisfaction, but their clinical relevance is still being examined. Challenges with a non–laxative-based preparation include inadequate images, altered colonic topography, and overtagging. In addition, same-day preparation increases the potential for optional same-day colonoscopy and biopsy.[15]

COLONIC DISTENTION

An important aspect of CTC is adequate distention of the colon. Adequate distention implies a balance between sufficient distention to provide visualization and too much distention, which increases the risk of perforation. Gaseous distention is achieved either by room air or CO_2 insufflation that is introduced automatically or manually via a flexible rectal catheter.[6] CO_2 provides quick distention and quick resorption after the procedure, allowing for improved comfort and decreased gas retention.[18] Automated CO_2 delivery systems have yielded improvements in distention and postprocedural discomfort.[19] Using automated CO_2 delivery, as with surgical laparoscopic insufflation units, allows the procedure to be tailored to the patient and reduces the risk of perforation.[18,19]

To distend the colon, the CT technologist places a rectal catheter and starts the automated CO_2 delivery at a low pressure to reduce colonic spasm. Sedation is not necessary because the rectal tube and CO_2 insufflation are generally well tolerated.[18–20] One key to the use of CO_2 is that images must be obtained during the infusion given the active reabsorption across the colonic mucosa. The lack of sedation and the marked decrease in invasiveness of CTC are the most notable benefits of CTC compared with colonoscopy.[20]

The disadvantages of colonic distention, including the possibility of perforation, have declined with improved methodology. Nearly all reported CTC perforations have involved the use of room air manual insufflation.[21–23] Protocols using automatic delivery of CO_2, combined with improvements in patient repositioning to allow complete gaseous filling, have led to decreased amounts of gas and pressure needed for CTC.[23] Repositioning also helps reduce bowel kinking or twisting, which could increase the risk of perforation.[6] Automated insufflators have programmed variable inflow and electronic pressure and volume cutoffs, which also improve safety.

CT PROTOCOL

Following colonic preparation and distention, CTC is performed in both the supine and prone positions, with the addition of a decubitus series if needed (about 10% of examinations).[7] Compared with traditional CT, colonography is straightforward, given that the colon is a static structure and, for most colon polyp screening protocols, the standard minimum target size is 6 mm. Therefore, submillimeter collimation is unnecessary, and 8- or 16-multidetector CT scanners are adequate. The increase in radiation dose and number of images needed for submillimeter collimation may offset any improved benefit for small (<6 mm) polyp detection and would not alter clinical management.[6]

CT INTERPRETATION

Following the scan, the radiologist will evaluate the colon using some combination of the 2D and 3D datasets. Many institutions use a primary 3D interpretation with 2D problem solving. The quality of 2D and 3D images, the sensitivity/specificity of the display, and the training of the radiologist all factor into the method and quality of interpretation.[9] One advantage of providing multiple modes (2D and 3D), and multiple views (polyp and abdominal windows, and tracking both proximal to distal and the reverse) is that the image redundancy allows accurate polyp detection and built-in quality control.[6] Despite an increased number of images, CTC can be interpreted quickly and accurately. A typical interpretation time of 10 minutes is possible; however, inadequate preparation or distention may prolong the interpretation time because of the need for additional problem solving.

Among large CTC trials with low-prevalence patient populations for colonic polyps or cancer, using only 2D imaging provided decreased accuracy of detection compared with using 3D imaging alone.[24–26] At our institution, radiologists perform a primary 3D approach for initial polyp detection and use 2D images for confirmation and further characterization of suspected lesions.[6] This method of interpretation has allowed a decreased rate of missed polyps, and provides more accurate polyp detection than traditional colonoscopy. For adenomas 6 mm or larger, 2D CTC sensitivity was 44.1% compared with 85.7% for 3D (P<.001). For adenomas 10 mm or larger, sensitivity of 2D CTC was 75.0% versus 92.2% at 3D (P = .027).[27] Gastroenterologists at our institution have commented that CTC has detected conspicuous polyps that may have otherwise been missed during endoscopy, and that the CTC images aid in efficient and effective colonoscopy.[6] In addition, patients with suspicious lesions via CTC are offered same-day optical colonoscopy, avoiding the need for additional bowel preparation.[6] In studies using segmental unblinding, CTC often discovered polyps that may have initially been missed at optical colonoscopy, thereby rendering the examination more effective, particularly in optical colonoscopic blind spots.[28]

CTC PERFORMANCE FOR POLYP DETECTION AND COLORECTAL CANCER
Current Colorectal Cancer Screening Modalities

Colorectal cancer (CRC) is the third most common cancer in the United States, with more than 150,000 new cases annually. It is the second leading cause of cancer deaths, with more than 52,000 deaths in the United States each year.[29] For patients of average risk (no personal of family history of polyps or cancer), screening standards are recommended at age 50 years. However more than 60% of adults older than 50 years are not being routinely screened. About 15% of US citizens are considered at moderate risk, and thus recommended to have colon screening at age 40 years.

There are multiple tests available for CRC screening. The least expensive and least invasive is the fecal occult blood test (FOBT). FOBT has been shown to be effective in CRC detection and in decreasing mortality from CRC.[29] Pitfalls of FOBT include high false-positive and false-negative rates and inability to detect precursor lesions to CRC.[30] The current gold standard for CRC screening is optical colonoscopy. However, colonoscopy is the most expensive and invasive compared with alternative screening tools. In addition, it is associated with limited, but well-described, morbidity and mortality.[31]

As with the options for evaluation and screening of colon discussed earlier, CTC has its own benefits and risks. It has been proved to be safe and is gaining in popularity as a screening tool for CRC. There are multiple studies comparing performance between CTC and colonoscopy with promising results, and these are discussed later.

CTC for Colon Cancer Screening

Numerous studies have been published in attempt to validate the use of CTC as a screening tool for polyp and CRC detection. Early trials comparing CTC with conventional colonoscopy showed promising results. An early trial by Pickhardt and colleagues[32] (DoD) evaluated the performance of CTC as a screening tool in asymptomatic adults at average risk. The sensitivity for CTC was 88.7% for polyps at least 6 mm in diameter, 93.9% for polyps at least 8 mm in diameter, and 93.8% for polyps at least 10 mm in diameter. These results compared favorably with those of conventional colonoscopy for similar-sized polyps (**Table 1**). The combined analysis by polyp and patient in this study showed a higher but nonsignificant difference compared with optical colonoscopy.

This DoD study also noted that 56 patients in the CTC group had extra colonic findings, with 5 patients diagnosed with extracolonic cancers. An example of an extracolonic neoplasm is seen in **Fig. 4**. The overall time spent by patients in the CT suite versus the colonoscopy suite was significantly shorter. More patients reported a recalled greater discomfort with CTC than with conventional colonoscopy, likely in part because patients undergoing CTC receive no sedation.

Cotton and colleagues[25] compared the sensitivity of CTC versus colonoscopy and reported the sensitivity of CTC for detecting 1 or more lesions of at least 6 mm in size to be 39%. The sensitivity of CTC to detect lesions 10 mm or greater was reported to be 55%. In contrast to the DoD study by Pickhardt and colleagues,[32] this was a nonrandomized multi-institutional report that did not use fecal tagging and uniform 3D fly through as an evaluation tool. This study included all diagnostic examinations and did not focus on a screening population for colon cancer.

Johnson and colleagues[33] analyzed CTC accuracy for the detection of medium to large adenomas and cancers in the American College of Radiology Imaging Network (ACRIN) trial. This study used similar imaging and tagging techniques, including 3D fly through analysis, as reported in the initial DoD study noted earlier. CTC sensitivity in detecting large polyps, 10 mm or greater, was comparable with conventional colonoscopy, with detection of 90% of these lesions. The sensitivity for detection of medium sized lesions (≥6 mm) was slightly lower at 78% (see **Table 1**).

Table 1
Sensitivity of CTC versus conventional colonoscopy from 2 major trials published in the New England Journal of Medicine

	Polyp Size ≥6 mm (%)	Polyp Size ≥10 mm (%)
Pickhardt et al[32]		
CTC	85.7	92.2
Colonoscopy	88.7	93.8
Johnson et al[33]		
CTC	70	84
Colonoscopy	78	90

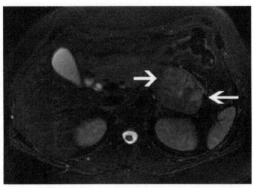

Fig. 4. Extra colonic pancreatic tail mass later proven to be an islet cell tumor (*white arrows*).

Multiple meta-analyses have been performed to summarize the data from various trials.[5,20,34] A recent meta-analysis showed overall per-polyp sensitivity for CTC to be 66%, with a per-polyp sensitivity of 83% for polyps 9 mm or larger.[34] Another meta-analysis concluded that CTC had a comparable sensitivity for detecting large polyps 10 mm or larger, but was less accurate for smaller polyps (<10 mm).[20] Earlier meta-analyses have published similar results to these studies.[5] These meta-analyses include studies in which important diagnostic tools that improve CTC sensitivity, such as stool tagging and 3D image analysis, may not have been used.

The overall sensitivity for CTC to detect colonic lesions has improved in recent years. Early studies showed some variability in CTC sensitivity, and the reasons for this variability in data are explained later. There are several distinct factors contributing to study variability. One problem is that conventional colonoscopy has been its own reference standard for many years. In the DoD trial, they used segmental unblinding; meaning that patients screened with CTC were sent for conventional colonoscopy without revealing the results of the CTC to the gastroenterologist. If the lesions seen at CTC were not initially found, the results were segmentally revealed, and polyps often were subsequently found. This method allowed for a different reference standard that revealed a 12% miss rate for conventional colonoscopy in the detection of adenomas larger than 10 mm. In addition, CTC may perform better in conventional colonoscopic blind spots such as the back side of folds and within 10 cm of the ano-rectal verge.

The experience level of individual radiologists is also an important determinant of CTC result interpretation and variability. Another factor that influences published CTC sensitivities is the reporting of data in certain studies that use a nonconsistent threshold for polyp size and grouping (ie, studies group polyps together by using by using the phrase "greater than or equal to"). This type of reporting can falsely increase the sensitivities of CTC in the smaller-lesion group. In spite of the variability in the early studies, improvements in technique and experience have resulted in increasing sensitivity of CTC. More importantly, CTC seems to have comparable sensitivities with colonoscopy, especially in the detection of larger colonic lesions. In addition, larger lesions are the most at risk for dysplastic or malignant transformation.[35]

Most studies focus on CTC as a screening tool for CRC in polyp detection, but recent studies have focused on CTC-aided diagnosis of CRC (see **Fig. 2**). Sabanli and colleagues[36] reported the overall sensitivity for CTC in the diagnosis of CRC to be 95%, which compares favorably with the sensitivities of double-contrast barium enema (92%) and colonoscopy (94%). Patients referred for CTC in this study tended to be older and had comorbidities that precluded colonoscopy, such as the need for anticoagulation therapy. Older studies have reported similar sensitivities for CTC to aid in the detection of advanced colonic neoplasia.[37] Advanced neoplasia of the large intestine consists of both adenocarcinomas and a subgroup of benign neoplasms referred to as advanced adenomas, but associated with a high risk of progression to cancer.

CTC IMPLEMENTATION: FACTORS AFFECTING ACCEPTANCE
Safety

The two main risks of CTC are colonic perforation and the risk of radiation exposure. Recent studies have estimated the risk of serious complications to range from 0.06% to 0.08%.[22,38] The perforation risk of CTC is less than that of conventional colonoscopy. CTC perforations that have been reported usually occur in patients who have underlying colonic disease or coexisting issues such as inguinal hernias affecting the colon. Another risk factor for colonic perforation is recent (within 2 weeks) colonoscopy with polypectomy or deep biopsy.[39] As a result, patients who have had a polypectomy are advised to wait at least 2 weeks before undergoing CTC, and sometimes even 4 to 6 weeks if the patient had deep biopsies.

CTC has a lower rate of perforation than traditional colonoscopy. A multicenter analysis of CTC showed the overall percentage of complication of CTC to be 0.02%. The percentage of asymptomatic and nontreated colonic perforations (found incidentally) was 0.009%, and that of symptomatic, treated colonic perforations was 0.005% (or 1 out of 21,923 patients who underwent CTC). In comparison, colonoscopy perforation rates are reported between 0.01% and 0.02%.[40] More importantly, colonic perforation resulting from colonoscopy may result in increased morbidity and mortality compared with the perforations caused by CTC, because of the higher probability of required intervention.[20,21,41]

Another important risk factor for patients undergoing CTC is radiation exposure, which is important when comparing CTC with colonoscopy, the latter test requiring no radiation. The current CTC radiation dose is low, although the cumulative dosage with multiple repeated scans may become significant.[42] Image quality may also be affected by radiation dose. The median radiation dose for institutions performing CTC research was 8.8 mSv.[7] For comparison, the traditional adult abdominal CT requires 15 to 20 mSv, and a barium enema requires 15 mSv.[20,43] Although there is no radiation risk with colonoscopy, the low dose of radiation used in CTC poses few disadvantages and offers limited morbidity and mortality.[6,8,20,21]

Cost

The cost-effectiveness of CTC versus conventional colonoscopy relies on a wide variety of factors including the frequency of recommended follow-up, the cost of the test, further work-up of extracolonic lesions, and indications for immediate colonoscopy following CTC.[30] There have been several reports analyzing the cost-effectiveness of CTC. One method that has been used is the use of decision analysis computer simulation studies. Pickhardt and colleagues[44] showed that CTC is the most cost-effective screening option when clinically insignificant (<6 mm) lesions were not included in the analysis. Although cost analysis studies are still ongoing, reports to date, such as that of Pickhardt and colleagues,[44] have shown a similar cost-benefit analysis in CRC prevention rates.[45,46]

The work-up of extracolonic lesions discovered during CTC may influence examination cost. Pickhardt and colleagues[41] reported that, if extracolonic findings are considered, the extracolonic cancer detection rate is 1:300. The United States Preventive Task Force[47] concluded that the benefits, risks, and value for working up extra colonic lesions could not be determined. One current proposal for follow-up intervals for CTC is based largely on polyp size,[44] although there are conflicting studies regarding patient comfort and physician compliance with this proposal.[48] Recently published CT colonography standards recommend referral for colonoscopy/polypectomy for any polyp found on CTC that is greater or equal to 10 mm in diameter.[9] Medium polyps (6–9 mm) can be either referred for polypectomy or surveyed by CTC in 3 years if there are less than 3 polyps identified. Diminutive polyps (<6 mm) can be followed by routine surveillance, defined as screening CTC performed at 5-year intervals. There are limited data for the acceptance by physicians and patients in following these guidelines, as shown by recent studies.[48,49] If CTC is used as a screening tool, the overall cost is affected by how strictly physicians follow the recommendations for immediate colonoscopy based on polyp size.

CTC Implementation and Payment

As described earlier, there are many reasons to consider CTC as a screening method for colon cancer. Most patient satisfaction studies have indicated that it is the preferred approach, even if the interval of CTC recommended by the American Cancer Society is 5 years, compared with 10 years between negative colonoscopies.[49] However, barriers to optimal use include training of CTC technicians and radiologists, educating primary care providers on CTC, standardizing ordering practices, and providing coverage for patients through health care reimbursement. Discussions concerning who should perform the test (radiologists experienced with CT, vs gastroenterologists experienced in patient contact, and who could test/counsel/treat simultaneously) will continue and will be linked to costs and patient satisfaction. Currently, a primary care physician may order CTC as a screening test. A radiologist then performs and interprets the test, and the results are relayed to the primary care physician.

However, the Centers for Medicare and Medicaid Services (CMS) in the United States have denied coverage of CTC in 2009, concluding that "the evidence is inadequate."[50] This opinion was based on concern that the study populations in CTC trials could not be generalized to the CMS population. In particular, they noted that the mean age of participants in the studies was lower than that of Medicare beneficiaries. Until CTC is reimbursed by Medicare, widespread coverage for, and use of, CTC in the United States may continue to be delayed.

Beyond Polyps and CRC Screening: Potential Uses for CTC

There have been numerous novel applications for CTC in the past few years. One such application is the use of CTC in the preoperative evaluation of patients with acute colonic obstruction secondary to CRC.[51] Results from recent studies have been promising, with CTC proving to be a useful adjunct in evaluation of the colon proximal to a stenosis or an obstructing lesion.[52] Surgeons can use the information from preoperative CTC to serve as a road map to help determine the extent of colonic resection and timing of postoperative colonic imaging. CTC may also have a role in inflammatory bowel disease as a diagnostic tool for Crohn disease and ulcerative colitis.[53] Potential applications of CTC to inflammatory bowel disease have ranged from detection of terminal ileitis in Crohn disease to characterizing the extent of colonic involvement in ulcerative colitis.

SUMMARY

CT colonography is rapidly emerging as a more recent option for colon cancer screening, and is endorsed by the American Cancer Society, the American College of Radiology, and the US Multisociety Task Force on Colorectal Cancer for early detection of colorectal cancer and adenomatous polyps.[54] The protocol for CTC is still evolving, with ongoing research aiming to improve the role of colon preparation, automated colonic insufflation, CTC software, and scan interpretation. Technology advancement, patient satisfaction, and payer systems will all influence CTC development and use. CTC is a robust colorectal alternative screening strategy that is safe and fast, with equal efficacy to conventional optical colonoscopy. CTC examination quality and reliability depend on uniform and tightly defined patient preparation, contrast tagging, and evaluation standards.

Even now, patients coming for surgical consultation may bring outside CTC records instead of, or in addition to, colonoscopy and biopsy records. Therefore, surgeons should become adept in reading CTC as well as knowing its limitations and pitfalls.

REFERENCES

1. Vining DJ, Hara AK, Johnson CD, et al. Technical feasibility of colon imaging with helical CT and virtual reality. AJR Am J Roentgenol 1994;162:S104.
2. Vining DJ. Virtual endoscopy: is it reality? Radiology 1996;200:30–1.
3. Dachman AH, Yoshida H. Virtual colonoscopy: past, present, and future. Radiol Clin North Am 2003;41:377–93.
4. Laghi A. Multislice CT colonography: technical developments. Semin Ultrasound CT MR 2001;22:425–31.
5. Mulhall BP, Veerappan GR, Jackson JL. Meta-Analysis: computed tomographic colonography. Ann Intern Med 2005;142(8):635–50.
6. Pickhardt PJ. Screening CT colonography: how I do it. AJR Am J Roentgenol 2007;189:290–8.
7. Brenner DJ, Hall EJ. Computed tomography – an increasing source of radiation exposure. N Engl J Med 2007;357:2277–84.
8. Brenner DJ, Georgsson MA. Mass screening with CT colonography: should radiation exposure be of concern? Gastroenterology 2005;129:328–37.
9. Burling D. CT colonography standards. Clin Radiol 2010;65:474–80.
10. Thomas J, Carenza J, McFarland E. Computed tomography colonography (virtual colonoscopy): climax of a new era of validation and transition into community practice. Clin Colon Rectal Surg 2008;21(3):220–31.
11. Pickhardt PJ, Kim DH. CT colonography: principles and practice of virtual colonoscopy. Philadelphia: Saunders Elsevier; 2010.
12. Kim DH, Pickhardt PJ, Hinshaw JL, et al. Prospective blinded trial comparing 45-ml and 90-ml doses of oral sodium phosphate for bowel preparation prior to CT colonography. J Comput Assist Tomogr 2007;31:53–8.
13. Yoon SH, Kim SH, Kim SG, et al. Comparison study of different bowel preparation regimens and different fecal-tagging agents on tagging efficacy, patients' compliance, and diagnostic performance of computed tomographic colonography: preliminary study. J Comput Assist Tomogr 2009;33(5):657–65.
14. Borden ZS, Pickhardt PJ, Kim DH, et al. Bowel preparation for CT colonography: blinded comparison of magnesium citrate and sodium phosphate for catharsis. Radiology 2010;254(1):138–44.
15. Pickhardt PJ, Choi JR. CT colonography without catharsis: the ultimate study or useful additional option? Gastroenterology 2005;128:521–2.

16. Markowitz GS, Stokes MB, Radhakrishnan J, et al. Acute phosphate nephropathy following oral sodium phosphate bowel purgative: an under recognized cause of chronic renal failure. J Am Soc Nephrol 2005;16:3389–96.
17. Taylor SA, Slater A, Burling DN, et al. CT colonography: optimization, diagnostic performance and patient acceptability of reduced-laxative regimens using barium-based fecal tagging. Eur Radiol 2008;18:32–42.
18. Burling D, Taylor SA, Halligan S, et al. Automated insufflation of carbon dioxide for MDCT colonography: distension and patient experience compared with manual insufflation. AJR Am J Roentgenol 2006;186:96–103.
19. Shinners TJ, Pickhardt PJ, Taylor AJ, et al. Patient-controlled room air insufflation versus automated carbon dioxide delivery for CT colonography. AJR Am J Roentgenol 2006;186:1491–6.
20. Rosman AS, Korsten MA. Meta-analysis comparing CT colonography, air contrast barium enema, and colonoscopy. Am J Med 2007;120:201–10.
21. Lin OS. Computed tomographic colonography: hope of hype? World J Gastroenterol 2010;12(8):915–20.
22. Burling D, Halligan S, Slater A, et al. Potentially serious adverse events at CT colonography in symptomatic patients: national survey of the United Kingdom. Radiology 2006;239:464–71.
23. Sosna J, Blachar A, Amitai M, et al. Colonic perforation at CT colonography: assessment of risk in a multicenter large cohort. Radiology 2006;239(2):457–63.
24. Johnson CD, Harmsen WS, Wilson LA, et al. Prospective blinded evaluation of computed tomographic colonography for screen detection of colorectal polyps. Gastroenterology 2003;125:311–9.
25. Cotton PB, Durkalski VL, Pineau BC, et al. Computed tomographic colonography (virtual colonoscopy): a multicenter comparison with standard colonoscopy for detection of colorectal neoplasia. JAMA 2004;291:1713–9.
26. Rockey DC, Paulson E, Niedzwiecki D, et al. Analysis of air contrast barium enema, computed tomographic colonography, and colonoscopy: prospective comparison. Lancet 2005;365:305–11.
27. Pickhardt PJ, Lee AD, Taylor AJ, et al. Primary 2D versus primary 3D polyp detection at screening CT colonography. AJR Am J Roentgenol 2007;189:1451–6.
28. Pickhardt PJ, Nugent PA, Mysliwiec PA, et al. Location of adenomas missed at optical colonoscopy. Ann Intern Med 2004;141:352–9.
29. Mandel JS, Bond JH, Church TR, et al. Reducing mortality from CRC by screening FOBT: MCCCS. N Engl J Med 1993;328:1365–71.
30. Otto Schiueh L. CTC: hope or hype? World J Surg 2010;16(8):915–20.
31. Rabeneck L, Paszat LF, Hilsden RJ, et al. Bleeding and perforation after outpatient colonoscopy and their risk factors in usual clinical practice. Gastroenterology 2008;153(6):1899–906.
32. Pickhardt PJ, Choi JR, Hwang I, et al. Computed tomographic virtual colonoscopy to screen for colorectal neoplasia in asymptomatic adults. N Engl J Med 2003;349:2191–200.
33. Johnson DC, Chen MH, Toledano AY, et al. Accuracy of CT colonography for detection of large adenomas and cancers. N Engl J Med 2008;359:1207–17.
34. Chaparro M, Gisbeert JP, del Campo L, et al. Accuracy of computed tomographic colonography for the detection of polyps and colorectal tumors: a systematic review and meta-analysis. Digestion 2009;80:1–17.
35. Bond JH. Clinical evidence for the adenoma-carcinoma sequence, and the management of patients with colorectal adenomas. Semin Gastrointest Dis 2000;11:176–84.

36. Sabanli M, Balasingam A, Bailey W, et al. Computed tomographic colonography in the diagnosis of colorectal cancer. Br J Surg 2010;97:1291–4.
37. Kim DH, Pickhardt PJ, Taylor AJ, et al. CT colonography versus colonoscopy for detection of advanced neoplasia. N Engl J Med 2007;357:1403–12.
38. Sosna J, Bar-Ziv J, Libson E, et al. Colonic perforation at CT colonography: assessment of risk in a multicenter large cohort. Radiology 2006;239:457–63.
39. Rockey D. Computed tomographic colonography: current perspectives and future directions. Gastroenterology 2009;137:7–17.
40. Pickhardt PJ. Incidence of colonic perforation at CT colonography: review of existing data and implications for screening of asymptomatic adults. Radiology 2006;239:313–6.
41. Pickhardt PJ. Noninvasive radiologic imaging of the large intestine: a valuable complement to optical colonoscopy. Curr Opin Gastroenterol 2010;26:61–8.
42. Brenner D. Radiation risks potentially associated with low dose CT screening of adult smokers for lung cancer. Radiology 2004;231:440–5.
43. Van Gelder RE, Venema HW, Serlie IW, et al. CT colonography at different radiation dose levels: feasibility of dose reduction. Radiology 2002;224:25–33.
44. Pickhardt PJ, Hassan C, Laghi A, et al. Cost-effectiveness of colorectal cancer screening with computed tomography colonography: the impact of not reporting diminutive lesions. Cancer 2007;109:2213–21.
45. Ladabaum U, Song K, Fredrick AM. Colorectal neoplasia screening with virtual colonoscopy: when, at what cost, and with what national impact? Clin Gastroenterol Hepatol 2004;2:554–63.
46. Hassan C, Pickhardt P, Laghi A. Computed tomographic colonography to screen for colorectal cancer, extracolonic cancer, and aortic aneurysm. Arch Intern Med 2008;168(7):696–705.
47. US Preventive Services Task Force. Screening for colorectal cancer: U.S. Preventive Services Task Force recommendation statement. Ann Intern Med 2008;149: 627–37.
48. Shah JP, Hynan LS, Rockey DC. Management of small polyps detected by screening CT colonography: patient and physician preferences. Am J Med 2009;687:1–9.
49. Pickhardt PJ, Taylor AJ, Kim DH, et al. Screening for colorectal neoplasia with CT colonography: initial experience from the 1st year of coverage by third-party payers. Radiology 2006;241:417–25.
50. Decision memo for screening computed tomography (CTC) for colorectal cancer. Centers for Medicare and Medicaid Services; 2009.
51. Cha EY, Park H, Lee SS, et al. CT colonography after metallic stent placement for acute malignant colonic obstruction. Radiology 2010;254:774–82.
52. Coccetta M, Migliaccio C, La Mura F, et al. Virtual colonoscopy in stenosing colorectal cancer. Ann Surg Innov Res 2009;3:11.
53. Ota Y, Matsui T, Ono H, et al. Value of virtual computed tomographic colonography for Crohn's colitis: comparison with endoscopy and barium enema. Abdom Imaging 2003;28(6):778–83.
54. Levin B, Lieberman DA, McFarland B, et al. Screening and surveillance for the early detection of colorectal cancer and adenomatous polyps, 2008: a joint guideline from the American Cancer Society, the US Multi-Society Task Force on Colorectal Cancer, and the American College of Radiology. CA Cancer J Clin 2008;58:130–60.

Update on Imaging for Acute Appendicitis

Nancy A. Parks, MD, Thomas J. Schroeppel, MD*

KEYWORDS

• Imaging • Acute • Appendicitis • CT • US • MRI

Acute appendicitis (AA) remains one of the most common surgical emergencies in the United States with over 250,000 cases diagnosed each year. Lifetime risk of developing AA is 8.6% in men and 6.7% in women, with an overall appendectomy rate of 12% in men and 23% in women.[1] The pathophysiology of AA is likely related to luminal obstruction of the vermiform appendix. This condition leads to rising intraluminal pressure, ischemia, and eventual perforation. Perforation increases the mortality rate of AA from 0.0002% to 3% and increases the morbidity from 3% to 47%.[2] This increase in complications associated with advanced appendicitis and perforation has led to the traditional surgical teaching that a negative appendectomy rate of 20% is acceptable to balance the need for early diagnosis and avoid perforation. Current negative appendectomy rates are lower because of the increasing use of imaging. A recent population-based review found the rate of negative appendectomy to be 4.5% in those with imaging and 9.8% in those with no imaging.[3]

Advances in imaging techniques over the past 20 years have changed the way suspected AA is evaluated. Traditionally, the diagnosis was made based solely on the history taking and physical examination. However, AA is known as the "great masquerader" and has highly variable presentations and findings on examination. The presentation of AA may be atypical, complicating the diagnosis and leading to delays in treatment, prolonged hospitalization, and unnecessary surgery. Diagnostic accuracy based on clinical findings alone is 80%. Based solely on history taking and physical examination, men are diagnosed correctly 78% to 92% of the time, whereas women are diagnosed correctly only 58% to 85% of the time.[4] This difference is because in women of childbearing age, the diagnosis of lower abdominal pain is difficult and may be secondary to gynecologic conditions, such as ovarian disease or pelvic inflammatory disease. Clinicians are able to use a variety of imaging techniques in the evaluation of suspected AA. In this article, ultrasonography (US), computed tomography

The authors have nothing to disclose.
Department of Surgery, University of Tennessee Health Science Center, 910 Madison Avenue, Suite 220, Memphis, TN 38163, USA
* Corresponding author.
E-mail address: tschroep@uthsc.edu

Surg Clin N Am 91 (2011) 141–154
doi:10.1016/j.suc.2010.10.017   **surgical.theclinics.com**

(CT), and magnetic resonance imaging (MRI) are reviewed with respect to their accuracy in the diagnosis of AA and their ability to reduce negative appendectomy rates.

PLAIN RADIOGRAPHS

Plain abdominal radiographs are not routinely recommended for the evaluation of suspected AA. If they are obtained in patients with acute abdominal pain, nonspecific findings suggestive of AA may be evident. A calcified density in the right lower quadrant, or appendicolith, suggests the diagnosis of AA in the appropriate clinical setting (**Fig. 1**). However, an appendicolith is visualized on plain radiographs in less than 5% of patients with AA.[4] Other findings on plain radiographs include abnormal gas patterns in the right lower quadrant, a thickened appendix with irregular walls, or a general haziness in the right lower quadrant. These findings are nonspecific and present infrequently, greatly limiting their reliability in the diagnosis of AA.[5]

Perforated appendicitis (PA) with abscess can occasionally be demonstrated on plain radiographs. Abscesses may appear as irregularly shaped, unilocular lucencies, which occasionally contain gas. An abscess can cause an obstructive pattern on radiograph, and in the correct clinical setting, PA should be considered as a possible cause. Although a small amount of air may be released with PA, it is typically not enough to be detected as pneumoperitoneum on plain radiographs.[6]

US

US has been used as a tool to aid in the diagnosis of AA since the 1980s. Over the last 30 years, advances in ultrasound technology and the graded compression technique

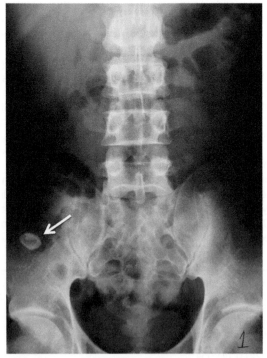

Fig. 1. Plain radiograph of the abdomen with arrow highlighting the calcified appendicolith.

have improved the ability to visualize the appendix. The graded compression technique involves applying steady, gradual pressure to the right lower quadrant in an effort to collapse the normal bowel and eliminate normal bowel gas to visualize the appendix. If AA is present, the appendix will be immobile, noncompressible, and thickened with a diameter of greater than 6 to 7 mm (**Figs. 2–4**).[7]

US is operator dependent, and therefore, the reported sensitivity and specificity of US in the diagnosis of AA is variable. US is most reliable in centers with considerable experience using this imaging modality. In 2 recent meta-analyses reviewing the utility of US, the sensitivity was reported as 78% and 83% and the specificity was 83% and 93%.[8,9] Although both of these meta-analyses reported higher sensitivity and specificity data for CT than for US, a prospective trial comparing US with CT showed that the diagnostic performance of both modalities was similar. In that trial, 94 adult patients suspected of having AA underwent US and CT scanning. Findings on US and CT were compared to clinical follow-up or surgical pathologic findings. The diagnostic accuracy of US and CT were not significantly different, but there were significantly more inconclusive findings with ultrasonography.[10]

Poortman and colleagues[11] have developed an imaging pathway to minimize radiation exposure from CT, while attempting to achieve a high accuracy in the diagnosis of AA. In their prospective trial, 151 adults with suspected AA were evaluated. All patients had an initial US. Of these patients, 79 (52%) were diagnosed with AA on US and proceeded directly to appendectomy. The remaining 72 patients had a subsequent CT scan. CT diagnosed AA in 21 patients and found an alternative diagnosis in 12 patients and no cause for the abdominal pain in 39 patients. This strategy yielded a negative appendectomy rate of 8%.

US has been particularly useful in the diagnosis of AA in children. Pediatric centers have gained a large experience in US because of the concerns with childhood exposure to ionizing radiation. A recent study of pediatric patients evaluated for acute abdominal pain underscored the value of ultrasonography. Of the 622 patients, 152 were evaluated clinically and discharged. Another 81 patients were taken directly to the operating room for appendectomy based on history taking and physical examination alone. Of these patients, 16 had a normal appendix on pathologic examination (20% negative appendectomy rate). The remaining 389 patients had imaging performed to evaluate their abdominal pain; 386 patients underwent US and 7 patients underwent CT scans. Of the 389 patients, 137 were diagnosed with AA; only 3% of

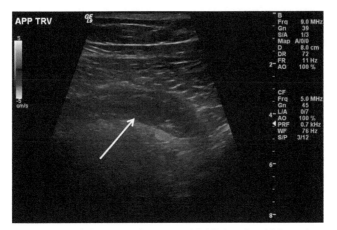

Fig. 2. Sagittal US image of the appendix. Arrow highlights the thickened appendix.

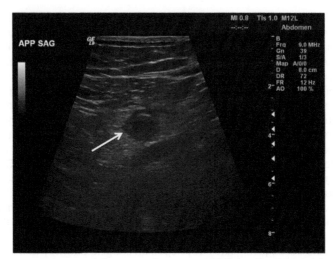

Fig. 3. Transverse US image of the appendix. Arrow highlights the thickened appendix.

this group had a negative appendectomy. No patients returned with a missed diagnosis of appendicitis. In this series, US was the primary imaging modality in children with abdominal pain, yielding a lower rate of negative appendectomy than clinical evaluation alone.[12]

US is also valuable in the diagnosis of AA in pregnant women. US is safe during all trimesters of pregnancy and therefore is the initial imaging study of choice in pregnant women with new-onset abdominal pain. US in pregnancy has a variable sensitivity, ranging from 66% to 100%, but a good specificity of 95% to 96%.[13] Because US is safe, easy to obtain, and widely available, it is a good imaging study for pregnant women with suspected AA. However, if the US result is negative or inconclusive, AA cannot be excluded and further imaging studies are recommended.

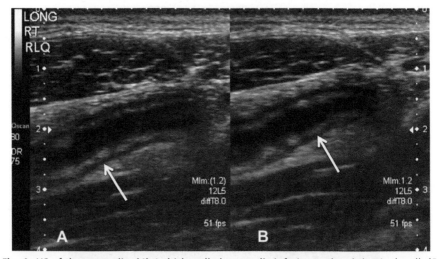

Fig. 4. US of the appendix. (A) A thick-walled appendix inferior to the abdominal wall. (B) Compression view demonstrating a noncompressible appendix. Arrows highlight the thickened wall of the appendix.

Advantages of US include the absence of ionizing radiation, low cost, and wide-spread availability. In addition, it is noninvasive, safe, and quick to obtain and can identify other causes of abdominal pain. A significant disadvantage of US is that it is operator dependent, relying both on the US technician and the interpretation by the radiologist. Also, if the appendix is not visualized, the study is inconclusive and no decision can be made about the cause of the abdominal symptoms.

CT

CT is a highly accurate and effective modality for the evaluation of patients with sus-pected AA. Modern helical CT scans have excellent resolution, are widely available, and are operator independent. CT scans are easy to interpret and can provide signif-icant information regarding alternative diagnoses. CT has been shown to have a sensi-tivity of 90% to 100%, specificity of 91% to 99%, positive predictive value of 92% to 98%, and negative predictive value of 95% to 100%.[14] This high accuracy is main-tained in large university and rural community hospitals.[15] However, in spite of the widespread use and high accuracy of CT scanning, there is still considerable debate regarding the true benefit of CT in patients with suspected AA.

CT diagnosis of AA is based on the appearance of a thickened, inflamed appendix and surrounding signs of inflammation. In AA, the appendix is usually greater than 7 mm in diameter with circumferential wall thickening and mural enhancement, which may give the appearance of a "target sign" on CT scan (**Fig. 5**).[14] A calcified appen-dicolith may be seen in up to 30% of cases (**Fig. 6**). Periappendiceal inflammation, such as fat stranding, periappendiceal fluid, and clouding of the adjacent mesentery, are common in AA. In PA, there may be a right lower quadrant abscess or extraluminal gas (see **Fig. 6; Figs. 7** and **8**).[16] If the appendix is not visualized and there are no find-ings of inflammation in the right lower quadrant, the diagnosis of AA can be excluded.[17]

Many possible protocols have been described for CT imaging in suspected AA. One of the original articles to show a benefit with routine CT scanning in the evaluation of suspected AA was done by Rao and colleagues[18] using a limited appendiceal

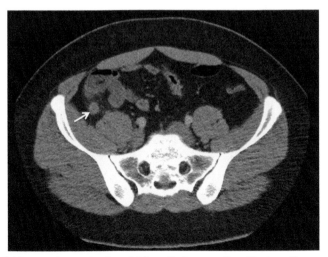

Fig. 5. CT axial image demonstrating thick-walled appendix with stranding and inflamma-tion. The arrow highlights the appendix with a "target sign."

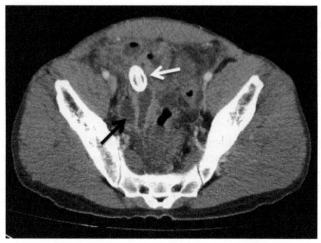

Fig. 6. CT axial image demonstrating PA. The white arrow highlights a calcified appendicolith. The black arrow highlights an abscess cavity with a bubble of air adjacent to the appendix.

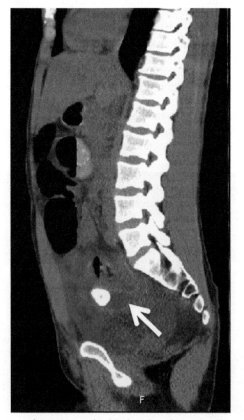

Fig. 7. CT sagittal image of PA. Arrow highlights the abscess cavity containing a calcified appendicolith.

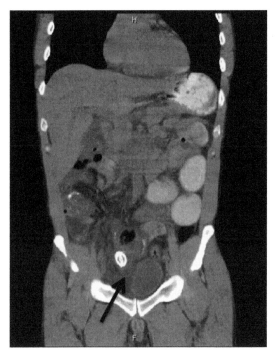

Fig. 8. CT coronal image of PA. Arrow highlights the abscess cavity containing a calcified appendicolith.

protocol. In this study, 100 consecutive patients with suspected AA underwent a limited scan through the region of the ileocecal valve after receiving enteric contrast injected per rectum. The field of the scan included a 15-cm region centered around the cecum as seen on the initial CT radiograph. The benefit of the limited scan is that it requires approximately one-third the radiation of a full CT scan of the abdomen and pelvis. Using this technique, the appendix was visualized in 94% of the patients. The CT scan had an accuracy of 94%, and hence, the treatment plan in 59 patients was changed, including preventing unnecessary appendectomy in 13 patients. A cost analysis demonstrated an overall savings with the increased use of CT scanning because of a decrease in the number of negative appendectomies and decreased inpatient observation for equivocal cases.

There continues to be controversy regarding the optimal extent of the CT scan and the need for contrast. A recent retrospective review of 100 consecutive, nonfocused abdominal CT scans obtained for suspected AA concluded that limited appendiceal CT scans should not be done because alternative diagnoses can be missed. The investigators identified 7 patients with abnormalities in the upper abdomen, and 4 of them required surgery. These findings would have been missed on a limited CT scan. Based on these findings, the investigators concluded that full-abdomen and pelvis CT scans should be obtained in the evaluation of suspected AA.[19]

There is also significant debate considering which, if any, contrast to administer with CT scanning. In a series of 300 consecutive patients with suspected AA, CT scans of the abdomen and pelvis were obtained without using any intravenous (IV) or enteric contrast material to rapidly scan the abdomen. Radiological findings were compared to clinical follow-up and surgical pathologic findings, yielding a sensitivity of 96%, a specificity of 99%, and an accuracy of 97%. There were 5 false-negative results in this series, 3 of which occurred in thin, young women with little intraperitoneal fat. The lack of intraperitoneal fat in a noncontrast CT scan was thought to lead to difficulty in identifying the inflammatory process.[20]

Other investigators have reported on the value of contrast-enhanced CT scans. A prospective randomized trial of 91 patients was done comparing the traditional triple-contrast CT of the abdomen and pelvis with a limited appendiceal CT with rectal contrast only. In this study, the limited scan with only rectal contrast was determined to be superior to the triple contrast scan because it was more specific for AA, was well tolerated by the patients, and quicker to perform.[21] Other investigators have stated that CT scans should be obtained with IV contrast to visualize the mild changes in the appendix associated with early appendicitis.[22]

The final major area of debate is regarding which patients suspected of having AA should have a CT scan before appendectomy. There are multiple articles in the literature, which argue against routine preoperative imaging of patients with suspected AA.[23–25] In these articles, the routine use of imaging has not been shown to decrease the rate of negative appendectomy. In addition, concerns have been raised that ordering routine imaging in the emergency department, before surgical consultation, may actually delay the diagnosis and appropriate intervention in cases of AA.[26] Early surgical consultation and involvement of the surgeon while deciding to obtain a CT scan may avoid an unnecessary delay.

Other studies have shown a benefit from preoperative imaging in suspected AA. Naoum and colleagues[27] showed that the development of a guideline to obtain a CT in patients with an equivocal presentation decreased the rate of negative appendectomy from 25% to 6%. Over the same time period, the use of preoperative CT scan increased from 32% to 84% and the rate of PA remained unchanged. A review of a large, prospectively gathered database of general surgical procedures in Washington State found the negative appendectomy rate to be 9.8% in patients with no preoperative imaging and only 4.5% in those who had a preoperative CT scan. This difference was statistically significant.[3] Based on these findings, CT scans seem to have significant benefit in the evaluation of patients with suspected AA.

MRI

MRI has had little role in the evaluation of acute abdominal pain. However, increasing concerns over the potentially hazardous effects of ionizing radiation associated with CT have made MRI the study of choice to evaluate pregnant women and children with symptoms of appendicitis and equivocal US findings.[28]

MRI has excellent resolution and has been shown to be highly accurate in diagnosing AA when based on standard criteria. A normal appendix is less than or equal to 6 mm in diameter and filled with air or oral contrast material. MRI is considered to provide positive results for AA when the appendix is enlarged (>7 mm), the appendiceal wall is thicker than 2 mm, or there are signs of inflammatory changes surrounding the appendix, such as fat stranding, phlegmon, or abscess formation (**Figs. 9–11**).[29]

Cobben and colleagues[30] have evaluated the accuracy of MRI in diagnosing AA. In this prospective study, 138 patients underwent both abdominal US and a limited, noncontrast MRI through the region of the ileocecal valve. Overall, 62 patients were found to have appendicitis, 42 had alternative diagnoses, and 34 did not have a cause for abdominal pain identified. Their imaging results were compared to surgical pathological findings or clinical follow-up in the patients not requiring surgery. US had a sensitivity of 88% and a specificity of 99%. MRI was highly accurate with a sensitivity of

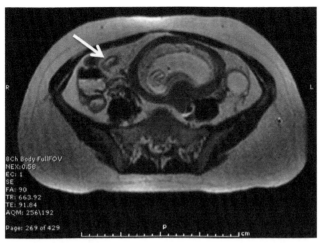

Fig. 9. MR scan with T1-weighted axial image of the abdomen in a gravid woman. Arrow highlights the thickened appendix.

100%, specificity of 98%, positive predictive value of 98%, and negative predictive value of 100%. MRI identified AA in 8 of the 36 patients with nondiagnostic US results. The cost of obtaining an MRI in patients with equivocal US results was compared to the cost of one day of inpatient hospital observation, and an overall cost savings was found with MRI because patients could be discharged home safely after negative MRI results.

Although MRI may be used in any patient with suspected AA, there is a special role for MRI in pregnant women with new-onset abdominal pain. AA is the most common

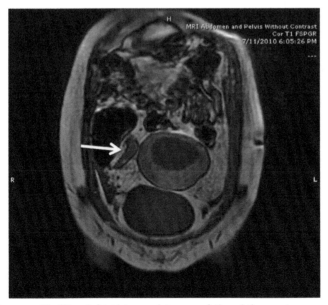

Fig. 10. MR scan with T1-weighted coronal image of the abdomen in a gravid woman. Arrow highlights the thickened appendix.

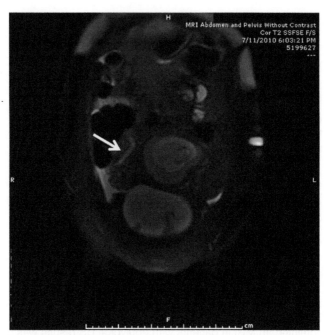

Fig. 11. MR scan with T2-weighted coronal image of the abdomen in a gravid woman. Arrow highlights the thickened appendix.

nonobstetric surgical emergency during pregnancy, complicating 1 in 766 births.[31] AA can be difficult to diagnose during pregnancy because the history and clinical presentation are often atypical. The location of abdominal pain associated with AA is highly variable during pregnancy, with the appendix being displaced superiorly and laterally by the enlarging uterus. Leukocytosis is a nonspecific finding during pregnancy.[32] Traditional surgical teaching had been aggressive in recommending that pregnant women with suspected AA undergo appendectomy because it was believed that the risk of appendiceal perforation and subsequent fetal loss was greater than the risk associated with negative appendectomy.[33] A recent review found that negative appendectomy rates were higher in pregnant women (23%) than in nonpregnant women (18%). However, in this review negative appendectomy was associated with fetal loss in 4% of cases and preterm delivery in 10% of cases. In comparison, rates of fetal loss after appendectomy were 2% in simple appendicitis and 6% in complicated appendicitis. Preterm delivery occurred in 4% of patients with simple appendicitis and 11% of patients with complicated appendicitis.[34] These data underscore the need for appropriate and timely diagnosis of AA in pregnancy.

MRI has been shown to reliably exclude the diagnosis of AA in pregnant women. In a study by Pedrosa and colleagues,[35] 51 consecutive pregnant women suspected of having AA underwent MRI. The patients were given oral contrast but no IV contrast. Based on clinical follow-up and pathology results, this study showed that MRI had a sensitivity of 100%, specificity of 93.6%, accuracy of 94%, and negative predictive value of 100% in diagnosing pregnant women with AA.

MRI has many advantages. It is highly valuable in the imaging of pregnant women and children because there is no exposure to ionizing radiation. Although MRI is safe during pregnancy, no IV contrast should be used during pregnancy because gadolinium is a category C drug and potentially teratogenic. However, noncontrast

MRI provides detailed images, which usually provide the correct diagnosis. MRI is operator independent and the results are highly reproducible. MRI is more useful than US in obese patients and in patients with a retrocecal appendix, which is difficult to visualize on US. Drawbacks of MRI are that it is more expensive than other imaging modalities and not as widely available. The examination itself takes longer to perform and may be degraded by motion artifact. There are concerns that, with the exception of trained radiologists, other health care providers are not comfortable interpreting MRI findings. As MRI becomes more available and faster protocols are developed, these limitations may become less of an issue.[36]

PA

The imaging of advanced appendicitis merits special discussion because the preoperative recognition of PA or a well-formed abscess associated with AA may alter treatment. US findings of PA are an irregular contour of the appendiceal wall or a periappendiceal fluid collection. However, the appendix decompresses with perforation, making PA more difficult to diagnose with US.[2] Surrounding inflammatory changes may be the most obvious findings on US after appendiceal perforation. A phlegmon may be seen as a hypoechoic region with surrounding inflammation. An abscess is seen as a fluid collection, possibly containing gas bubbles.[14] Pickuth and colleagues[37] obtained both CT and US in 120 consecutive patients suspected of having appendicitis and found that CT was superior to US in assessing periappendiceal inflammation. On CT, 15% of the patient population had an identifiable abscess or phlegmon, whereas on US, the abscess or phlegmon in only 9% of the patients was identified.

Horrow and colleagues[38] studied the ability of CT to differentiate PA and AA. By retrospectively reviewing the CT scans of 94 patients with appendicitis, the investigators were able to evaluate the sensitivity and specificity of the following findings, abscess, phlegmon, extraluminal air, extraluminal appendicolith, and focal defect in the appendiceal wall. Although the sensitivity for any one finding was low, using the presence of any 1 of the 5 findings together increased the sensitivity to 94.9%. The overall specificity was 94.5%. A similar study by Bixby and colleagues[39] retrospectively reviewed the CT scans of 244 patients with proven appendicitis. The specificity for PA was as follows: abscess 99%, extraluminal gas 98%, and ileus 93%, but the sensitivities were 34%, 35%, and 53%, respectively. Only the visualization of a defect in the enhancing appendiceal wall has been shown to have both a high sensitivity (95%) and specificity (96.8%) for PA.[40]

TYPHLITIS

Typhlitis, or neutropenic colitis, is an inflammatory condition of the cecum, ascending colon, and occasionally the terminal ileum and appendix, which can easily be mistaken for AA. Patients are typically immunocompromised, and imaging studies show bowel wall thickening with intramural edema and surrounding inflammatory changes. Radiographic studies showing colonic thickening greater than 0.3 cm, fluid or fat stranding surrounding the colon, or edematous bowel wall are consistent with typhlitis. AA and typhlitis can be differentiated by a clinical history of neutropenia as well as imaging findings. The finding of symmetric thickened cecum and ascending colon strongly suggests typhlitis; in addition, the extent of bowel involvement is usually much greater in typhlitis than in AA.[41]

Both US and CT have been used in the evaluation of suspected typhlitis. McCarville[42] has evaluated 92 children being treated for cancer who developed typhlitis. In this study, US measurements of bowel wall thickness correlated with duration of

Table 1
Statistics of imaging modalities for AA

	Sensitivity (%)	Specificity (%)	PPV (%)	NPV (%)
US[8,9,13,14]	66–100	83–96	91–94	89–97
CT[14]	90–100	91–99	92–98	95–100
MRI[30,35,36]	97–100	92–98	57–98	96–100

Abbreviations: NPV, negative predictive value; PPV, positive predictive value.

symptoms, whereas CT measurements did not, which may be because of overestimation of bowel wall thickness on CT. Although CT may overestimate the edema of the bowel wall, it provides additional information about the extent of inflammatory changes in the right lower quadrant. Findings on CT associated with typhlitis include pericolonic fluid collections, fat stranding, pneumatosis coli, or low-attenuation regions within the colon wall indicative of possible necrosis.[43]

SUMMARY

Appendicitis is one of the most common surgical emergencies in the United States, but it remains a diagnostic challenge in many patients who may present with atypical clinical findings. Traditionally, negative appendectomy rates of approximately 20% have been considered acceptable to avoid delayed diagnosis and increased rates of PA. Imaging studies aid in the evaluation of suspected AA and reduction of negative appendectomy rate. US is readily available and inexpensive, but it is highly operator dependent and has lower overall sensitivity and specificity than CT or MRI. US is a good screening test particularly in children, pregnant women, and centers with an established US program. CT is widely available, is not operator dependent, and has excellent accuracy in the diagnosis of appendicitis. However, care must be taken to select patients with an equivocal clinical presentation and to involve the surgical consultant early to yield the full benefits of CT scanning. CT scans are highly valuable in the diagnosis of abdominal pain in women of childbearing age. Although CT scans provide significant information about the inflammatory process associated with appendicitis, only a CT scan result showing a defect in the appendiceal wall is diagnostic of PA. MRI is another highly accurate tool in evaluating suspected AA. The drawbacks to MRI include its expense, longer time to obtain the study, and limited availability compared with other imaging modalities. MRI is of the greatest value in evaluating patients, such as children and pregnant women, who should not be exposed to additional ionizing radiation and who have equivocal or nondiagnostic findings on US. The respective sensitivities, specificities, and positive and negative predictive values of US, CT, and MRI in the evaluation of suspected AA are seen in **Table 1**. AA remains a disease that is diagnosed first and foremost with the initial history and physical examination. If there is diagnostic uncertainty, then imaging studies can improve negative appendectomy rates and diagnose alternatives, including PA and typhlitis. CT remains the diagnostic study of choice for most patients requiring imaging to aid in the diagnosis of AA.

REFERENCES

1. Addiss DG, Shaffer N, Fowler BS, et al. The epidemiology of appendicitis and appendectomy in the United States. Am J Epidemiol 1990;132:910–25.

2. Rybkin AV, Thoeni RF. Current concepts in imaging of appendicitis. Radiol Clin North Am 2007;45:411–22.
3. Cuschieri J, Florence M, Flum DR, et al. The SCOAP Collaborative. Negative appendectomy and imaging accuracy in the Washington State Surgical Care and Outcomes Assessment Program. Ann Surg 2008;248:557–63.
4. Old JL, Dusing RW, Yap W, et al. Imaging for suspected appendicitis. Am Fam Physician 2005;71:71–8.
5. Rypins EB, Evans DG, Hinrichs W, et al. Tc-99m-HMPAO white blood cell scan for diagnosis of acute appendicitis in patients with equivocal clinical presentation. Ann Surg 1997;226:58–65.
6. Baker SR. Acute appendicitis: plain radiographic considerations. Emerg Radiol 1996;3:63–9.
7. Prystowsky JB, Pugh CM, Nagle AP. Appendicitis. Curr Probl Surg 2005;42: 694–742.
8. Van Randen A, Bipat S, Zwinderman AH, et al. Acute appendicitis: meta-analysis of diagnostic performance of CT and graded compression US related to prevalence of disease. Radiology 2008;249:97–106.
9. Doria AS, Moineddin R, Kellenberger CJ, et al. US or CT for diagnosis of appendicitis in children and adults? A meta-analysis. Radiology 2006;241:83–94.
10. Keyzer C, Zalcman M, De Maertelaer V, et al. Comparison of US and unenhanced multi-detector row CT in patients suspected of having acute appendicitis. Radiology 2005;236:527–34.
11. Poortman P, Oostvogel HJM, Bosma E, et al. Improving diagnosis of acute appendicitis: results of a diagnostic pathway with standard use of ultrasonography followed by selective use of CT. J Am Coll Surg 2009;208:434–41.
12. Hernandez JA, Swischuk LE, Angel CA, et al. Imaging of acute appendicitis: US as the primary imaging modality. Pediatr Radiol 2005;35:392–5.
13. Patel SJ, Reede DL, Katz DS, et al. Imaging the pregnant patient for nonobstetric conditions: algorithms & radiation dose considerations. Radiographics 2007; 27(6):1705–22.
14. Birnbaum BA, Wilson SR. Appendicitis at the millennium. Radiology 2000;215: 337–48.
15. Holloway JA, Westerbuhr LM, Chain J, et al. Is appendiceal computed tomography in a community hospital useful? Am J Surg 2003;186:682–4.
16. Whitley S, Sookur P, McLean A, et al. The appendix on CT. Clin Radiol 2009;64: 190–9.
17. Brown MA. Imaging acute appendicitis. Semin Ultrasound CT MR 2008;29: 293–307.
18. Rao PM, Rhea JT, Novelline RA, et al. Effect of computed tomography of the appendix on treatment of patients and use of hospital resources. N Engl J Med 1998;338:141–6.
19. Kamel IR, Goldberg SN, Keogan MT, et al. Right lower quadrant pain and suspected appendicitis: nonfocused appendiceal CT—review of 100 cases. Radiology 2000;217:159–63.
20. Lane MJ, Liu DM, Huynh MD, et al. Suspected acute appendicitis: nonenhanced helical CT in 300 consecutive patients. Radiology 1999;213:341–6.
21. Mittal VK, Goliath J, Sabir M, et al. Advantages of focused helical computed tomographic scanning with rectal contrast only vs triple contrast in the diagnosis of clinically uncertain acute appendicitis. Arch Surg 2004;139:495–500.
22. Birnbaum BA, Jeffrey RB. CT and sonographic evaluation of acute right lower quadrant abdominal pain. AJR 1998;170:361–71.

23. Perez J, Barone JE, Wilbanks TO, et al. Liberal use of computed tomography scanning does not improve diagnostic accuracy in appendicitis. Am J Surg 2003;185:194–7.
24. Vadeboncoeur TF, Heister RR, Behling CA, et al. Impact of helical computed tomography on the rate of negative appendicitis. Am J Emerg Med 2006;24:43–7.
25. Morris KT, Kavanagh M, Hansen P, et al. The rational use of computed tomography scans in the diagnosis of appendicitis. Am J Surg 2002;183:547–50.
26. Lee SL, Walsh AJ, Ho HS. Computed tomography and ultrasonography do not improve and may delay the diagnosis and treatment of acute appendicitis. Arch Surg 2001;136:556–62.
27. Naoum JJ, Mileski WJ, Daller JA, et al. The use of abdominal computed tomography scan decreases the frequency of misdiagnosis in cases of suspected appendicitis. Am J Surg 2002;184:587–90.
28. Singh A, Danrad R, Hahn PF, et al. MR imaging of the acute abdomen and pelvis: acute appendicitis and beyond. Radiographics 2007;27:1419–31.
29. Tkacz JN, Anderson SA, Soto J. MR imaging in gastrointestinal emergencies. Radiographics 2009;29:1767–80.
30. Cobben L, Groot I, Kingma L, et al. A simple MRI protocol in patients with clinically suspected appendicitis: results in 138 patients and effect on outcome of appendectomy. Eur Radiol 2009;19:1175–83.
31. Andersen B, Nielsen TK. Appendicitis in pregnancy: diagnosis, management and complications. Acta Obstet Gynecol Scand 1999;78:758–62.
32. Gjelsteen AC, Ching BH, Meyermann MW, et al. CT, MRI, PET/CT, and ultrasound in the evaluation of obstetric and gynecologic patients. Surg Clin North Am 2008; 88:361–90.
33. Freeland M, King E, Safcsak K, et al. Diagnosis of appendicitis in pregnancy. Am J Surg 2009;198:753–8.
34. McGory ML, Zingmond DS, Tillou A, et al. Negative appendectomy in pregnant women is associated with a substantial risk of fetal loss. J Am Coll Surg 2007; 205:534–40.
35. Pedrosa I, Levine D, Eyvazzadeh AD, et al. MR imaging evaluation of acute appendicitis in pregnancy. Radiology 2006;238:891–9.
36. Lam M, Singh A, Kaewlai R, et al. Magnetic resonance of acute appendicitis: pearls and pitfalls. Curr Probl Diagn Radiol 2008;37:57–66.
37. Pickuth D, Heywang-Kobrunner SH, Spielmann RP. Suspected acute appendicitis: is ultrasonography or computed tomography the preferred imaging technique? Eur J Surg 2000;166:315–9.
38. Horrow MM, White DS, Horrow JC. Differentiation of perforated from nonperforated appendicitis at CT. Radiology 2003;227:46–51.
39. Bixby SD, Lucey BC, Soto JA, et al. Perforated versus nonperforated acute appendicitis: accuracy of multidetector CT detection. Radiology 2006;241:780–6.
40. Tsuboi M, Takase K, Kaneda I, et al. Perforated and nonperforated appendicitis: defect in enhancing appendiceal wall—depiction with multi-detector row CT. Radiology 2008;246:142–7.
41. Hoeffel C, Crema MD, Belkacem A, et al. Multi-detector row CT: spectrum of disease involving the ileocecal area. Radiographics 2006;26:1373–90.
42. McCarville MB. Evaluation of typhlitis in children: CT versus US. Pediatr Radiol 2006;36:890–1.
43. Yu J, Fulcher AS, Turner MA, et al. Helical CT evaluation of acute right lower quadrant pain: part II, uncommon mimics of appendicitis. AJR 2005;184:1143–9.

Bariatric Surgery and Postoperative Imaging

Shanu N. Kothari, MD

KEYWORDS

• Bariatric surgery • Laparoscopic gastric bypass • Imaging
• Complications

The field of bariatric surgery has expanded rapidly over the last decade and it remains one of the fastest growing surgical disciplines in the United States. In 2001, an estimated 40,000 bariatric procedures were performed in the United States. By 2008, this number has increased to approximately 220,000.[1] At present, there are several bariatric surgical procedures available. The most common are the Roux-en-Y gastric bypass, laparoscopic adjustable gastric banding, sleeve gastrectomy, and biliopancreatic diversion/duodenal switch. The single most commonly performed bariatric procedure in the United States is the gastric bypass, which is increasingly being performed with a laparoscopic approach.[2,3] Although not necessarily required to perform bariatric surgery, general surgeons are required by the American Board of Surgery to be able to manage bariatric patients and their postoperative complications.[4] Radiological imaging provides significant information on a variety of surgical procedures. This article discusses imaging and management in the post–bariatric surgery patient, focusing on the gastric bypass procedure (**Fig. 1**).

THE ROLE OF IMAGING MODALITIES
Plain Film

Plain films have a somewhat limited role in the evaluation of the post–gastric bypass patient. Obviously, a patient presenting with a remote history of gastric bypass and free air on a film warrants immediate surgical exploration. A general view of the intestinal gas pattern can be ascertained from reviewing plain films. However, life-threatening obstruction may be present, despite a normal-appearing radiograph (**Fig. 2**). Presence of multiple air-fluid levels is most likely consistent with a distal bowel obstruction in the common channel near the terminal ileum. This obstruction may not be directly related to the gastric bypass per se but may be related to adhesions from the gastric bypass or other previous abdominal or pelvic surgeries. Another

Covidien provides fellowship grant support. Dr Kothari serves as a consultant for Covidien, Valleylab and LifeCell.
Department of General and Vascular Surgery, Gundersen Lutheran Health System, 1900 South Avenue C05-001, La Crosse, WI 54601, USA
E-mail address: snkothar@gundluth.org

Surg Clin N Am 91 (2011) 155–172
doi:10.1016/j.suc.2010.10.013   **surgical.theclinics.com**
0039-6109/11/$ – see front matter © 2011 Elsevier Inc. All rights reserved.

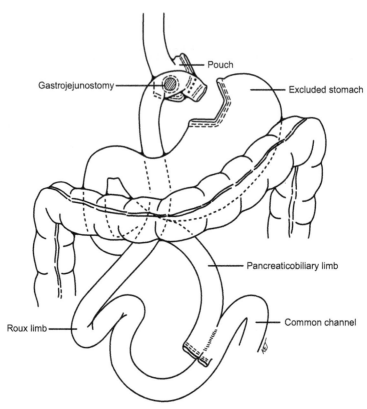

Fig. 1. Roux-en-Y gastric bypass anatomy.

subtle clue that should not be overlooked on a plain film is an air-fluid level in the left upper quadrant under the left hemidiaphragm, consistent with a significant amount of distention and fluid in the excluded stomach (**Fig. 3**). Vomiting does not provide relief in this patient because of the division of the stomach. This finding often warrants immediate surgical intervention to prevent a gastric remnant blowout.

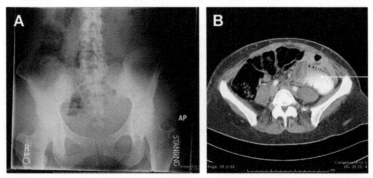

Fig. 2. Normal radiograph (*A*) and CT image indicating obstruction (*arrow, B*) in the same patient.

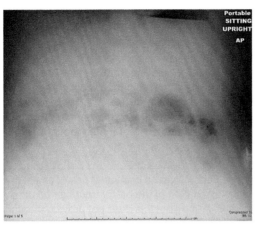

Fig. 3. Radiograph illustrating a distended excluded stomach.

Upper Gastrointestinal Tract Imaging

Upper gastrointestinal tract imaging (UGI) plays a valuable role in the evaluation of the post–gastric bypass patient. The author routinely performs UGI on postoperative day 1 in all gastric bypass patients. A solution of meglumine diatrizoate and sodium diatrizoate (Gastrografin) may be used alone or followed by barium at the radiologist's discretion. The advantages of performing UGI on postoperative day 1 include the following:

1. It documents the size of the pouch postoperation. Patients may have significant weight regain in the future and a repeat UGI may show an enlarged pouch. It also documents that a correctly sized pouch was made during the initial operation and that the patient has stretched it over time.
2. It can assess for nonemptying of the pouch itself, consistent with either edema of the gastrojejunal anastomosis, which is treated conservatively, or technical narrowing and/or backwalling of the anastomosis, which would warrant surgical revision.
3. It can assess for Roux limb distention and/or stricture or narrowing at the mesocolic defect or jejunojejunostomy. Despite obtaining a normal UGI result on postoperative day 1, if the patient has inability to tolerate liquids, it is typically because the patient is drinking too much or too fast as opposed to an obstructive process.
4. If a patient re-presents with signs and symptoms suspicious for a gastrojejunal anastomotic leak, the originally obtained negative UGI result provides a comparison film to assess for radiographic clues of a leak.

Computed Tomographic Scan

Computed tomographic (CT) scan provides a significant amount of information regarding intra-abdominal pathology in the post–gastric bypass patient. CT scans can be used to assess for intra-abdominal versus intraluminal bleeding, abdominal wall bleeds, as well as a variety of obstructive processes including internal herniation with subsequent obstruction and they may help ascertain the level of intestinal obstruction.

Ultrasonography

Transabdominal ultrasonography has a role in assessing gallstone formation in the post–gastric bypass patient. Another option is intraoperative laparoscopic ultrasonography. Both techniques can document the presence of gallstones at the time of surgery. The post–gastric bypass patient is at a high risk of forming gallstones in the rapid weight-loss phase (within the first 6 months postoperation). This risk can be significantly reduced with the use of ursodeoxycholic acid.[5] The role of observation versus routine versus selective cholecystectomy in the face of asymptomatic cholelithiasis in the bariatric patient is a matter of controversy, particularly in the minimally invasive era. Although many bariatric surgeons in the open era routinely removed the gallbladder, it is not without potential for significant added morbidity during a laparoscopic gastric bypass, in part, because of the suboptimal port location.[6,7]

Cholangiopancreatography

The post–gastric bypass patient is at an increased risk of cholelithiasis and symptomatic choledocholithiasis. Evaluation of the biliary tract can be done via magnetic resonance cholangiopancreatography but this does not provide therapeutic options. Other approaches include traditional endoscopic retrograde cholangiopancreatography (ERCP), but based on the Roux limb and biliopancreatic limb lengths, the likelihood of successfully reaching the duodenum in a retrograde fashion is low. New angled scopes that are under investigation are specifically designed to gain access to the excluded stomach via the traditional endoscopic route.[8] However, many post–gastric bypass patients undergo laparoscopic-assisted transgastric ERCP (**Fig. 4**) for interrogation of the biliary tree.[9] This procedure allows not only for diagnostic intervention but also for therapeutic intervention, if necessary. Laparoscopic cholecystectomy with intraoperative cholangiography and laparoscopic transcystic common duct exploration should be attempted before entering the gastric remnant, based on the surgeon's comfort and tortuosity of the cystic duct.

Hepatobiliary Iminodiacetic Acid Scan

Hepatobiliary iminodiacetic acid (HIDA) scan is useful in the post–gastric bypass patient to aid in diagnosing acute versus chronic cholecystitis. HIDA scans may

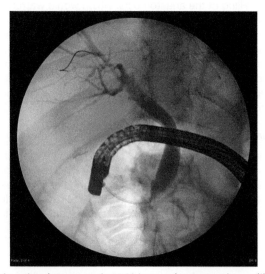

Fig. 4. Laparoscopic-assisted transgastric ERCP image demonstrating a dilated common bile duct.

also play a role in the rare patient with superior mesenteric artery (SMA) syndrome, demonstrating nonpassage of the radioactive tracer past the third portion of the duodenum. In the early post–gastric bypass patient with bile present in the intra-abdominal drain despite a negative UGI result, HIDA scan can aid in ascertaining the level of potential injury. This condition could be from a liver capsule tear (**Fig. 5**), an injury to the common bile duct or duodenum, or an early dehiscence of the excluded stomach staple line.

IMAGING OF POSTOPERATIVE COMPLICATIONS
Leaks

An anastomotic leak is one of the most feared and potentially lethal complications following gastric bypass.[10] The patient can rapidly deteriorate to florid sepsis and death in a short period. Anastomotic leak rates for gastric bypass range from 0% to 6%.[11–14] Both UGI and CT are useful adjuncts in the assessment of a patient with a possible anastomotic leak. However, ultimately one's index of suspicion and clinical judgment must be used in any patient with unexplained tachycardia because this is considered a leak until proven otherwise. A negative imaging result does not rule out a leak with 100% certainty because it may not be apparent radiographically. If laparoscopy or laparotomy shows negative results, it should not be considered an inappropriate intervention or complication in a patient with a suspected anastomotic leak despite a radiographic study with negative results.[15] **Fig. 6** is an UGI demonstrating a leak at the gastrojejunal anastomosis in a post–gastric bypass patient. The linear streaking from the anastomosis itself can be seen. Follow-up CT in the same patient shows an air-contrast level consistent with an abscess (**Fig. 7**). This patient was hemodynamically stable and underwent percutaneous drainage of the abscess cavity for source control. A repeat UGI 1 week later did not show evidence of a leak, and the percutaneous drain was removed. **Fig. 8** shows the author's algorithm for the management of a patient with an anastomotic leak. As seen in the decision tree, the default position is always reexploration. The objective of any reexploration for presumed leak is directed drainage and source control. Attempts

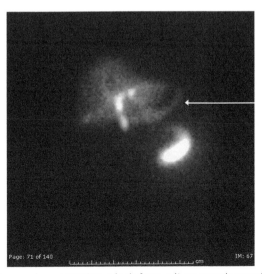

Fig. 5. HIDA scan image demonstrating a leak from a liver capsule tear (*arrow*).

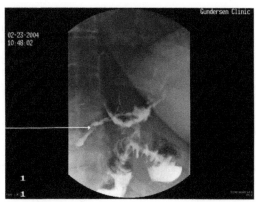

Fig. 6. Image obtained by UGI demonstrates a leak at the gastrojejunal anastomosis (*arrow*).

may be made to resuture the defect, but often the tissue is edematous and friable and has the potential to worsen the anastomotic leak. Although UGI and CT are useful adjuncts in this clinical scenario, a leak must also be suspected from the jejunojejunostomy, which is not as easily visualized because of the dilution of the Gastrografin downstream. Furthermore, a leak from the excluded stomach staple line must be considered in any patient with clinical deterioration in the face of a negative UGI result, because this study will be unable to assess the integrity of the staple line of the excluded stomach.

Hemorrhage

Postoperative hemorrhage can occur following any bariatric surgical procedure. There are several sources of bleeding to consider specifically in the post–gastric bypass patient: the abdominal wall (trocar sites, **Fig. 9**), solid organs (liver or spleen), the gastrojejunal or jejunojejunal anastomoses, the stump of the Roux limb, or the excluded stomach staple. In addition, injury to the mesentery during construction of the Roux

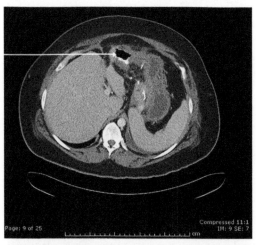

Fig. 7. CT image demonstrating an air-contrast level consistent with an abscess (*arrow*) in a patient with a gastrojejunal anastomotic leak.

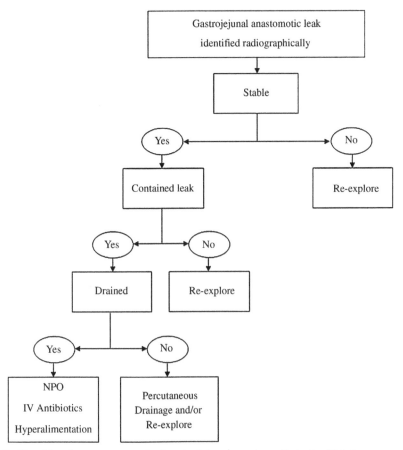

Fig. 8. Algorithm for management of gastrojejunal anastomotic leaks. IV, intravenous.

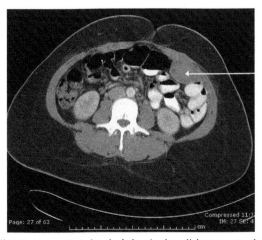

Fig. 9. CT image illustrating a contained abdominal wall hematoma (*arrow*), presumably from a trocar site bleed.

limb can cause hemorrhage. Any patient in the immediate postoperative period who has hemodynamic instability warrants immediate resuscitation and exploration and should forego any imaging. CT provides a useful adjunct in the patient who remains hemodynamically stable but has a declining hemoglobin level. **Fig. 10** shows the CT image of a patient who presented with an intra-abdominal bleed, presumably along the excluded stomach staple line and lesser sac, on postoperative day 5. In stable patients, serial examinations, serial hemoglobin levels, withholding the use of nonsteroidals (ie, ketorolac), and holding the use of any prophylactic agents for anticoagulation, such as heparin or enoxaparin, compose the initial management. Most bleeding subsides spontaneously. Some patients may require blood transfusion and, occasionally, reexploration.[16] If a drainage tube is still in place from the original operation, it can also act as a useful adjunct in the management of the patient, but one must be cautious because the tube can become plugged, giving a false sense that the bleeding has stopped. Also, the source of bleeding may not be near the location of the drain, giving a false sense of security that the patient is not actively bleeding. Some patients may present with hematemesis and the source would typically be intraluminal bleeding at the gastrojejunal anastomosis. Most bleeds stop with conservative management, but the thrombus may cause stomal outlet obstruction. If conservative treatment options fail, endoscopy can be performed in an attempt to stop the bleeding at the gastrojejunal anastomosis, but one must be careful with cautery and epinephrine because these hemostatic interventions may predispose the anastomosis to a leak.[17] Reexploration with revision of the anastomosis is an option as well. Some patients present with bright red blood per rectum on postoperative day 1. Many of these patients can be treated conservatively as well, as long as they are hemodynamically stable. The source of this type of hemorrhage is typically the jejunojejunostomy. However, one of the most feared complications in a patient with intraluminal bleeding after gastric bypass is obstruction of the jejunojejunostomy because of thrombus, resulting in biliopancreatic limb obstruction and blowout of the excluded stomach. This is a potentially lethal complication.[18] CT scan plays a role in evaluation of the excluded stomach to assess the degree of distension. In this case, there is a role for reexploration, either by laparoscopy or laparotomy with evacuation of the

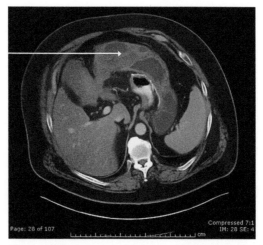

Fig. 10. CT image demonstrating an intra-abdominal bleed (*arrow*) along the excluded stomach staple line.

thrombus in the stomach; oversewing of the excluded stomach staple line; and gastrostomy tube placement. The jejunojejunostomy may need to be reexplored as well and oversewn because it, too, may have been the source of bleeding. **Fig. 11** shows an image obtained by UGI in a patient with obstruction of the jejunojejunostomy due to intraluminal thrombus. This patient was treated with a fluoroscopically placed nasogastric tube for decompression and close observation, and the thrombus passed spontaneously.

Intestinal Obstructions

A variety of intestinal obstructions can occur following laparoscopic gastric bypass. These complications are more commonly noted in laparoscopy than in open gastric bypass.[14,19] Radiological imaging provides a useful adjunct in the management of the patient with obstructive symptoms. Plain films can often appear benign, despite the presence of potentially life-threatening intestinal obstruction. In addition, there are reported series with up to 20% of CT scan results being negative despite clinical evidence of intestinal obstruction.[20] As a result, sound surgical judgment should be used and diagnostic laparoscopy or laparotomy performed as needed to rule out occult intestinal obstruction that is not apparent radiographically.

There are a variety of methods to perform the Roux-en-Y reconstruction. The most common technique is to take the Roux limb antecolic/antegastric, although a retrocolic/retrogastric approach is used as well. Both techniques have a unique set of advantages and disadvantages.[21–23] Less common forms are antecolic/retrogastric and retrocolic/antegastric reconstructions.

There are 3 internal hernias that can develop in a post–gastric bypass patient **(Fig. 12)**. One hernia occurs at the transverse mesocolic defect, resulting in herniation into the lesser sac, another occurs in the Petersen space where the Roux limb mesentery intersects the mesentery of the transverse colon, and the other develops between the mesenteric leaflets of the jejunojejunostomy. Most surgeons think that the internal mesenteric defects should be closed to prevent internal herniation and subsequent bowel obstruction.[21,24,25] Some investigators dispute this thought and have demonstrated similar obstruction rates when not closing the defects.[26] Despite adequate closure, after the patients lose weight, their mesenteric fat is reduced as well, and the adequate closure results in opening up of the mesenteric spaces allowing internal

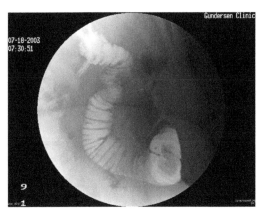

Fig. 11. UGI in a patient with obstruction of the jejunojejunostomy caused by intraluminal thrombus.

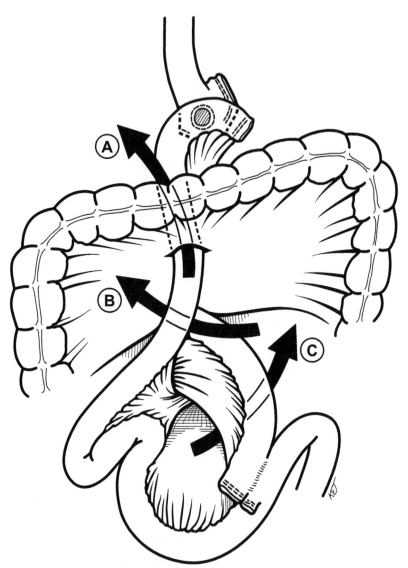

Fig. 12. Mesenteric defects: (A) transverse mesocolic, (B) Petersen space, and (C) jejunojejunostomy mesentery.

herniation to develop. Crampy abdominal pain in the post–gastric bypass patient should be taken seriously and often warrants surgical exploration.

Petersen hernia

Fig. 13 shows a fluid-filled excluded stomach without rugal folds. This is an abnormal radiographic finding and indicates an obstruction distally with backflow of gastric and intestinal contents into the excluded stomach. If left untreated, this could lead to blowout of the excluded stomach, with resulting sepsis and death. **Fig. 14** shows the same patient with a Petersen hernia. Of note is the swirl (hurricane) sign seen in the mesentery, requiring immediate surgical intervention. On exploration, often the

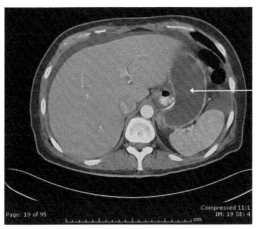

Fig. 13. CT image depicting fluid-filled excluded stomach (*arrow*) with no rugal folds present.

limbs are indistinguishable near the mesentery of the transverse colon, and manipulation can result in worsening the hernia and possibly even rupture of the distended intestine, resulting in subsequent spillage of intestinal contents. If an internal hernia is suspected, the terminal ileum should be identified and gently grasped and run proximally, and in doing so, the herniated contents are often passively detorsed in the mesenteric defect, reestablishing the normal anatomy and allowing reclosure of the Petersen space with minimal injury to the bowel.

Jejunojejunostomy hernia
Fig. 15 demonstrates a similar swirl pattern in a patient with an internal hernia at the jejunojejunostomy defect. This finding, too, warrants immediate surgical exploration.

Mesocolic hernia
For patients with a retrocolic/retrogastric limb, the Roux limb itself can migrate into the lesser sac causing obstruction of the Roux limb (**Fig. 16**) or other intestinal contents

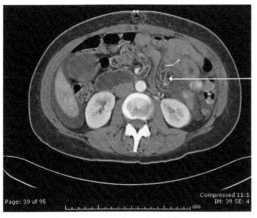

Fig. 14. CT image demonstrating Petersen hernia with a swirl sign (*arrow*) seen in the mesentery.

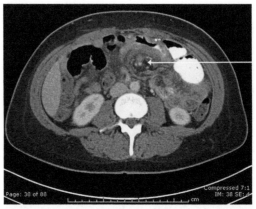

Fig. 15. CT of an internal hernia at the jejunojejunostomy defect demonstrates a swirl pattern (*arrow*).

can migrate through this defect as well. This migration can be caused by inadequate suture fixation of the Roux limb and Petersen space at the time of operation or occasionally by postoperative vomiting that can tear the sutures allowing migration of the Roux limb into the lesser sac. In addition, closure of the mesocolic defect over the Roux limb in a retrocolic/retrogastric route may result in too tight a closure, causing obstruction of the outflow of the Roux limb. **Fig. 17** demonstrates an image obtained by UGI, in which there is a sharp cutoff sign of the Roux limb, a distended blind tip of the Roux limb, and retained contrast within the gastric pouch. These findings warrant surgical revision to release the Roux limb that is under tension. An advantage of the antecolic/antegastric Roux limb is that there is no chance of kinking of the Roux limb through the retrocolic tunnel. However, there is still a potential Petersen space defect behind the Roux limb on top of the colon, which can result in herniation and obstruction. In addition, there are case reports of colonic obstructions from the Roux limb over the transverse colon.[26]

Jejunojejunostomy obstruction
Another cause of intestinal obstruction can occur at the jejunojejunostomy. In the early postoperative phase, this obstruction can be caused by technical narrowing of the

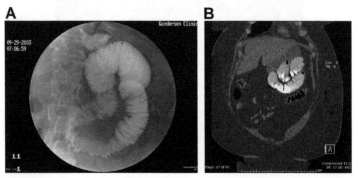

Fig. 16. Roux limb migration into lesser sac causing Roux limb obstruction as viewed by UGI (*A*) and CT (*B*).

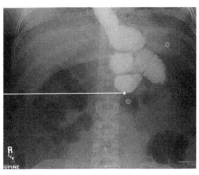

Fig. 17. Image obtained by UGI, demonstrating a sharp cutoff sign (*arrow*) of the Roux limb, a distended blind tip of the Roux limb, and retained contrast within the gastric pouch.

jejunojejunostomy, resulting in distension of the Roux limb and/or biliopancreatic limb. A patient with this condition typically has not left the hospital, and this situation warrants reexploration and revision of the jejunojejunostomy. Other causes include strictures or external adhesions from the epiploic appendages of the transverse colon, adhering to the staple line of the jejunojejunostomy and resulting in kinking of the bowel at this site (**Fig. 18**). Another source of intestinal obstruction that can occur postoperation is from a thrombus at the jejunojejunostomy.[27] Hidalgo and colleagues[28] have proposed a schematic classification for intestinal obstructions following laparoscopic gastric bypass.

Intussusception

Another rare cause of small bowel obstruction in the post–gastric bypass patient is intussusception. This obstruction most commonly occurs at the jejunojejunostomy (**Fig. 19**).[29] Typically, the common channel intussuscepts into either the Roux limb or the pancreaticobiliary limb. Physical examination findings reveal a palpable mass,

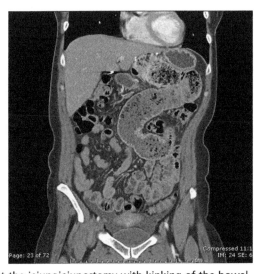

Fig. 18. Stricture at the jejunojejunostomy with kinking of the bowel.

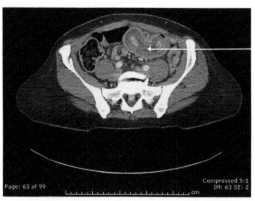

Fig. 19. CT image demonstrating intussusception at jejunojejunostomy (*arrow*).

and CT scan can show a target sign consistent with a lumen within a lumen.[29] A variety of theories have been proposed to explain this phenomenon. The theories range from altered peristalsis to increased intestinal mobility caused by loss of mesenteric fat.[30] The intussusception typically occurs in a retrograde fashion, although antegrade has been described as well.[30] This diagnosis is a surgical emergency and warrants urgent exploration. If the bowel is viable, the intussusception can be milked back. If ischemia is present, resection and reconstruction of the Roux limb, pancreaticobiliary limb, and common channel is necessary. Plication of the common channel to the Roux limb has been described to prevent the reoccurrence of intussusception following surgical intervention.[29]

Other Conditions

There are 2 rare conditions that can occur in the post–gastric bypass patient and they warrant discussion.

SMA syndrome

SMA syndrome can develop in a post–gastric bypass patient who loses a significant amount of weight and has resulting changes in the aortomesenteric angle. Unlike other patients with SMA syndrome, the post–gastric bypass patient cannot vomit for relief of symptoms because the stomach has been divided. This syndrome can be a challenging diagnosis to make and is probably underreported in the post–gastric bypass patient population.[31] CT scan is a useful adjunct to measure the aortomesenteric angle.[32,33] In **Fig. 20**, it can be seen that the SMA compresses the duodenum over the aorta, with subsequent proximal duodenal dilation. A percutaneous gastrostomy tube placed in the excluded stomach of the same patient shows inability of passage of the contrast on UGI via the gastrostomy tube while the patient is in the supine position but free flow in the prone position (**Fig. 21**). Weight gain is the initial treatment of choice, but for obvious reasons, the post–gastric bypass patient is reluctant to proceed down this course and the surgical treatment is a duodenojejunostomy of the common channel to the proximal dilated duodenum, performed either laparoscopically or open.[34] A HIDA scan could also be a useful adjunct in this situation because it could potentially show nonpassage of the radioactive tracer past the third portion of the duodenum and would preclude the need for a gastrostomy tube in the excluded stomach.[35]

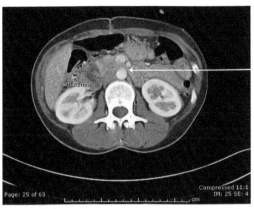

Fig. 20. CT image demonstrating the SMA compressing the duodenum over the aorta (*arrow*), with subsequent proximal duodenal dilation.

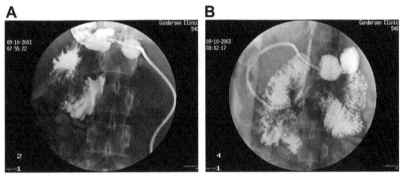

Fig. 21. UGI with contrast in a patient with a gastrostomy tube placed in the excluded stomach demonstrates inability of passage of the contrast via the gastrostomy tube with the patient in supine position (*A*) but free flow in the prone position (*B*).

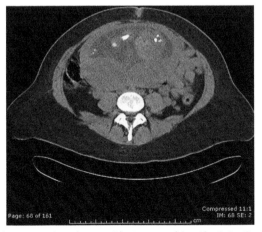

Fig. 22. CT image demonstrating the gravid uterus pushing the intestinal contents into the left upper quadrant.

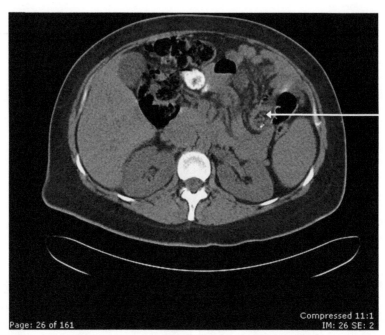

Fig. 23. CT image showing Petersen hernia (*arrow*) in a pregnant patient.

Pregnancy in the post–gastric bypass patient

In the pregnant patient who has undergone gastric bypass, crampy abdominal pain in addition to nausea and vomiting should not be attributed to pregnancy-induced nausea because mechanical causes may be a factor. There are case reports of intestinal obstructions resulting in significant morbidity and even mortality of the fetus and the mother.[36] Prompt diagnosis, a high index of suspicion, and early intervention prevent a poor outcome in this scenario.[37] The gravid uterus tends to push the intestinal contents into the left upper quadrant (**Fig. 22**), resulting in Petersen hernia (**Fig. 23**) or other internal hernia and subsequent bowel obstructions. This condition is a surgical emergency that warrants prompt intervention to increase the likelihood of bowel viability and survival of the fetus and the mother.

SUMMARY

Radiological imaging provides a useful adjunct in the management of the post–gastric bypass patient. When abnormalities are present, a thorough understanding of the reconstructed anatomy is critical to interpret radiological images. Radiological imaging can help guide the surgeon's decisions on management in these challenging situations but does not supersede prompt surgical intervention based on patients' presenting signs and symptoms.

REFERENCES

1. American Society for Metabolic and Bariatric Surgery (ASMBS) fact sheet. www. asmbs.org. Available at: http://www.asbs.org/Newsite07/media/asmbs_fs_surgery. pdf. Accessed July 12, 2010.

2. Samuel I, Mason EE, Renquist KE, et al. Bariatric surgery trends: an 18-year report from the International Bariatric Surgery Registry. Am J Surg 2006;192(5): 657–62.
3. Buchwald H, Oien DM. Metabolic/bariatric surgery Worldwide 2008. Obes Surg 2009;19(12):1605–11.
4. The American Board of Surgery. Booklet of Information, Surgery, 2009–2010. www.absurgery.org. Available at: http://home.absurgery.org/xfer/BookletofInfo-Surgery.pdf. Accessed July 12, 2010.
5. Sugerman HJ, Brewer WH, Shiffman ML, et al. A multicenter, placebo-controlled, randomized, double-blind, prospective trial of prophylactic ursodiol for the prevention of gallstone formation following gastric-bypass-induced rapid weight loss. Am J Surg 1995;169(1):91–6 [discussion: 96–7].
6. Hamad GG, Ikramuddin S, Gourash WF, et al. Elective cholecystectomy during laparoscopic Roux-en-Y gastric bypass: is it worth the wait? Obes Surg 2003; 13(1):76–81.
7. Tucker ON, Fajnwaks P, Szomstein S, et al. Is concomitant cholecystectomy necessary in obese patients undergoing laparoscopic gastric bypass surgery? Surg Endosc 2008;22(11):2450–4.
8. Lopes TL, Wilcox CM. Endoscopic retrograde cholangiopancreatography in patients with Roux-en-Y anatomy. Gastroenterol Clin North Am 2010;39(1): 99–107.
9. Nguyen NT, Hinojosa MW, Slone J, et al. Laparoscopic transgastric access to the biliary tree after Roux-en-Y gastric bypass. Obes Surg 2007;17(3):416–9.
10. Gonzalez R, Sarr MG, Smith CD, et al. Diagnosis and contemporary management of anastomotic leaks after gastric bypass for obesity. J Am Coll Surg 2007;204(1): 47–55.
11. Bellorin O, Abdemur A, Sucandy I, et al. Understanding the significance, reasons and patterns of abnormal vital signs after gastric bypass for morbid obesity. Obes Surg 2010 [Online].
12. Fullum TM, Aluka KJ, Turner PL. Decreasing anastomotic and staple line leaks after laparoscopic Roux-en-Y gastric bypass. Surg Endosc 2009;23(6):1403–8.
13. Podnos YD, Jimenez JC, Wilson SE, et al. Complications after laparoscopic gastric bypass: a review of 3464 cases. Arch Surg 2003;138:957–61.
14. Kothari SN, Kallies KJ, Mathiason MA, et al. Excellent laparoscopic gastric bypass outcomes can be achieved at a community-based training hospital with moderate case volume. Ann Surg 2010;252(1):43–9.
15. ASMBS Clinical Issues Committee. ASMBS guideline on the prevention and detection of gastrointestinal leak after gastric bypass including the role of imaging and surgical exploration. Surg Obes Relat Dis 2009;5(3):293–6.
16. Kothari SN, Lambert PJ, Mathiason MA. Best Poster Award. A comparison of thromboembolic and bleeding events following laparoscopic gastric bypass in patients treated with prophylactic regimens of unfractionated heparin or enoxa-parin. Am J Surg 2007;194:709–11.
17. Nguyen NT, Longoria M, Chalifoux S, et al. Gastrointestinal hemorrhage after laparoscopic gastric bypass. Obes Surg 2004;14:1308–12.
18. Helling T. The lethality of obstructing hematoma at the jejunojejunostomy following Roux-en-Y gastric bypass. Obes Surg 2005;15:290–3.
19. Capella RF, Iannace VA, Capella JF. Bowel obstruction after open and laparoscopic gastric bypass surgery for morbid obesity. J Am Coll Surg 2006;203(3):328–35.
20. Higa KD, Ho T, Boone KB. Internal hernias after laparoscopic Roux-en-Y gastric bypass: incidence, treatment and prevention. Obes Surg 2003;13(3):350–4.

21. Carmody B, Demaria EJ, Jamal M. Internal hernia after laparoscopic Roux-en-Y gastric bypass. Surg Obes Relat Dis 2005;188:543–8.
22. Miyashiro LA, Fuller WD, Ali MR. Favorable internal hernia rate achieved using retrocolic, retrogastric alimentary limb in laparoscopic Roux-en-Y gastric bypass. Surg Obes Relat Dis 2010;6(2):158–62.
23. Bauman RW, Pirrello JR. Internal hernia at Petersen's space after laparoscopic Roux-en-Y gastric bypass: 6.2% incidence without closure—a single surgeon series of 1047 cases. Surg Obes Relat Dis 2009;5:565–70.
24. Comeau E, Gagner M, Inabnet WB, et al. Symptomatic internal hernias after laparoscopic bariatric surgery. Surg Endosc 2005;19:34–9.
25. Felsher J, Brodsky J. Small bowel obstruction after laparoscopic Roux-en-y gastric bypass. Surgery 2003;134:501–5.
26. Cho M, Pinto D, Carrodeguas L, et al. Frequency and management of internal hernias after laparoscopic antecolic antegastric Roux-en-Y gastric bypass without division of the small bowel mesentery or closure of mesenteric defects: review of 1400 consecutive cases. Surg Obes Relat Dis 2006;2(2):87–91.
27. Awais O, Raftopoulos I, Luketich JD, et al. Acute, complete proximal small bowel obstruction after laparoscopic gastric bypass due to intraluminal blood clot formation. Surg Obes Relat Dis 2005;1(4):418–22.
28. Hidalgo JE, Ramirez A, Rosenthal R, et al. Small bowel complication after malabsorptive procedures: internal hernias, obstructions, and intussusception. Bariatric Times 2009 March. Available at: http://bariatrictimes.com/2009/03/06/small-bowel-complication-after-malabsorptive-procedures-internal-hernias-obstructions-and-intussusception. Accessed July 13, 2010.
29. Simper SC, Erzinger JM, McKinlay RD, et al. Retrograde (reverse) jejuna intussusception might not be such a rare problem: a single group's experience of 23 cases. Surg Obes Relat Dis 2008;4:77–83.
30. Coster DD, Sundberg SM, Kermode DS, et al. Small bowel obstruction due to antegrade and retrograde intussusception after gastric bypass: three case reports in two patients, literature review, and recommendations for diagnosis and treatment. Surg Obes Relat Dis 2008;4:69–72.
31. Schroeppel TJ, Chilcote WS, Lara MD, et al. Superior mesenteric artery syndrome after laparoscopic Roux-en-Y gastric bypass. Surgery 2005;137(3):383–5.
32. Konen E, Amitai M, Apter S, et al. CT angiography of superior mesenteric artery syndrome. AJR Am J Roentgenol 1998;171(5):1279–81.
33. Applegate GR, Cohen AJ. Dynamic CT in superior mesenteric artery syndrome. J Comput Assist Tomogr 1988;12(6):976–80.
34. Baker MT, Lara MD, Kothari SN. Superior mesenteric artery syndrome after laparoscopic Roux-en-Y gastric bypass. Surg Obes Relat Dis 2006;2(6):667.
35. Goitein D, Gagné DJ, Papasavas PK, et al. Superior mesenteric artery syndrome after laparoscopic Roux-en-Y gastric bypass for morbid obesity. Obes Surg 2004;14(7):1008–11.
36. Maggard MA, Yermilov I, Li Z, et al. Pregnancy and fertility following bariatric surgery: a systematic review. JAMA 2008;300(19):2286–96.
37. Baker MT, Kothari SN. Successful surgical treatment of a pregnancy-induced Petersen's hernia after laparoscopic gastric bypass. Surg Obes Relat Dis 2005; 1(5):506–8.

The Use of Ultrasound in Vascular Procedures

Steven W. Khoo, MD[a], David C. Han, MD, MS[b],*

KEYWORDS
- Ultrasound • Vascular access • Vena cava filter
- Pseudoaneurysm

Advances in ultrasound (US) technology and the advent of smaller more portable units have made this imaging modality more accessible to the surgeon and have expanded the role of US in clinical practice. The sonographic characteristics of the vascular system, and the blood which courses through it, have made US an invaluable tool for vascular-based interventions. Its ease of use and ability to provide real-time imaging of the vascular system have significantly improved the safety, comfort, and success of various vascular procedures. Although the basic principles of US imaging are described in greater detail elsewhere in this monograph, there are several concepts that are key to understanding its unique role and limitations in vascular imaging. The concepts include a basic understanding of ultrasound physics and in particular, the Doppler equation.

ULTRASOUND PHYSICS

Sound is simply the propagation of an energy wave through a medium. Unlike an electromagnetic wave that may travel through vacuum, a sound wave is transmitted by the vibration of the particles composing the medium through which it travels. It proceeds as a succession of areas of high pressure (compression) interspersed with areas of low pressure (rarefaction). The distance between pressure peaks (or troughs) is the familiar term wavelength. Frequency refers to the number of these pulses (cycles) that pass in a given period of time. Pitch is a function of frequency, and the human ear is tuned to detect a frequency of between approximately 20 and 20,000 cycles per second, or hertz (Hz). Ultrasound frequencies commonly used in medical applications are far beyond the detectable range of human hearing and typically fall between 2 and 20 MHz.

[a] Penn State Hershey Heart and Vascular Institute, Penn State Hershey Medical Center, Penn State College of Medicine, Hershey, PA, USA
[b] Department of Surgery, Penn State Hershey Heart and Vascular Institute, Penn State Hershey Medical Center, Penn State College of Medicine, Hershey, PA, USA
* Corresponding author.
E-mail address: dhan@hmc.psu.edu

Surg Clin N Am 91 (2011) 173–184
doi:10.1016/j.suc.2010.10.009
0039-6109/11/$ – see front matter © 2011 Published by Elsevier Inc.

Frequency and wavelength are inversely proportional, that is, as frequency increases, wavelength decreases and vice versa.

The speed of transmission of sound waves is independent of both frequency and wavelength and is determined by the characteristics of the medium through which the sound waves travel. Denser materials propagate sound at a much faster rate than less-dense media. The speed of sound through air is approximately 343 m/s. Sound travels through water at approximately 1482 m/s, reflecting the significant increase in density of the medium. A basic assumption is that sound travels through soft tissue at a speed of 1540 m/s but it actually travels through various human tissues at varying rates. This variability is a significant cause of imaging artifacts.[1]

As sound waves travel through the body, they encounter interfaces between tissues of varying density and a proportion will be reflected back toward the probe. This proportion depends on the change in density such that small changes (ie, a tumor within soft tissues) reflect a small proportion of the beam, whereas a significant change (ie, bone interface) reflects most of the beam. By calculating the timing of these reflections and taking into account the relatively constant speed of sound in tissue, an image can be created. The standard gray-scale imaging refers to the display of bright lines corresponding to the depth of returned echoes (hence the term brightness mode, or B-mode).

The Doppler effect refers to the shift in frequency of a sound wave when it encounters a moving object. In the blood stream, the red blood cells act as the spectral reflectors. The Doppler equation is used to calculate this frequency shift, which is directly proportional to the velocity of the moving object. The Doppler equation also takes into account the angle of the sound beam relative to the moving object. Practically, this angle is determined by the sonographer, who defines the line of the ultrasound beam and estimates the longitudinal axis of the vessel. By applying the Doppler equation that correlates frequency change (between the sent and the received signal) to velocity of the object encountered, blood flow velocity may be calculated, and this method forms the basis of noninvasive vascular imaging. It is the combination of B-mode imaging with superimposed Doppler equation–derived velocities that composes duplex imaging.

APPLICATION OF US FOR VASCULAR PROCEDURES

Blood, being primarily a fluid, is nearly anechoic causing it to appear dark on an US image. This characteristic has led to US being a very useful modality for imaging vascular structures. Furthermore, as mentioned earlier, the flow of blood allows the vasculature to be readily visualized and interrogated using Doppler US. In addition to simply obtaining diagnostic information, these characteristics lend themselves to the use of US imaging for a variety of vascular interventions.

Central Venous Access

Central venous catheterization (CVC) is an extremely useful clinical adjunct in the perioperative period and in the management of the critically ill patient. It provides excellent reliable venous access for high-volume resuscitation and is a method of invasive monitoring of hemodynamics. It is also the preferred method for long-term venous cannulation for administration of chemotherapeutics, antibiotics, nutrition supplements, or other ongoing intravenous infusions. Because of the broad range of clinical applications of CVC, its use has become more and more prevalent.

However, like all invasive procedures, CVC does not come without certain inherent risks. Potential complications include inadvertent arterial puncture, pneumothorax, nerve injury, hematoma, and inability to appropriately position the catheter. Although the complication rate and the total number of CVCs that occur are difficult to estimate, the patient safety problem of morbidity caused by CVC was recognized by the Agency for Healthcare Research and Quality as early as 2001. Recommendations for the use of US guidance during central line insertion were noted to have the "greatest strength of evidence regarding their impact and effectiveness."[2]

The traditional landmark method of catheter placement relies on anatomic associations and surface anatomy to guide the operator. However, anatomy is not constant, and the relationship of the vein to the artery can be highly variable. Real-time US imaging has been extremely valuable in decreasing CVC complications and in increasing the success rate of venous cannulation.[3–7] Complication rates have been shown to be significantly decreased with US guidance compared to the landmark method.[7] One study has demonstrated a 0% rate of pneumothorax using US to access the internal jugular (IJ) vein as opposed to 2.4% using the landmark method.[4] The same study showed a 100% success rate in CVC with US guidance versus a 94.4% success rate when relying on the landmark method.

Although a variety of US technology is available, venous access usually relies simply on B-mode imaging to identify the vessel of interest. Simple systems that strictly use B-mode imaging and are primarily designed for venous access are available and they often come with a needle guide (**Fig. 1**). The guide is an appropriately angled attachment through which the needle is passed such that the needle crosses the plane of the ultrasound wave at a specified depth (**Fig. 2**). Although this system makes access somewhat easier, it is not a necessity, and any machine capable of rendering a B-mode image can be used. A higher frequency probe is used, given the superficial location of the structure being imaged, and a small footprint probe is also helpful.

Much of what has been published regarding US guidance for CVC describes IJ vein access. Although the IJ vein typically lies lateral to the carotid artery, its actual position may vary significantly. One study identified 5 variations in its location relative to the

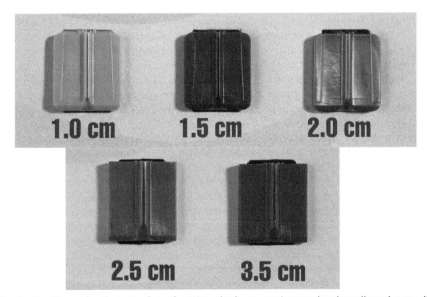

Fig. 1. Needle guides that attach to the US probe have varying angles that allow the needle to cross the path of the ultrasound beam at various depths.

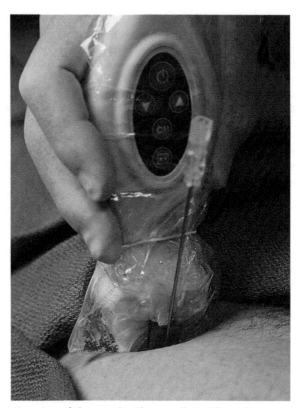

Fig. 2. Transverse imaging of the vessel with a needle guide in place.

carotid artery, with the vein actually being anterior and medial or directly medial to the artery in 16.3% of cases.[4] Although Doppler color imaging is helpful in properly identifying the vein because of the pulsatile flow characteristics of the artery, there are other reliable methods of making this distinction, which do not require Doppler capability. Location (medial vs lateral) of the vein can be a clue but should be verified by other maneuvers. The vein should be nonpulsatile and compressible with gentle pressure (**Fig. 3**). In addition, it should increase in size in the Trendelenburg position or with Valsalva.

When performing CVC, it is often helpful to initially interrogate the vein before establishing a sterile field. If it is of too small a caliber, if it is noncompressible (implying thrombosis), or if a thrombus is visualized, another target should be considered. Once a suitable access site has been identified, the patient is prepared and draped in the usual fashion. A sterile sleeve is used to cover the US probe, and a generous amount of coupling gel should be placed inside the sleeve (it may be sterile or unsterile gel). The probe is then inserted into the sleeve, which is then drawn over probe and the cord. Sterile coupling gel is then placed directly on the patient. The vein can be visualized in either the cross-sectional or longitudinal view. The cross-sectional view has the advantage of being easier to obtain and should suffice for most purposes. The longitudinal view typically requires more expertise with using US but is useful if attempting a low IJ vein access (eg, for tunneled catheter placement) in that it allows better visualization of the vessel closer to the level of the clavicle.

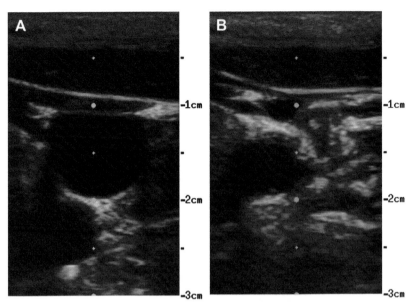

Fig. 3. (*A*) B-mode image of right IJ vein (1–2 cm deep) and common carotid artery located deep (2.0–2.5 cm) and medial to the jugular vein. (*B*) Compression of right IJ vein (1 cm deep).

The US probe should be held in the nondominant hand, and once the vessel is appropriately visualized, the access site can be anesthetized. The needle can be visualized in the subcutaneous tissues, and the infiltration of local anesthetic can be observed as an expanding area of echolucency. Once local anesthetic has been administered, the dominant hand can then be used to advance the access needle under real-time direct visualization. The needle first encounters the anterior wall and likely indents it before puncturing it. The anterior wall may then be seen to recoil, implying that the needle has pierced it, and the tip should then be located within the lumen of the vessel. In the case of a small or flat vein, the needle may actually collapse the vein and pierce both walls simultaneously. In this event, slow withdrawal of the needle while applying gentle negative pressure with a syringe should provide a return of blood when the needle tip is safely within the lumen of the vessel.

Once the vessel has been accessed, the US probe should be placed on the sterile field (in the event it is required again), access should then be secured with a guidewire, and the catheter is placed using the standard Seldinger technique. The access needle should be the only needle required to puncture the vein; US guidance obviates the need for a finder needle. In addition, real-time direct visualization is essential. The benefits of US are lost if it is simply used to identify and mark the vein and access then proceeds blindly using those markings.

The advantages of US guidance extend beyond IJ vein access and are applicable to the puncture of the subclavian and femoral veins. Complication rates from subclavian vein access are typically somewhat higher given its proximity to the lung and greater depth (**Fig. 4**). The subclavian vein can usually be readily visualized with US, despite its depth and relative degree of protection by the clavicle.[8] Depending on the patient's body habitus, the femoral vein can be a relatively deep vessel to access and likewise, its identification by US may be advantageous.

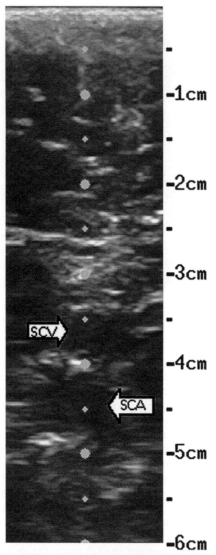

Fig. 4. US image of subclavian vein and artery in transverse view. Subclavian vein is 3.5 to 4.0 cm deep. SCA, subclavian artery; SCV, subclavian vein.

Arterial Access

Arterial access, although not as common as central venous access, is another extremely valuable clinical adjunct for the surgical patient. It allows for continuous hemodynamic monitoring and access for frequent blood gas analysis to monitor pulmonary function. Furthermore, arterial access is the gateway for a variety of endovascular interventions. Typically, a palpable pulse provides a reliable landmark for arterial puncture; however, image guidance can be of particular benefit in a variety of circumstances. Patients with a weakly palpable pulse pose a particular problem as well as the patient with relatively small arteries, which may be difficult to access.

Obese patients whose pulses may be diminished or made difficult to find by the intervening soft tissues also pose a challenge. In all of these situations, US imaging can be vital in obtaining arterial access.

Again, B-mode imaging may be all that is required, given the characteristic appearance of arteries on US. An artery is typically uniformly round with a thick muscular wall. It is a pulsatile structure, which does not readily compress. Despite these characteristic findings, the vessel may be difficult to identify for a variety of reasons. In these situations, using color flow can help to identify where the vessel lies. Once it has been identified with color, the color flow can be turned off and the artery visualized on B-mode.

Accessing the artery is performed in a similar manner to venous access. Again, prior to creating a sterile field the target vessel should be visualized to ensure that it is suitable for access. The patient and the US probe are then sterilely prepared. Imaging the vessel in cross section is typically easier as it allows the operator to see the artery and the vein side by side. A needle access guide is also helpful, after measuring the distance to the vessel on the US unit. The vessel is identified and the access needle is advanced under direct visualization. Due to the thicker less deformable wall, the vessel should be accessed in the center because a tangential approach often results in the needle slipping alongside the vessel. This situation is not only frustrating to the operator but also irritating to the vessel and may cause the vessel to spasm, which may, in turn, make it virtually inaccessible at that point.

Inferior Vena Cava Filter Placement

The indications for inferior vena cava (IVC) filter placement remain a topic of great debate.[9] The advent of retrievable IVC filters has led to more IVC filters being placed in increasingly sick patient populations. Although caval venography remains the gold standard for filter placement, US has found a niche in this application as well. Contrast venography carries with it certain inherent risks such as radiation exposure, contrast administration, and, for the most critically ill patients, the simple risk of transport from an intensive care setting to the angiography suite. Now that relatively sophisticated duplex US capability can be brought to the bedside, IVC filters can be placed without having to expose the patient to any of these risks. Intravascular US (IVUS) serves as another modality to assist with anatomic visualization and bedside filter placement.

Several techniques have been described for using US visualization for IVC filter deployment.[10–14] Initial experiences were with transabdominal duplex US.[10,12] With this technique, the junction of the IVC and the right renal vein is first visualized because it serves as the landmark for deployment (the right renal vein is typically the lowest renal vein). The right renal artery courses posteriorly to the IVC and also serves as a landmark. The IVC is then measured at that level to ensure that its diameter is suitable for the proposed device. Finally, the planned access site is examined for patency. If this initial evaluation is suitable, then placement of the filter proceeds using US guidance.

With the advent of IVUS, newer methods have been developed for guiding filter deployment.[13] In patients in whom surface scanning does not provide adequate visualization of the appropriate landmarks, the IVUS catheter can be used to determine appropriate placement. With this method, initial groin access is obtained and the IVUS catheter is passed through the IVC to the level of the atrium. The catheter is withdrawn and several landmarks are observed including the right atrium, the hepatic veins, both the renal veins, and finally, the confluence of the iliac veins. Contralateral wire access may make identification of the iliac confluence more readily visible. The IVUS catheter is then used to visualize the lowest renal vein, and the filter is advanced to this level and deployed. Alternatively, if single access is preferred, the IVUS catheter can be measured against the delivery device to identify the appropriate insertion depth for deployment. Following filter deployment, the IVC is evaluated again with US to confirm appropriate positioning. Finally, positioning can be further confirmed with plain abdominal radiographs, although this is not necessarily a requirement.

In one retrospective analysis directly comparing bedside US-guided IVC filter placement to contrast venography, technical success was noted to be similar in the 2 groups.[15] Venography had a minor advantage with a technical success rate of 99.7% versus 97.4% ($P = .018$) of US. All the technical failures in this study were filter maldeployments (iliac vein deployment, suprarenal deployment, filter angulation >15°) and their rate was consistent with other published reports, which typically fall in the 2% to 4% range.[10–13] Taking into account the near-equivalency of the 2 methods, the investigators concluded that the small benefit afforded by venography could be compensated in the critically ill patient by the benefit of bedside placement with US.

Diagnosis and Treatment of Femoral False Aneurysm

In most settings, duplex US is the standard initial examination in the workup and identification of femoral false aneurysms. Other modalities include computed tomography, magnetic resonance imaging, and catheter-based angiography. In addition to a high level of sensitivity and specificity, duplex US holds several advantages in terms of quickness, cost, and portability, as well as the avoidance of ionizing radiation and the toxicity associated with radiographic contrast agents. The use of US also allows for guidance of therapy in the form of either US-guided compression or thrombin injection.

US-guided compression therapy has been used for more than 2 decades with variable success.[16] The technique involves placement of the US probe directly over the neck of the pseudoaneurysm, with subsequent compression until inflow into the pseudoaneurysm ceases. The compression is maintained for up to 10 minutes and is then released with reimaging performed to document thrombosis of the pseudoaneurysm. If unsuccessful, the technique may be repeated several times usually for a total of 40 to 60 minutes.[17] The technique has been shown to have initial failure rates as high as 27%.[18] Contraindications include the presence of infection, large hematomas with impending compartment syndrome, limb or skin ischemia, excessive patient discomfort, and unsuitable anatomy. Most success is predicted for pseudoaneurysms measuring 4 cm or less.[18,19] If initially successful, recurrence rates on the order of 4% have been documented.[20]

Since its first description in 1986, US-guided thrombin injection has proven to be an even more successful tool in the treatment of pseudoaneurysms.[21] Original applications of thrombin included transarterial as well as percutaneous injections with balloon protection.[22] More recently, percutaneous injection without balloon occlusion is the more commonly used technique. Duplex US is used to first identify the pseudoaneurysm and its anatomy (**Fig. 5**). Distal pulses and vascular status are carefully documented. The skin is sterilely prepared. Relationships of the pseudoaneurysm, its neck, and the native circulation are identified. Access from a lateral approach parallel to the ultrasound beam is preferred. If desired, a needle guide can also be used (**Fig. 6**). A 18-gauge or 20-gauge needle is inserted into the pseudoaneurysm cavity (**Fig. 7**). Small increments of thrombin ($\cong$ 0.2 mL or 200 units) are injected using a 1-mL syringe under US guidance. Therapy is continued until thrombosis of the pseudoaneurysm occurs and cessation of flow is identified (**Fig. 8**). In most cases, no more than 1 or 2 injections are required. For appropriately selected cases, success rates of 95% to 100% have been documented in randomized trials.[17] Complications include

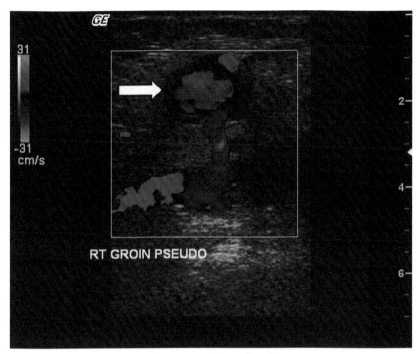

Fig. 5. US image of femoral pseudoaneurysm (*arrowhead*).

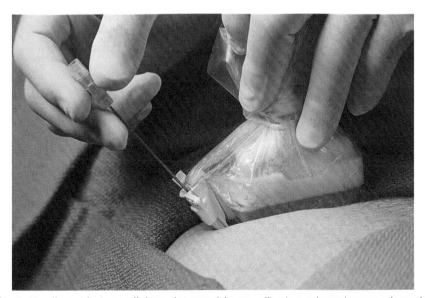

Fig. 6. Needle guide is parallel to ultrasound beam, allowing a lateral approach to the pseudoaneurysm.

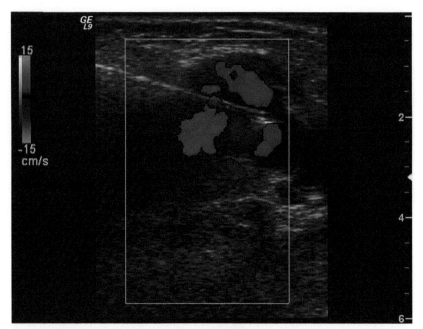

Fig. 7. US image of a needle inserted into a pseudoaneurysm.

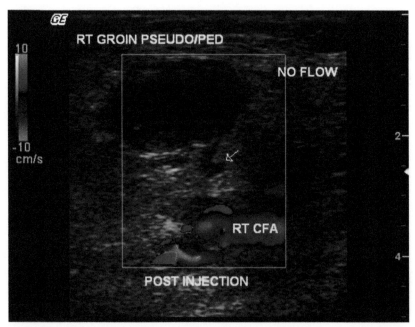

Fig. 8. US view of thrombosed pseudoaneurysm and pedicle (*arrow*), with preserved flow in the common femoral artery.

a risk of arterial thrombosis or embolization, as well as a small risk of anaphylaxis. Although the largest body of data describes its application in peripheral pseudoaneurysms, US-guided thrombin injection has been used in other abdominal arterial beds successfully.[23,24]

SUMMARY

Although the use of US in the past has conjured thoughts of grainy, ill-defined, black-and-white images with relatively specific applications, advances in technology and sharper resolution have dramatically expanded its clinical utility. With the addition of Doppler analysis, US has become an extremely powerful tool for the clinician performing vascular interventions. The use of US has become the standard of care when performing CVC and has improved success rates and decreased complications of CVC, a frequently performed procedure. Although a palpable landmark often makes arterial access somewhat easier, visualization of the vessel can be invaluable when circumstances make palpation difficult. US management of iatrogenic pseudoaneurysms can avoid the morbidity of an open groin exploration and pseudoaneurysm repair. Modern portable US and IVUS technology have made IVC filter placement a potential bedside procedure, eliminating the need to transport critically ill patients away from an intensive care setting. As this technology continues to improve, it will open the door to a potentially ever-increasing number of vascular interventions.

REFERENCES

1. Cosgrove DO, Meire HB, Lim A. Ultrasound: general principles. In: Adam A, Dixon AK, editors. Grainger & Allison's diagnostic radiology a textbook of medical imaging. 5th edition. Philadelphia: Elsevier; 2008. p. 55–77.
2. Shojania KG, Duncan BW, McDonald KM, et al, editors. Making health care safer: a critical analysis of patient safety practices. Evidence report/technology assessment no. 43. (Prepared by the University of California at San Francisco-Stanford Evidence-based Practice Center under Contract No. 290-97-0013), AHRQ publication no. 01-E058. Rockville (MD): Agency for Healthcare Research and Quality; 2001. p. 620.
3. Feller-Kopman D. Ultrasound-guided internal jugular access a proposed standardized approach and implications for training and practice. Chest 2007;132: 302–9.
4. Karakitsos D, Labropoulos N, De Groot E, et al. Real-time ultrasound-guided catheterisation of the internal jugular vein: a prospective comparison with the landmark technique in critical care patients. Crit Care 2006;10:R162.
5. Keenan SP. Use of ultrasound to place central lines. J Crit Care 2002;17:126–37.
6. Mallory DL, McGee WT, Shawaker TH, et al. Ultrasound guidance improves the success rate of internal jugular vein cannulation. A prospective, randomized trial. Chest 1990;98:157–60.
7. Randolph AG, Cook DJ, Gonzales CA, et al. Ultrasound guidance for placement of central venous catheters: a meta-analysis of the literature. Crit Care Med 1996; 24:2053–8.
8. Sakamoto N, Arai Y, Takeuchi Y, et al. Ultrasound-guided radiological placement of central venous port via the subclavian vein: a retrospective analysis of 500 cases at a single institute. Cardiovasc Intervent Radiol 2010;33: 989–94.

9. Geerts WH, Bergqvist D, Pineo GF, et al. Prevention of venous thromboembolism: American College of Chest Physicians evidence-based clinical practice guidelines (8th edition). Chest 2008;133:381S–453S.

10. Conners MS, Becker S, Guzman RJ, et al. Duplex scan-directed placement of inferior vena cava filters: a five-year institutional experience. J Vasc Surg 2002; 35:286–91.

11. Garrett JV, Passman MA, Guzman RJ, et al. Expanding options for bedside placement of inferior vena cava filters with intravascular ultrasound when transabdominal duplex ultrasound imaging is inadequate. Ann Vasc Surg 2004;18: 329–34.

12. Neuzil DF, Garrard CL, Berkman RA, et al. Duplex-directed vena caval filter placement: report of initial experience. Surgery 1998;123:470–4.

13. Passman MA, Dattilo JB, Guzman RJ, et al. Bedside placement of inferior vena cava filters by using transabdominal duplex ultrasonography and intravascular ultrasound imaging. J Vasc Surg 2005;42:1027–32.

14. Wellons ED, Matsuura JH, Shuler FW, et al. Bedside intravascular ultrasound-guided vena cava filter placement. J Vasc Surg 2003;38:455–8.

15. Corriere MA, Passman MA, Guzman RJ, et al. Comparison of bedside transabdominal duplex ultrasound versus contrast venography for inferior vena cava filter placement: what is the best imaging modality? Ann Vasc Surg 2005;19:229–34.

16. Fellmeth BD, Roberts AC, Bookstein JJ, et al. Postangiographic femoral artery injuries: nonsurgical repair with US-guided compression. Radiology 1991;178: 671–5.

17. Tisi PV, Callam MJ. Treatment for femoral pseudoaneurysms [review]. Cochrane Database Syst Rev 2009;2:CD004981.

18. Dean SM, Olin JW, Piedmonte M, et al. Ultrasound-guided compression closure of postcatheterization pseudoaneurysms during concurrent anticoagulation: a review of seventy-seven patients. J Vasc Surg 1996;23:28–35.

19. Demirbas O, Guven A, Batyraliev T. Management of 28 consecutive iatrogenic femoral pseudoaneurysms with ultrasound-guided compression. Heart Vessels 2005;20:91–4.

20. Hajarizadeh H, LaRosa CR, Cardullo P, et al. Ultrasound-guided compression of iatrogenic femoral pseudoaneurysm failure, recurrence, and long-term results. J Vasc Surg 1995;22:425–33.

21. Cope C, Zeit R. Coagulation of aneurysms by direct percutaneous thrombin injection. Am J Roentgenol 1986;147:383–7.

22. Loose HW, Haslam PJ. The management of peripheral arterial aneurysms using percutaneous injection of fibrin adhesive. Br J Radiol 1998;71:1255–9.

23. Reus M, Morales D, Vazquez V. Ultrasound-guided percutaneous thrombin injection for treatment of extrarenal pseudoaneurysm after renal transplantation. Transplantation 2002;74:882–4.

24. Sparrow P, Asquith J, Chalmers N. Ultrasonic-guided percutaneous injection of pancreatic pseudoaneurysm with thrombin. Cardiovasc Intervent Radiol 2003; 26:312–5.

Computed Tomography for the Diagnosis and Management of Abdominal Aortic Aneurysms

Clark A. Davis, MD

KEYWORDS

• Abdominal aortic aneurysm • Endovascular aneurysm repair
• Aortic aneurysm imaging
• Computed tomography of abdominal aortic aneurysms

COMPUTED TOMOGRAPHY AND ABDOMINAL AORTIC ANEURYSMS

The use of computed tomography (CT) scanning in the diagnosis and treatment of abdominal aortic aneurysms (AAAs) is continuing to expand. Advances in technology with the use of rapid spiral CT scanning, CT angiography (CTA), multiplanar reconstruction, and 3-dimensional (3-D) reconstruction are now readily available. CT has allowed for the incidental diagnosis of AAA when being performed for various abdominal symptoms. CT allows the diagnosis of inflammatory AAA, ruptured AAA, and mycotic AAA to be determined with relative certainty. Determination of rupture risk of AAA is enhanced with CT. Operative planning for surgery is also aided with CT by delineating anatomic factors that may impair open surgery. Since the expansion of endovascular aneurysm repair (EVAR), CT has become essential for determining the anatomic suitability for EVAR.

CT AND AAA DIAGNOSIS

With the increasing use of CT imaging in the diagnosis and treatment of abdominal disorders, the incidental finding of AAA is more commonplace. Chervu and colleagues[1] reviewed 243 patients undergoing elective AAA repair, and found that 38% of AAAs were found initially on physical examination whereas 62% were found incidentally by radiological examinations. Furthermore, AAAs become increasingly

The author has nothing to disclose.
Department of General and Vascular Surgery, Gundersen Lutheran Health System, 1900 South Avenue C05-001, La Crosse, WI 54601, USA
E-mail address: cadavis@gundluth.org

Surg Clin N Am 91 (2011) 185–193
doi:10.1016/j.suc.2010.10.007   surgical.theclinics.com

more common with age, as does a patient's exposure to radiological imaging for diagnostic and other screening examinations. Pickhardt and colleagues,[2] in 2009, suggested a cost benefit with the use of screening CT colonography versus optical colonoscopy used for the screening of colorectal cancer in patients older than 65 years. With the use of optical colonoscopy at 10-year periods versus CT colonography at 5- and 10-year periods, a hypothetical cohort of patients was examined using a Markov computer model for the development of colorectal cancer as well as AAA. Because of the theoretical ability to diagnose AAA incidentally with CT colonography (thus reducing AAA-related mortality), Pickhardt and colleagues concluded that CT colonography is a cost-effective screening test for the Medicare population. However, this does not take into account AAA diagnosis with physical examination or by other imaging that is frequently ordered for the Medicare population.

Incidental findings on CT done for both preoperative planning and postoperative surveillance have been found to be significant. Indes and colleagues[3] followed 82 consecutive patients undergoing EVAR who had both preoperative and postoperative CT data. Fourteen of 82 patients (19%) were found to have clinically significant primary incidental findings, the most common of which was a lung mass (n = 4). Secondary clinically significant incidental findings found on postoperative surveillance CT included lung mass (n = 6), liver mass (n = 6), and pancreatic mass (n = 3).

During the diagnosis of AAA it is occasionally necessary to determine whether the etiology is more than that of a simple degenerative aneurysm. Inflammatory AAAs are found to have extensive thickening of the periaortic tissues and retroperitoneum, referred to as an "inflammatory rind" (**Fig. 1**). This "rind" is enhanced with intravenous contrast and has a distinct appearance. Mycotic aneurysms appear more irregular in shape and may have eccentric, saccular outpouchings seen on CT scanning. Pseudoaneurysms as a result of trauma or iatrogenic interventions can also be identified on CT (**Fig. 2**). Aortoenteric fistulae cause extensive air to be seen within the aortic sac and typically occur in patients with previous open AAA repair (**Fig. 3**). CT also helps to determine aneurysm extent, involvement of renal and iliac arteries, and determination of saccular or fusiform shape. Horseshoe kidney may be evident on CT, requiring careful operative planning for renal preservation, and a retroaortic left renal vein may make proximal aortic clamping dangerous. This anatomic variant is depicted in **Fig. 4**.

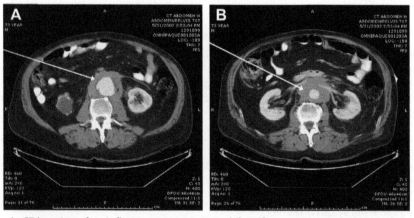

Fig. 1. CT imaging of an inflammatory AAA. Note (*A*) uniform periaortic thickening (*arrow*) and (*B*) displacement of the left renal vein (*arrow*).

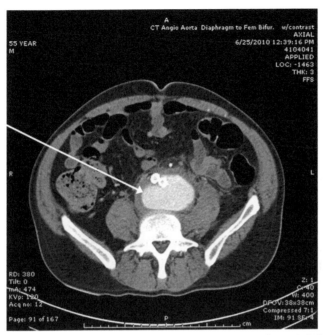

Fig. 2. CT demonstrating contrast in an aortic pseudoaneurysm (*arrow*) following stent placement for chronic iliac occlusion.

CT AND AAA RUPTURE RISK

AAA diameter has been shown to help determine rupture risk. The use of multiplanar CT with and without 3-D reconstruction allows the clinician to most accurately determine true diameter. Precise transverse measurements can be made, with 91% of studies showing interobserver variability as low as 5 mm.[4] Current research to better determine rupture risk involves the use of CT and measurement of actual wall stress.

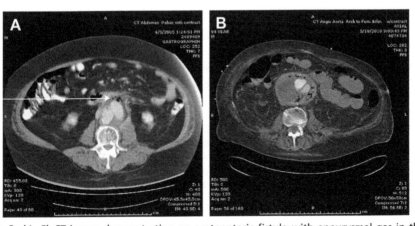

Fig. 3. (*A, B*) CT image demonstrating an aortoenteric fistula with aneurysmal gas in the setting of a previous open AAA repair. (*A*) Duodenal fistula with extensive intra-aneurysmal air; note duodenum adherent to aneurysm (*arrow*).

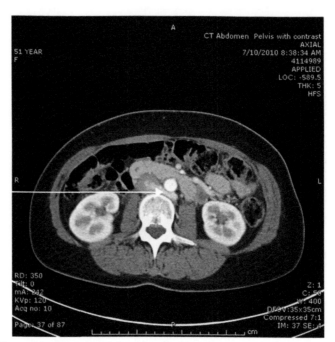

Fig. 4. CT illustrating retroaortic left renal vein (*arrow*).

"Finite element analysis" uses mathematical models, 3-D CT reconstruction, and blood pressure values to measure multiple areas of the aneurysm for wall stress. Fillinger and colleagues[5] analyzed 48 patients (10 ruptured AAA, 8 symptomatic AAA, and 30 elective AAA) using "finite element analysis" and concluded that wall stresses were significantly higher in the ruptured and symptomatic group than in the elective group. The same investigators analyzed 103 patients with AAA who were scheduled for at least 6 months of observation. Those patients who went on to repair after growth or rupture had significantly greater initial diameter as well as wall stresses.[6] Peak wall stress was felt to be superior to diameter measurements in differentiating patients who would go on to experience catastrophic outcome. Similar results using finite element analysis and determination of rupture risk have since been published, and an assertion for multicenter validation is under way.[7,8]

Fillinger and colleagues[9] reviewed the CT scans of 122 ruptured and 137 elective AAA patients, and evaluated them for infrarenal neck length, maximum thrombus thickness, and aortic tortuosity. When matched for gender, age, and diameter, those with rupture had less aortic tortuosity.

The extent of intramural thrombus may also be determined on CTA, and has been implicated in rates of growth and rupture of AAA. Speelman and colleagues[10] recently found that a larger thrombus reduced wall stress but was shown to result in higher AAA diameter growth rate. The thrombus caused weakening of the wall, resulting in increasing growth. However, others debate the effect of thrombus on aneurysm rupture risk, as they describe a benefit associated with thrombus, arising from reduction in wall tension.[11]

CT AND RUPTURE DIAGNOSIS

Once AAA rupture has occurred, CT scan may be diagnostic. Frequently a noncontrast CT for ureteral lithiasis or nephrolithiasis will reveal extensive retroperitoneal blood and an AAA (**Fig. 5**). Contrast CTA can also show active aneurysmal leak (**Fig. 6**). Contrast CTA may show active extravasation or the findings of a "crescent sign" may indicate impending rupture. Crescent sign (bleeding into the aneurysm thrombus; **Fig. 7**) was the focus of a study by Roy and colleagues[12] in 2008, in which CT scans from patients with ruptured AAAs were reviewed and compared with similar-sized aneurysms without rupture. The crescent sign was present in 38% of those with rupture versus 14% without rupture. The crescent sign was predictive of the site of rupture and was shown to be associated with AAA rupture. Also, those aneurysms with greater bleeding into the thrombus were more likely to have ruptured.[12]

OPEN SURGICAL PLANNING

Once the need for surgery is established, CT is very helpful in determining suitability for open surgery or EVAR. Open repair requires proximal aortic clamp placement above the aneurysm in noncalcified vessels to avoid arterial tearing and to achieve adequate vascular control. Circumferential calcifications are easily seen on nonintravenous contrast CT and, if extensive at the infrarenal level, clamp placement will need to be suprarenal or the use of balloon control may be needed. Other anatomic considerations seen on CTA for proximal control include the presence of a retroaortic left renal vein, accessory renal arteries, or duplication of the inferior vena cava. Evidence of renal artery stenosis present on CTA may allow for consideration of renal artery bypass at the time of open repair or for renal artery angioplasty.

Distal arterial control during repair also requires knowledge of the extent of the aneurysm and whether the iliac arteries are involved. Evidence of inferior mesenteric artery patency on CTA alerts the surgeon to the need for possible reimplantation to avoid colonic ischemia.

PLANNING FOR EVAR

Anatomic considerations for determining whether a patient is a candidate for EVAR are readily evaluated with CTA. Current approved endovascular grafts require an infrarenal aortic neck length of 1 to 1.5 cm, measured from the lowest renal artery to the start of the aneurysm. Cross-sectional measurements as well as coronal views are used to

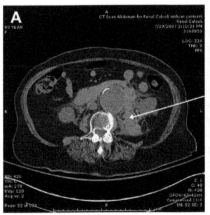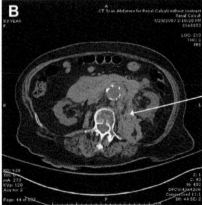

Fig. 5. (*A, B*) Noncontrast CTA demonstrating large retroperitoneal hematoma (*arrow*) associated with ruptured AAA.

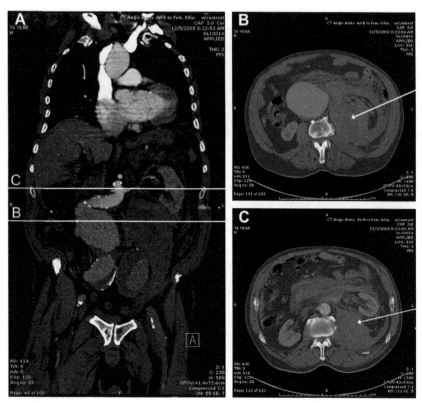

Fig. 6. Contrast CTA demonstrating large retroperitoneal hematoma associated with ruptured AAA. (*A*) Coronal view, with lines indicating locations of views for (*B*) and (*C*). (*B*) Cross-sectional view with retroperitoneal hematoma (*arrow*). (*C*) Hematoma (*arrow*) extending above renal artery origin, displacing the left kidney anteriorly.

accurately determine neck length. The presence of neck thrombus or extensive calcification may affect suitability for EVAR and can also be seen on CT. In cases of renal insufficiency, noncontrast CT can be used to obtain a good recognition of the anatomy; however, thrombus extent and precise measurements can be more difficult.

Accurate measurements of neck diameter are vital to appropriate graft sizing. Cross-sectional measurements are most commonly used at the level of the lowest renal artery for graft sizing. Oversizing of 10% to 20% is recommended to ensure graft seal and to avoid late-term proximal graft leak in cases of infrarenal aortic neck enlargement. Neck angulation can be determined from the coronal and sagittal views, and severe angulation can make graft placement difficult. Less than 60° angulation of the aortic neck in relation to the long axis of the aneurysm is ideal. **Fig. 8** depicts how neck angulation is measured. Conical neck morphology in which the diameter enlarges, moving from lowest renal artery to aneurysm, may also make EVAR difficult. By using the cross-sectional diameters and fine-cut CT (1-mm slices), almost all necessary neck measurements can be made for safe EVAR planning. 3-D reconstructions are available with the use of TeraRecon (TeraRecon Inc, San Mateo, CA, USA) and other available software programs.

It is also important to know distal landing zones in the iliac arteries preoperatively. Iliac landing zones of greater than 10 mm are optimal. If the common iliac arteries

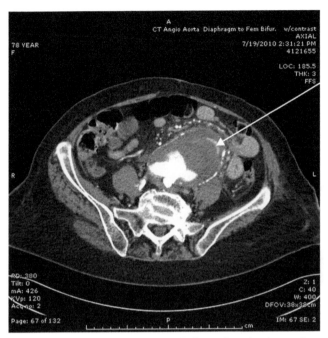

Fig. 7. Contrast CTA illustrating crescent sign (*arrow*) of intrathrombus hemorrhage within AAA.

are aneurysmal, the graft may need to be extended into the external iliacs. If the internal iliac arteries are patent, preoperative embolization may be necessary to prevent retrograde flow into the aneurysm sac, which results in occlusion of the internal iliac arteries and the potential risk of pelvic intestinal and muscle ischemic injury. Compromise of both internal iliac vessels greatly increases this risk and should be avoided. Severe iliac calcification and tortuosity can make delivery of the endograft difficult and can place the patient at risk of arterial tearing or rupture. Retroperitoneal conduit placement for endograft access may be needed if the external iliac arteries measure less than 7.5 mm in diameter.

Postoperative follow-up after EVAR can be done with scheduled CT scanning or color duplex ultrasound (CDU). Initial recommendations after the original approval of EVAR by the Food and Drug Administration required serial CT follow-up data. Advocates of CT surveillance cite a greater sensitivity of endoleak detection when compared with CDU. AbuRahma[13] followed postoperative patients with both CDU and CTA. Two hundred and thirty-two patients were followed for 5 years after EVAR, and only those with endoleaks were analyzed (n = 35 [15%]). CDU failed to identify 11 of 39 endoleaks identified by CT scan, with potential consequences to treatment occurring in 2 patients. This report suggests that CDU is not as sensitive as CTA in endoleak detection and that CDU should not be used as the sole method in surveillance.

Due to repeated radiation exposure and contrast toxicity with surveillance CTA, others have advocated CDU surveillance. Dias and colleagues[14] evaluated 279 consecutive asymptomatic patients treated with EVAR who were followed with CT scanning. Twenty-six (9.3%) of the 279 patients undergoing yearly CT scans under-went an intervention for treatment of CT findings such as AAA diameter expansion (n = 18), kink in the stent graft (n = 4), component separation (n = 2), isolated common

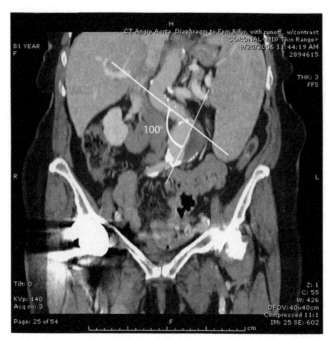

Fig. 8. Angle measurement determined from long axis of aneurysm in relation to long axis of the infrarenal aortic neck. This patient's anatomy is less suitable for EVAR due to the angle of 100°.

iliac artery expansion (n = 1), and partial malperfusion of the superior mesenteric artery due to partial fabric coverage (n = 1). Their conclusion was that only one patient would have had a delay in reintervention if only simple diameter measurements were used instead of routine CT. Less frequent CT follow-up will help reduce cost and radiation exposure to patients. However, if reintervention is planned, CT is vital in operative planning. Color flow duplex scanning has been found to be efficacious in post-EVAR follow-up of aortic sacs that are stable in size.[15] Examination of the United States Zenith (Cook Inc, Bloomington, IN, USA) Endovascular graft trials led to the recommendation that in all patients without early endoleak, the 6-month surveillance study could be eliminated and that CDU should be done at 1 year and yearly thereafter. However, these recommendations need to be validated by a randomized, prospective trial.[16] Mills and colleagues[17] reviewed 223 patients who underwent open or endovascular AAA repair. Both groups experienced a drop in glomerular filtration rates, and this decline was greater and persistent in the EVAR group. Due to contrast-induced nephropathy, radiation toxicity, and the need for post-EVAR surveillance, many advocate CDU with selective CTA.[14–17]

SUMMARY

CTA is useful in the incidental detection and early diagnosis of AAA. A patient's risk of AAA rupture can be assessed by accurately measuring diameter, tortuosity, thrombus extent, and wall stress. Anatomic variants as well as AAA etiology are determined with CTA. Suitability for EVAR and open surgery is made by close examination of AAA morphology as well as anatomic features.

REFERENCES

1. Chervu A, Clagett GP, Valentine RJ, et al. Role of physical examination in detection of abdominal aortic aneurysms. Surgery 1995;117:454–7.
2. Pickhardt PJ, Hassan C, Laghi A, et al. CT colonography to screen for colorectal cancer and aortic aneurysm in the Medicare population: cost-effectiveness analysis. Am J Roentgenol 2009;192:1332–40.
3. Indes JE, Lipsitz EC, Veith FJ, et al. Incidence and significance of nonaneurysmal-related computed tomography scan findings in patients undergoing endovascular aortic aneurysm repair. J Vasc Surg 2008;48:286–90.
4. Jaakkola P, Hippeläinen M, Farin P, et al. Interobserver variability in measuring the dimensions of the abdominal aorta: comparison of ultrasound and computed tomography. Eur J Vasc Endovasc Surg 1996;12:230–7.
5. Fillinger MF, Raghavan ML, Marra SP, et al. In vivo analysis of mechanical wall stress and abdominal aortic aneurysm rupture risk. J Vasc Surg 2002;36:589–97.
6. Fillinger MF, Marra SP, Raghavan ML, et al. Prediction of rupture risk in abdominal aortic aneurysm during observation: wall stress versus diameter. J Vasc Surg 2003;37:724–32.
7. Venkatasubramaniam AK, Fagan MJ, Mehta T, et al. A comparative study of aortic wall stress using finite element analysis for ruptured and nonruptured abdominal aortic aneurysms. Eur J Vasc Endovasc Surg 2004;28:168–76.
8. Truijers M, Pol JA, Schultzekool LJ, et al. Wall stress analysis in small asymptomatic, symptomatic and ruptured abdominal aortic aneurysms. Eur J Vasc Endovasc Surg 2007;33:401–7.
9. Fillinger MF, Racusin J, Baker RK, et al. Anatomic characteristics of ruptured abdominal aortic aneurysm on conventional CT scans: Implications for rupture risk. J Vasc Surg 2004;39:1243–52.
10. Speelman L, Schurink GW, Bosboom EM, et al. The mechanical role of thrombus on the growth rate of an abdominal aortic aneurysm. J Vasc Surg 2010;51:19–26.
11. Mower WR, Quiñones WJ, Gambhir SS. Effect of intraluminal thrombus on abdominal aortic aneurysm wall stress. J Vasc Surg 1997;26:602–8.
12. Roy J, Labruto F, Beckman MO, et al. Bleeding into the intraluminal thrombus in abdominal aortic aneurysms is associated with rupture. J Vasc Surg 2008;48:1108–13.
13. AbuRahma AF. Fate of endoleaks detected by CT angiography and missed by color duplex ultrasound in endovascular grafts for abdominal aortic aneurysms. J Endovasc Ther 2006;13:490–5.
14. Dias NV, Riva L, Ivancev K, et al. Is there a benefit of frequent CT follow-up after EVAR? Eur J Vasc Endovasc Surg 2009;37:425–30.
15. Chaer RA, Gushchin A, Rhee R, et al. Duplex ultrasound as the sole long-term surveillance method post-endovascular aneurysm repair: a safe alternative for stable aneurysms. J Vasc Surg 2009;49:845–9.
16. Sternbergh WC 3rd, Greenberg RK, Chuter TA, et al. Redefining postoperative surveillance after endovascular aneurysm repair: recommendations based on 5-year follow-up in the US Zenith multicenter trial. J Vasc Surg 2008;48:278–84.
17. Mills JL Sr, Duong ST, Leon LR, et al. Comparison of the effects of open and endovascular aneurysm repair on long term renal function using chronic kidney disease staging based on glomerular filtration rate. J Vasc Surg 2008;47:1141–9.

Focused Assessment with Sonography for Trauma: Methods, Accuracy, and Indications

Nirav Y. Patel, MD[a],*, Jody M. Riherd, MD[b]

KEYWORDS

- Focused assessment with sonography • Ultrasound
- Abdominal trauma • Cardiac tamponade

The use of ultrasound in the evaluation of abdominal trauma was first described in 1971 by Kristensen and colleagues.[1] However, it was not until the 1990s that ultrasound was incorporated into the acute resuscitative environment. In 1996, Rozycki and colleagues[2] coined the term FAST (focused assessment with sonography for trauma), an acronym that has since persisted for trauma ultrasonographic evaluation. FAST has been considered the most important advance in the initial evaluation of patients with blunt abdominal trauma since the introduction of diagnostic peritoneal lavage (DPL) and has recently been included in the eighth edition of the Advanced Trauma Life Support (ATLS) course[3] as an adjunct to abdominal examination. Its increased use has been driven primarily by the advantages it affords over other diagnostic modalities (**Box 1**).

A FAST examination can typically be completed in 5 minutes and encompasses 4 to 6 views (3–5 intra-abdominal, 1 cardiac), with the intent of identifying free fluid within the peritoneal cavity or pericardial sac. Experience with the use of FAST has transformed its original intent from being a method of detection of free intra-abdominal fluid to that of specific injury identification and from being an adjunct for other screening/diagnostic modalities to an exclusive diagnostic modality in an effort to decrease cost and invasiveness. Over the past 2 decades, FAST has been applied for many different indications, and in varied settings, making recommendations for its optimal use and effectiveness less clear.

The authors have nothing to disclose.

[a] Department of General and Vascular Surgery, Gundersen Lutheran Health System, 1900 South Avenue C05-001, La Crosse, WI 54601, USA

[b] Department of Diagnostic Radiology, Gundersen Lutheran Health System, 1900 South Avenue C02-002, La Crosse, WI 54601, USA

* Corresponding author.

E-mail address: nypatel@gundluth.org

Box 1
Advantages and limitations of FAST

Advantages

Portable

Noninvasive

Serial application

Accessibility

Bedside

Cost

Lack of ionizing radiation

Real-time imaging

Multiplanar capability

Limitations

Operator dependent

Patient habitus

Poor penetration through air (bowel gas, subcutaneous)

Specific injury identification

ANATOMIC REVIEW

Intra-abdominal views on FAST are based on 3 dependent areas within the peritoneal cavity in which free fluid is most likely to accumulate when the patient is in the supine position: (1) perihepatic, subphrenic and hepatorenal recess/Morrison pouch; (2) perisplenic, splenorenal fossa/subphrenic; and (3) pelvis. The minimum volume of free intraperitoneal fluid required for detection by FAST has been reported to range from 100 to 620 mL (**Table 1**).[4–8] Volumes at the lower end of the spectrum seem to have a higher likelihood of accumulating within the pelvis or adjacent to the site of injury.

From a clinical standpoint, how much fluid is significant with respect to guiding patient management? Semiquantitative measures such as small, moderate, and large based on the number of views in which fluid is detected have been reported, but the clinical significance has not been addressed. Multiple scoring systems have been developed in an effort to enable quantification of free fluid with minimal interrater variability and guide patient care. Huang and colleagues[9] reported a system that assigned 1 point for each

Table 1
Minimum volume of free fluid detection

Authors	View/Position	Volume (mL)
Goldberg et al[6]	Right lateral decubitus	100
Branney et al[4]	Morrison pouch/supine	619
Paajanen et al[7]	Perihepatic/perisplenic	>500
Abrams et al[8]	Morrison pouch	
	Supine	668
	5° Trendelenburg	443

of 4 anatomic sites (hepatorenal recess, pouch of Douglas, perisplenic space, paracolic gutter) in which fluid was detected by FAST. Fluid with a depth of more than 2 mm in the hepatorenal recess or pouch of Douglas was assigned 2 points. Floating loops of bowel were given 2 points. Scores ranged from 0 to 8. About 96% of patients with scores greater than 3 required exploratory laparotomy. Conversely, 38% of patients with score less than 3 also required laparotomy. McKenney and colleagues[10,11] developed and prospectively evaluated a scoring system that measured the depth of the largest fluid level, to the nearest tenth of a centimeter, in an anterior (near the surface of the abdomen) to posterior fashion and subsequently added 1 point for each of the other areas in which fluid was detected (4 areas maximum) to arrive at the final score. About 87% of patients with a score of 3 or more required a therapeutic operation, as opposed to 8 of 54 patients (15%) with a score of less than 3. Although these scoring systems enable some standardization of fluid quantification, they currently lack validation and fail to incorporate other associated clinical variables. As a result, although serving as a valuable parameter, they do not enable exclusive clinical decision making.

TECHNIQUE
Patient Position

The patient is preferably examined in the supine position. Other positions (Trendelenburg, reverse Trendelenburg, and decubitus) may facilitate pooling of fluid in dependent regions, thereby potentially increasing detection yield, and should be considered if the clinical scenario permits.

Transducer

Transducer selection depends on the size of the patient. For a typical adult, sound wave penetration must be at least 20 cm. Therefore, a lower-frequency transducer is selected, such as 3.5 to 5 MHz curved array.[12] The curved face on this transducer allows for a wider far field of view but does have limited resolution. In pediatric patients, a higher-frequency linear array transducer has better resolution and may still produce sound waves with adequate depth penetration.

FAST EXAMINATION VIEWS

A typical FAST examination incorporates a minimum of 4, but up to 6, views (**Fig. 1**).[13] When imaging a patient, the left side of the display screen should always be the patient's right side (**Fig. 2**). The screen should reflect cranial to caudal going from left to right when displaying a longitudinal view (**Fig. 3**).

Transverse Subxiphoid

The subxiphoid view (**Fig. 4**) is best obtained by moving the hand over the top of the transducer. Direct manual pressure is applied downward, and the transducer is then angled cranially. The transducer is held almost horizontally. It is ideal to also image portions of the left lobe of the liver to absorb scatter artifact in the near field. Rocking the probe toward the right shoulder or occasionally toward the left shoulder can provide a view of the right ventricle.

Longitudinal Right Upper Quadrant

The right upper quadrant sonographic window (**Fig. 5**) may vary depending on patient size. The kidney-liver interface can be visualized most often by placing the transducer at the midaxillary line in the subcostal region, with the probe placed along the longitudinal axis. An intercostal window is necessary in obese patients, requiring placement

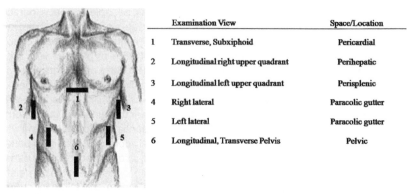

	Examination View	Space/Location
1	Transverse, Subxiphoid	Pericardial
2	Longitudinal right upper quadrant	Perihepatic
3	Longitudinal left upper quadrant	Perisplenic
4	Right lateral	Paracolic gutter
5	Left lateral	Paracolic gutter
6	Longitudinal, Transverse Pelvis	Pelvic

Fig. 1. FAST examination views. (*Adapted from* Rose JS. Ultrasound in abdominal trauma. Emerg Med Clin North Am 2004;22:581–99; with permission.)

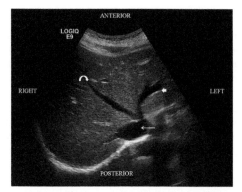

Fig. 2. FAST display for cross-sectional view demonstrating a transverse image of the liver. The patient's right is the left of the image. The anterior abdominal wall is at the top of the image. Note the intrahepatic inferior vena cava (*arrow*) and the left (*filled arrow*) and middle (*curved arrow*) hepatic veins. This is similar to the transverse plane of a CT scan.

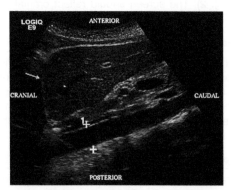

Fig. 3. FAST display for longitudinal view of the liver. Cranial aspect of the patient is on the left of the image. Anterior abdominal wall is seen at the top of the image. Note the aorta (*calipers*) and right hemidiaphragm (*arrow*). This is a similar plane to a sagittal CT image.

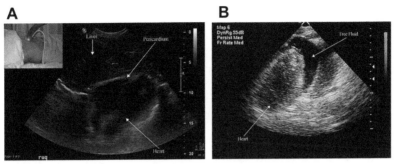

Fig. 4. Transverse subxiphoid views of a (*A*) normal transverse subxiphoid view of pericardium, with patient and transducer positioning (*inset*) and (*B*) pericardial effusion.

of the transducer parallel to the intercostal space. In this situation, using a transducer with a smaller footprint (but still using a lower frequency) may be helpful.

Longitudinal Left Upper Quadrant

To evaluate the splenorenal recess, the transducer is placed posterior to the midaxillary line (**Fig. 6**). Scanning parallel to multiple intercostal spaces may be required to fully evaluate the left upper quadrant. Failure to find the appropriate window is usually caused by not scanning far enough posteriorly or superiorly.

Longitudinal, Transverse Pelvis

Suprapubic views (**Fig. 7**) are obtained by placing the transducer just above the pubic symphysis in the transverse plane. The bladder should be in view as a well-circumscribed anechoic structure in the midline of the pelvis. The pouch of Douglas, or vesicorectal space, is superior to the prostate or cervix, which can be seen deep to the bladder on the transverse images. If these structures are in view, the transducer should be moved superiorly. Once the transverse image is captured, skin contact is maintained while turning the probe in the longitudinal direction to obtain an image of the suprapubic region. If there is fluid in the pelvis, additional scanning in the right and left lower quadrants and paracolic gutters may help estimate volume.

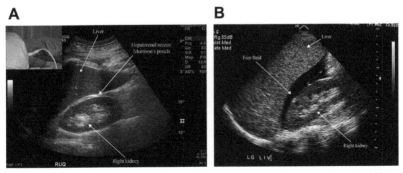

Fig. 5. Longitudinal view demonstrating a (*A*) normal view of hepatorenal interface, with patient and transducer positioning (*inset*) and (*B*) the presence of free fluid at hepatorenal interface.

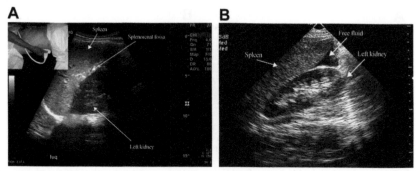

Fig. 6. Longitudinal view demonstrating a (*A*) normal view of the splenorenal interface, with patient and transducer positioning (*inset*) and (*B*) the presence of free fluid at the splenorenal interface.

IMAGE OPTIMIZATION

Image quality and overall sensitivity of the examination may be optimized by manipulation of factors influencing signal strength and image acquisition.

SIGNAL OPTIMIZATION
Gain

Gain refers to the amplification of receiver signals from deeper tissues to compensate for increased attenuation compared with near-field structures. Gain can be adjusted to

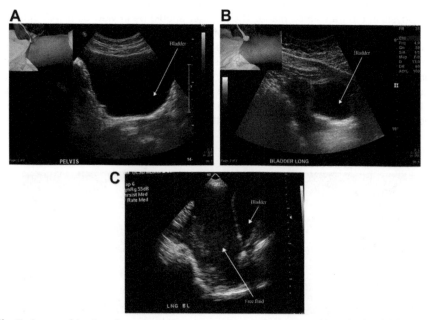

Fig. 7. Suprapubic view demonstrating a normal transverse (*A*) and longitudinal (*B*) suprapubic view, with patient and transducer positioning (*inset*) and (*C*) longitudinal suprapubic view demonstrating free fluid.

brighten or darken the whole image. The time gain compensation (TGC) curve can also be adjusted to brighten or darken segments of the image. The TGC curve requires frequent adjustments because different structures attenuate sound differently.

Focal Zone

The focal zone is the depth at which the sound waves have narrowed, resulting in the best lateral resolution at this level. This depth can be adjusted up and down to focus at the area of interest.

Field of View

The field of view can be adjusted to increase the width or depth to view more of the abdomen on one screen. Decreasing the field of view allows concentration on one area and eliminates scatter and artifact in the image.[14]

Image Acquisition

The operator needs to be in a comfortable position close to the patient, with the portable ultrasound machine immediately adjacent to the bedside. If the operator is uncomfortable, it may hinder the ability to find appropriate sonographic windows. Dimming the lights, if possible, can provide better visualization of findings. Trendelenburg or reverse Trendelenburg positioning can improve conspicuity of fluid in the upper quadrants or pelvis, respectively. Having the patient hold the breath on deep inspiration or a respiratory pause at the end of inspiration if mechanically ventilated can move the liver and spleen inferiorly and allow for subcostal visualization. Because of rib shadows in the right and left upper quadrant, acquisition of more than 1 image is often necessary to confirm positive or negative findings.

A full bladder provides an acoustic window enabling visualization of free fluid posteriorly. If a bladder catheter is in place, it should be clamped before beginning the examination, or if required, sterile fluid can be instilled into the bladder to optimize the view. Clotted blood does not look like simple anechoic fluid. It may be complex or diffusely hyperechoic. Alternatively, free fluid is not always blood. Ascites or physiologic fluid from menstruation are alternative types of fluid in the abdomen or pelvis.

CLINICAL APPLICABILITY

Two decades after the incorporation of ultrasonography in trauma, its precise role remains unclear. Much of this can be attributed to the comparative reference standards (DPL, computed tomography [CT], laparotomy, clinical observation) and end points (fluid detection, intervention), by which its effectiveness has been judged. In addition, advances in skills and technology have confounded the simple initial intent "detection of free fluid" and use as an "adjunct, not substitute" for preexisting modalities (DPL, CT).

The literature is rife with studies reporting the efficacy of FAST.[2,15–21] Sensitivity of the technique has been confounded by multiple variables, accounting for a wide range of 67% to 80%. In contrast, specificity and accuracy have been reported to range from 98% to 100% and 98% to 99%,[2,15–21] respectively.

Positivity has been based on a spectrum of findings, including, but not limited to, absence or presence of free fluid, actual quantity of fluid present, specific injuries identified, and interventions undertaken (therapeutic vs nontherapeutic). These inconsistencies in comparative standards have resulted in a significant variation of reported results and arguments for and against the effectiveness and role of ultrasound in the immediate evaluation of abdominal trauma.

An International Consensus Conference in 1999 examined the question "what does a positive or negative FAST study mean, and how should it affect patient management?"[22] It was acknowledged that to put sensitivity, specificity, and accuracy of ultrasonography in perspective, it was critical to examine the definitions of positivity and negativity used to calculate these numbers. It was noted that these definitions had been extremely variable and loosely applied in the literature and acknowledged that positivity and negativity often depended on the question being asked, such as whether it was being performed for the identification of free fluid only or free fluid and parenchymal lesions. When performed for the identification of free fluid only, the detection of free fluid would constitute a positive result. Conversely, when performed for any evidence of free fluid or parenchymal lesions, the detection of either yields a positive result and the absence a negative. Ultrasonographic views that were not clearly positive or negative would be termed indeterminate. A true positive study result, therefore, was one in which free fluid was detected and had been confirmed by CT, DPL, or laparotomy. A false-positive study result was one in which free fluid was found on ultrasonography but the criterion standard method had failed to confirm fluid. Similarly, a false-negative study result was one in which negative ultrasonographic results were not confirmed by the criterion standard. The category of true-negative results was recognized as being the most difficult. From a pure statistical standpoint, all true-negative results should be confirmed by standard tests, which, however, may be impractical in many clinical situations in which no additional testing was performed. Therefore, many true-negative results were based simply on successful patient observation with lack of adverse clinical events. The Consensus recommendation regarding positive and negative study results was as follows: (1) In hemodynamically unstable patients, a positive FAST examination result should generally be followed by laparotomy. A negative FAST examination result should prompt a search for extra-abdominal sources of hemorrhage. (2) In hemodynamically stable patients, a positive FAST result should be followed by CT to better define the nature of the injuries. Termed under "a majority viewpoint" was also a recommendation that a negative FAST result in hemodynamically stable patients be followed by a period of observation of at least 6 hours and a follow-up FAST. Also, a caution was issued about blindly proceeding to laparotomy in hemodynamically unstable patients without taking into consideration the quantity of free fluid present. For instance, a patient with a pelvic fracture and a small amount of free fluid may not require laparotomy.

At present, it would seem that FAST has the greatest utility in circumstances in which detection of free fluid (pericardial, intraperitoneal) would affect initial management directly, while avoiding diagnostic duplication and optimizing sensitivity and specificity. Studies that have looked at the sensitivity and specificity of ultrasonography with respect to the presence or absence of free fluid have reported sensitivities to range from 69% to 90% and specificity from 24% to 55% (**Table 2**).[23–27] Multiple studies have also evaluated the sensitivity in hypotensive patients with ranges from 79% to 100%. In the authors' personal series of 1277 patients who underwent FAST, 147 had hypotension, with an associated incidence of free fluid of 40%. Sensitivity and specificity of FAST in this specific subgroup were 68% and 90%, respectively.[27]

The hepatorenal interface has been reported to be the most sensitive intra-abdominal view for the detection of free fluid, consistent with the propensity of free fluid to preferentially flow to the right side of the abdomen.[28–30] Ma and colleagues[28] compared a single view of Morrison pouch with a 5-view FAST examination for detection of hemoperitoneum and reported a sensitivity of complete examination versus single view of 87% and 51%, respectively. Although a single hepatorenal view has been advocated in certain situations,[31] a multiple view FAST examination is recommended given its greater sensitivity.[30,31]

Table 2
Reported sensitivity, specificity, and predictive value

Author	N	Mechanism of Injury	End Point	Reference CT	DPL	OR	Clinical Observation	Sensitivity	Specificity	Predictive Value Positive	Negative	Accuracy
McGahan et al,[23] 1997	500	Blunt, penetrating	Fluid, intervention	X			X	63	95	—	—	85
Healey et al,[24] 1996	800	Blunt	Fluid, intervention	X	X			88	98	72	99	97
Tiling et al,[25] 1990	808	Blunt						89	100	—	—	98
Gaarder et al,[26] 2009	104	Blunt, penetrating	Fluid, intervention	X	X	X	X	62	96	84	88	88
Patel et al,[27] 2007	1277	Blunt	Fluid	X	X	X		69	95	69	95	—

Abbreviations: OR, patient taken to operating room; X, reported interventions.

Patients who benefit most from a multiview FAST examination are those who are hemodynamically unstable and in whom cardiac tamponade or sufficient free intra-abdominal fluid is present, which would account for the patient's instability. In unstable patients, the absence of sufficient intraperitoneal fluid to explain hemodynamic instability mandates a search for alternate sources of extraperitoneal hemorrhage.

The optimal use of FAST seems to be based on a combination of hemodynamic status and clinical findings. Based on a series experience with 1277 FAST examinations, the authors propose a treatment algorithm based on hemodynamic stability of patients (**Fig. 8**).

PEDIATRIC TRAUMA

Few studies on the efficacy of ultrasonography in children with abdominal injury have been reported. Scaife and colleagues[32] conducted an electronic survey of the use of FAST at American College of Surgeons (ACS) level 1 trauma centers, National Association of Children's Hospitals, and freestanding children's hospitals. FAST examinations were used in 96% adult-only institutions, 85% combined adult and pediatric centers, and 15% children's hospitals. The largest impediment to the use of FAST in children's hospitals seemed to be its limited sensitivity, 45% to 55%. This limitation was attributed to approximately 40% of abdominal injuries not being associated with free fluid.[33–36] As with adults, FAST seems to have a role as a diagnostic adjunct in hemodynamically unstable children. The eighth edition of ATLS[3] recognizes FAST as a diagnostic adjunct option for abdominal trauma in pediatric patients.

ACCREDITATION

After an initial 8-hour course that included didactic and hands-on training with FAST, Thomas and colleagues[37] reported a sensitivity of 81%, specificity of 91%, and overall accuracy of 98%.

At The International Consensus Conference in 1999,[22] the majority viewpoint supported an 8-hour (4 theoretical, 4 practical) minimum training period to learn the

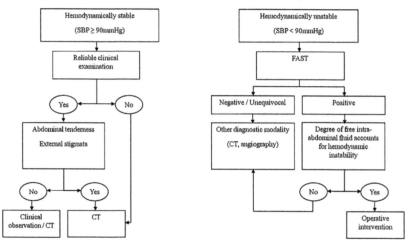

Fig. 8. Proposed algorithm for use of FAST with blunt abdominal trauma based on the authors' experience with 1277 FAST examinations. SBP, systolic blood pressure.

FAST procedure, with a minimum of 200 supervised patient examinations. A minority viewpoint was that as few as 50 examinations were sufficient. The sensitivity and specificity seems to plateau after 25 to 50 examinations.[5,37,38]

In addition to the overall number of examinations performed regarding proficiency in FAST, a critical variable is the presence of an adequate number of examinations with positive results. The rate of FAST studies with positive results has varied from 9% to 13%. Thus, with 50 sequential examinations, a provider may have less than 10 examinations with positive results. No current set number of examinations with positive results has been defined by the ACS. The American College of Emergency Physician's ultrasonography guidelines specify that 50% of proctored examinations should have positive results.[39]

FUTURE DIRECTIONS

Recent technological advancements in sonography can improve and expand the FAST examination in appropriate clinical settings. Three-dimensional sonography allows for multiplanar imaging, enabling acquisition of a plane through a desired point of interest that may not be accessible with conventional sonography because of size or location of the acoustic window. It also provides a new display of the images that can improve the ability to determine spatial relationships between normal and abnormal structures. Three-dimensional sonography is currently limited by the need for special equipment, additional postprocessing time, and added expertise.

Another advanced technique is contrast-enhanced sonography. Conventional sonography has limited ability to characterize the free fluid found in the abdomen in the setting of trauma. Intravenous contrast specific to sonography can offer the added benefit of identifying active bleeding from a solid organ in the abdomen or retroperitoneum. Promising results have been noted in animal studies and case reports.[40–42] Ultrasonography contrast agents are widely used in Europe and are currently under investigation in the United States.

SUMMARY

FAST has had a significant effect in the management of abdominal trauma, with its ease of rapid performance, portability, and noninvasive nature, resulting in a significant increase in its use over the past 2 decades. Extending its use from the original intent as a diagnostic adjunct for detection of free intraperitoneal fluid and pericardial effusion to a stand-alone diagnostic modality has raised questions regarding its validity and optimal role. FAST remains an invaluable adjunct in the management of abdominal trauma when used selectively based on a combination of hemodynamic status and clinical findings.

REFERENCES

1. Kristensen JK, Buemann B, Kühl E. Ultrasonic scanning in the diagnosis of splenic haematomas. Acta Chir Scand 1971;137:653–7.
2. Rozycki GS, Ochsner MG, Schmidt JA, et al. A prospective study of surgeon-performed ultrasound as the primary adjuvant modality for injured patient assessment. J Trauma 1995;39:492–8.
3. American College of Surgeons Committee on Trauma. Advanced trauma life support. 8th edition. Chicago: American College of Surgeons; 2008.
4. Branney SW, Wolfe RE, Moore EE, et al. Quantitative sensitivity of ultrasound in detecting free intraperitoneal fluid. J Trauma 1995;39:375–80.

5. Gracias VH, Frankel HL, Gupta R, et al. Defining the learning curve for the focused abdominal sonogram for trauma (FAST) examination: implications for credentialing. Am Surg 2001;67:364–8.

6. Goldberg BB, Goodman GA, Clearfield HR. Evaluation of ascites by ultrasound. Radiology 1970;96:15–22.

7. Paajanen H, Lahti P, Nordback I. Sensitivity of transabdominal ultrasonography in detection of intraperitoneal fluid in humans. Eur Radiol 1999;9:1423–5.

8. Abrams BJ, Sukumvanich P, Seibel R, et al. Ultrasound for the detection of intra-peritoneal fluid: the role of Trendelenburg positioning. Am J Emerg Med 1999;17:117–20.

9. Huang MS, Liu M, Wu JK, et al. Ultrasonography for the evaluation of hemoperitoneum during resuscitation: a simple scoring system. J Trauma 1994;36:173–7.

10. McKenney KL, McKenney MG, Cohn SM, et al. Hemoperitoneum score helps determine need for therapeutic laparotomy. J Trauma 2001;50:650–4.

11. Ong AW, McKenney MG, McKenney KA, et al. Predicting the need for laparotomy in pediatric trauma patients on the basis of the ultrasound score. J Trauma 2003; 54:503–8.

12. Goodman TR, Traill ZC, Phillips AJ, et al. Ultrasound detection of pneumothorax. Clin Radiol 1999;54:736–9.

13. Rose JS. Ultrasound in abdominal trauma. Emerg Med Clin North Am 2004;22:581–99.

14. Middleton WD, Kurtz AB, Hertzberg BS. Ultrasound: the requisites. 2nd edition. St Louis: Mosby; 2004.

15. Miller MT, Pasquale MD, Bromberg WJ, et al. Not so FAST. J Trauma 2003;54:52–9.

16. Rose JS, Levitt MA, Porter J, et al. Does the presence of ultrasound really affect computed tomographic scan use? A prospective randomized trial of ultrasound in trauma. J Trauma 2001;51:545–50.

17. Ma OJ, Mateer JR, Ogata M, et al. Prospective analysis of a rapid trauma ultrasound examination performed by emergency physicians. J Trauma 1995; 38:879–85.

18. Luks FI, Lemire A, St-Vil D, et al. Blunt abdominal trauma in children: the practical value of ultrasonography. J Trauma 1993;34:607–10.

19. McKenney M, Lentz K, Nunez D, et al. Can ultrasound replace diagnostic perito-neal lavage in the assessment of blunt trauma? J Trauma 1994;37:439–41.

20. Tso P, Rodriguez A, Cooper C, et al. Sonography in blunt abdominal trauma: a preliminary progress report. J Trauma 1992;33:39–43.

21. Jehle D, Guarino J, Karamanoukian H. Emergency department ultrasound in the evaluation of blunt abdominal trauma. Am J Emerg Med 1993;11:342–6.

22. Scalea TM, Rodriguez A, Chiu WC, et al. Focused assessment with sonography for trauma (FAST): results from an international consensus conference. J Trauma 1999;46:466–72.

23. McGahan JP, Rose J, Coates TL, et al. Use of ultrasonography in the patient with acute abdominal trauma. J Ultrasound Med 1997;16:653–62.

24. Healey MA, Simons RK, Winchell RJ, et al. A prospective evaluation of abdominal ultrasound in blunt trauma: is it useful? J Trauma 1996;40(6):875–83.

25. Tiling T, Boulion B, Schmid A. Ultrasound in blunt abdomino-thoracic trauma. In: Border Allgoewer M, Hanson ST, editors. Blunt multiple trauma: comprehensive pathophysiology and care. New York: Marcel Decker; 1990. p. 415–33.

26. Gaarder C, Kroepelien CF, Loekke R, et al. Ultrasound performed by radiologists-confirming the truth about FAST in trauma. J Trauma 2009;67:323–7.

27. Patel NY, Cogbill TH, Mathiason MA, et al. To FAST or not to FAST: that is the question [poster #64] [abstract]. In: American Association for the Surgery of Trauma Annual Meeting. Las Vegas (NV): 2007. p. 64. Available at: http://www.aast.org/AnnualMeeting/PastAbstracts.aspx. Accessed August 20, 2010.

28. Ma OJ, Kefer MP, Mateer JR, et al. Evaluation of hemoperitoneum using a single- vs multiple-view ultrasonographic examination. Acad Emerg Med 1995;2:581–6.

29. Ingeman JE, Plewa MC, Okasinski RE, et al. Emergency physician use of ultrasonography in blunt abdominal trauma. Acad Emerg Med 1996;3:931–7.

30. Rozycki GS, Ochsner MG, Feliciano DV, et al. Early detection of hemoperitoneum by ultrasound examination of the right upper quadrant: a multicenter study. J Trauma 1998;45:878–83.

31. Rose JS, Bair AE, Mandavia D, et al. The UHP ultrasound protocol: a novel ultrasound approach to the empiric evaluation of the undifferentiated hypotensive patient. Am J Emerg Med 2001;19:299–302.

32. Scaife ER, Fenton SJ, Hansen KW, et al. Use of focused abdominal sonography for trauma at pediatric and adult trauma centers: a survey. J Pediatr Surg 2009; 44:1746–9.

33. Coley BD, Mutabagani KH, Martin LC, et al. Focused abdominal sonography for trauma (FAST) in children with blunt abdominal trauma. J Trauma 2000;48:902–6.

34. Emery KH, McAneney CM, Racadio JM, et al. Absent peritoneal fluid on screening trauma ultrasonography in children: a prospective comparison with computed tomography. J Pediatr Surg 2001;36:565–9.

35. Suthers SE, Albrecht R, Foley D, et al. Surgeon-directed ultrasound for trauma is a predictor of intra-abdominal injury in children. Am Surg 2004;70:164–7.

36. Miller D, Garza J, Tuggle D, et al. Physical examination as a reliable tool to predict intra-abdominal injuries in brain-injured children. Am J Surg 2006;192:738–42.

37. Thomas B, Falcone RE, Vasquez D, et al. Ultrasound evaluation of blunt abdominal trauma: program implementation, initial experience, and learning curve. J Trauma 1997;42:384–8.

38. Shackford SR, Rogers FB, Osler TM, et al. Focused abdominal sonogram for trauma: the learning curve of nonradiologist clinicians in detecting hemoperitoneum. J Trauma 1999;46:553–62.

39. American College of Emergency Physicians. American College of Emergency Physicians. Use of ultrasound imaging by emergency physicians. Ann Emerg Med 2001;38:469–70.

40. Luo W, Zderic V, Carter S, et al. Detection of bleeding in injured femoral arteries with contrast-enhanced sonography. J Ultrasound Med 2006;25:1169–77.

41. Glen P, MacQuarrie J, Imrie CW, et al. A novel application of ultrasound contrast: demonstration of splenic arterial bleeding. Br J Radiol 2004;77:333–4.

42. Liu JB, Merton DA, Goldberg BB, et al. Contrast-enhanced two- and three-dimensional sonography for evaluation of intra-abdominal hemorrhage. J Ultrasound Med 2002;21:161–9.

Imaging of the Cervical Spine in Injured Patients

James T. Quann, MD[a], Richard A. Sidwell, MD[b,c],*

KEYWORDS

• Trauma • Cervical spine • Computed tomography

Assessment for cervical spine injury is an important component in the evaluation of the injured patient. The cervical spine should be immobilized with a semirigid cervical collar while immediate life-threatening injuries are identified and treated. The physician must then exclude or diagnose injury to the cervical spine, including ligamentous and cervical vascular injuries. In this article, the authors discuss the roles of imaging techniques of the cervical spine in injured patients, with particular attention to the evidence behind the best practices.

CLINICAL EVALUATION OF THE CERVICAL SPINE

The patient with potential injury to the cervical spine should be considered to have such an injury until proved otherwise; immobilization with a semirigid cervical collar should be maintained during resuscitation and evaluation. Once life-threatening injuries have been identified and treated, the physician should evaluate the condition of the patient's cervical spine. Clearance of the cervical spine can frequently be accomplished on the basis of clinical evaluation alone, without the need for radiographic studies. Two different clinical rules have been developed, validated, and published to aid the physician in clinically excluding injury to the cervical spine.

The National Emergency X-Radiography Utilization Study (NEXUS) was published in 2000.[1] This decision instrument was based on 5 clinical criteria: no midline cervical spine tenderness, no focal neurologic deficit, normal alertness, no intoxication, and no painful or distracting injury. Patients meeting these criteria were classified as

The authors have nothing to disclose.

[a] Department of Surgical Education, Iowa Methodist Medical Center, 1415 Woodland Avenue, Suite 140, Des Moines, IA 50309, USA

[b] Iowa Methodist Medical Center, 1200 Pleasant Street, Des Moines, IA 50309, USA

[c] Department of Surgery, University of Iowa Carver College of Medicine, 200 Hawkins Drive, Iowa City, IA 52245, USA

* Corresponding author. Iowa Methodist Medical Center, 1200 Pleasant Street, Des Moines, IA 50309.

E-mail address: rsidwell@iowaclinic.com

Surg Clin N Am 91 (2011) 209–216

doi:10.1016/j.suc.2010.10.016

surgical.theclinics.com

0039-6109/11/$ – see front matter © 2011 Elsevier Inc. All rights reserved.

having a low probability of injury. In the United States, 34,069 patients were evaluated at 21 centers. Eight hundred eighteen patients had an identified cervical spine injury. The clinical criteria correctly excluded injury in all of the remaining patients but incorrectly excluded injury in 8 patients with a proved cervical spine injury, yielding a sensitivity of 99% and a negative predictive value of 99.8%.

The Canadian C-Spine Rule (CCR) used 3 high-risk criteria (age >65 years, dangerous mechanism, paresthesias in extremities), 5 low-risk criteria (simple rear-end motor vehicle collision, sitting position in the emergency department, ambulatory at any time, delayed onset of neck pain, absence of midline cervical spine tenderness), and the ability to actively rotate the neck 45° left and right.[2] When compared with the NEXUS criteria, the CCR seemed superior in terms of sensitivity and specificity for cervical spine injury.[3]

Clearing the neck by clinical examination alone has recently been questioned in a study published in 2007 by Duane and colleagues.[4] This prospective study evaluated 534 blunt trauma patients, comparing clinical examination with computed tomography (CT). The clinical examination, based essentially on NEXUS criteria, failed to identify 10 of 17 patients with fractures, 4 of whom required intervention.

At the authors' institution, their practice is to perform a clinical evaluation of the patient's cervical spine, somewhat modified from the NEXUS criteria. The cervical spine is considered "cleared" if the patient is (1) awake, alert, oriented, and free of intoxication; (2) with normal neurologic examination; (3) without significant distracting pain or injury; (4) without pain with palpation of the cervical spine, including axial loading; and (5) without pain with full active range of motion of the neck, including flexion and extension. Patients who fail any of these criteria are subjected to radiologic evaluation. This approach is consistent with the most recent guidelines established by the Practice Guidelines Committee of the Eastern Association for the Surgery of Trauma (EAST) (Table 1).[5]

PLAIN FILM RADIOGRAPHY

A good-quality 3-view (cross-table lateral, anteroposterior, open-mouth odontoid) cervical spine series was once the mainstay of the radiographic evaluation of the cervical spine. The usefulness of plain film radiography in the exclusion of cervical spine injury is now considered more limited. As a part of the NEXUS analysis, Mower and colleagues[6] reported a prospective study on the reliability of standard plain film screening of the cervical spine. Among 34,069 blunt trauma patients, the negative predictive value of normal screening films was 99.9% for any cervical spine injury. The negative predictive value was 99.99% for unstable injuries. Unfortunately, of the 818 patients with cervical spine injury, only 498 (61%) were accurately identified by plain film. Looked at differently, there were 581 patients with cervical spine injury who had adequate plain films; 47 of these patients (8%) had normal studies and 36 had studies that were abnormal, but a specific injury could not be identified.

Plain cervical spine radiographs are also an inefficient method of evaluation of the cervical spine after blunt trauma. In 2005, Gale and colleagues[7] reported on 848 consecutive blunt trauma patients treated at a level I trauma center, 640 of whom had cervical spine radiographs performed. These radiographs provided inadequate visualization of the cervical spine in 72% of the patients, most of whom required supplemental CT scan of the cervical spine.

In summary, the traditional 3-view cervical spine series adds little to the clinical examination decision rules for exclusion of cervical spine injury in blunt trauma patients. The studies are frequently inadequate, and the sensitivity for injury is not

Table 1
Summary of practice management guidelines regarding imaging of the cervical spine from the EAST Practice Management Guidelines Committee

Clinical Situation	Recommendation	Level of Recommendation
Awake, alert trauma patients without neurologic deficit or distracting injury who do not have neck pain or tenderness with full range of motion of the cervical spine	Cervical spine imaging is not necessary, and the cervical collar may be removed	Level 2
All other patients in whom cervical spine injury is suspected must have radiographic evaluation. This applies to patients with pain or tenderness, neurologic deficit, altered mental status, and distracting injury	The primary screening modality is axial CT from the occiput to T1 with sagittal and coronal reconstructions	Level 2
	Plain radiographs contribute no additional information and should not be obtained	Level 2
Neurologically intact awake and alert patient complaining of neck pain with a negative CT result	Option 1: Continue cervical collar	N/A
	Option 2: Cervical collar may be removed after negative MRI result	Level 3
	Option 3: Cervical collar may be removed after negative and adequate flexion-extension films	Level 3
Obtunded patient with a negative CT result and gross motor function of extremities	Flexion-extension radiography should not be performed	Level 2
	The risk/benefit ratio of obtaining MRI in addition to CT is not clear, and its use must be individualized in each institution	Level 3
	If MRI result is negative, the cervical collar may safely be removed	Level 2

Abbreviations: CT, computed tomography; MRI, magnetic resonance imaging.
Recommendations are classified as level 1, 2, or 3. A level 1 recommendation is convincingly justifiable based on the available scientific information alone. A level 2 recommendation is reasonably justifiable by the available scientific evidence and strongly supported by expert opinion. A level 3 recommendation is supported by available data but adequate scientific evidence is lacking.
  Data from Como JJ, Diaz JJ, Dunham CM, et al. Practice management guidelines for identification of cervical spine injuries following trauma: update from the Eastern Association for the Surgery of Trauma Practice Guidelines Committee. J Trauma 2009;67:651–9.

as good as CT. At this institution, the trauma service no longer uses plain film radiographs of the cervical spine for the evaluation of blunt trauma patients, a position that is supported by the most recent guidelines established by the Practice Guidelines Committee of the EAST (see **Table 1**).[5]

COMPUTED TOMOGRAPHY

Axial CT with sagittal and coronal reconstructions is currently the best modality to screen for injury to the cervical spine.[5] Several investigators have addressed this, a full review of which is beyond the scope of this article. Two studies illustrate the current weight of evidence.

Brown and colleagues[8] reported a retrospective review of 3537 blunt trauma patients evaluated at a level I trauma center over a 2-year period. These authors used axial CT with reconstructions in the sagittal and coronal planes to screen for injury to all areas of the spine (cervical, thoracic, and lumbar). CT identified 99 of 100 (99%) injuries to the cervical spine. The missed injury was a minor compression fracture at C7 that was treated with a rigid cervical collar. Overall, CT identified 276 of 278 (99.3%) of spine fractures at all levels. This study supports the use of CT over plain film radiography.[9]

In a meta-analysis reported in 2005, Holmes and Akkinepalli[10] report a pooled sensitivity of 52% for plain radiography in the detection of cervical spine injury. This rate is compared to a pooled sensitivity of 98% for CT scan in the detection of cervical spine injury. The accumulated data led the EAST Practice Guidelines Committee to conclude that "CT cervical spine has supplanted plain radiography as the primary modality for screening suspected cervical spine injury after trauma."

The authors routinely use axial CT scan with sagittal and coronal reconstructions to evaluate for the presence of cervical spine injury in patients who we are unable to clear on the basis of the clinical evaluation. This scan has been found accurate for both diagnosis and treatment planning for a full range of injuries. Some injuries are obvious and would not be difficult to detect on plain film radiography (**Fig. 1**). Other injuries are subtle and not easily visualized with standard radiography (**Figs. 2 and 3**).

SPECIAL SITUATIONS
Neck Pain with Normal CT

Some patients have neck pain without demonstrable injury on CT scan. These patients may have significant ligamentous injury that would require some type of treatment. An evidence-based approach to this situation is difficult to establish, and several treatment options are available.

Flexion-extension (FE) radiographs can be used to establish dynamic stability of the cervical spine; however, studies evaluating the utility of FE radiographs antedate modern CT scanning techniques. One report in 2002 evaluated 106 FE studies[11] of which 74 (70%) were considered to be adequate studies; the remaining 30% were inadequate because of limited FE motion. Of the 74 adequate studies, 5 (6%) demonstrated a cervical spine injury. There were no false-negative examinations. Only 7 of the 106 patients had complete cross-sectional imaging of the cervical spine with CT scan; so it is unknown how many of these injuries would have been detected with modern CT imaging. The authors selectively use FE radiographs in the setting of persistent neck pain with a normal CT scan. The FE study is done under the supervision of a radiologist. Patients are asked to actively flex and extend their neck, stopping for significant pain or neurologic symptoms. If both studies are normal, the use of the cervical collar is discontinued.

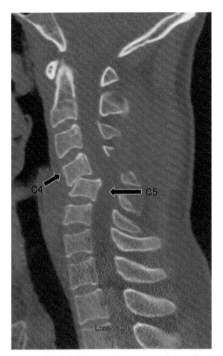

Fig. 1. Sagittal reconstruction of axial CT scan demonstrating a fracture or dislocation at the C4-C5 level, grade 2 spondylolisthesis of C4 on C5.

Magnetic resonance imaging (MRI) can also be used to evaluate the patient with neck pain and a normal CT scan. Data evaluating this practice are also limited. In 2005, Schuster and colleagues[12] reported on 93 awake patients with a normal motor examination. All patients had persistent neck pain with a normal CT of the cervical spine. All were evaluated with MRI of the cervical spine; none of these studies revealed clinically important injuries. The authors use MRI of the cervical spine on a limited basis in this situation, an example of which is shown in **Fig. 4**.

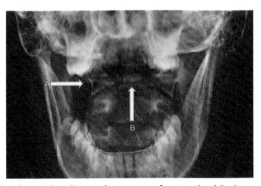

Fig. 2. Open-mouth odontoid radiograph, as part of a standard 3-view cervical spine radiograph series. (A) Arrow indicates right lateral mass of C1. (B) Arrow indicates dens of C2. This series was interpreted as normal, not visualizing the fracture of the right lateral mass of C1 seen on a subsequent CT scan (see **Fig. 3**).

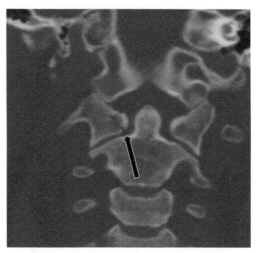

Fig. 3. Coronal reconstruction of axial CT scan demonstrating a fracture involving the right lateral mass of C1 (*arrow*). The standard 3-view cervical spine radiograph series did not visualize the fracture (see **Fig. 2**).

A final option for the patient with persistent cervical spine pain and a normal CT examination is to continue immobilization with a cervical collar until the pain has resolved. Patient at the author's institution are frequently managed in this manner, admittedly without supportive evidence. If the patient has continued midline pain at the time of follow-up (generally 2 weeks), either F-E radiographs or MRI of the cervical spine is obtained.

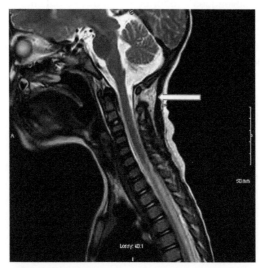

Fig. 4. MRI of the cervical spine. The arrow indicates edema of the posterior cervical soft tissues at the C1-C2 level consistent with tearing of the posterior atlantoaxial membrane. Axial CT scan with sagittal reconstruction was normal, but the patient had persistent midline neck pain.

The Obtunded Patient

There is, perhaps, no more controversial area in the evaluation for cervical spine injury than the issue of how to manage the obtunded patient who has a normal CT of the cervical spine. The central question is the risk of clinically significant injury when a neurologic examination cannot be reliably performed or the patient is unable to communicate neck pain.

In 2007, Como and colleagues[13] reported a prospective evaluation of obtunded blunt trauma patients whose initial CT cervical spine result was negative for acute injury. Of 115 patients, 6 (5.2%) were identified as having acute injury by MRI, none of whom required a change in management or continued use of the cervical collar. Interestingly, 6 patients also developed decubitus ulceration related to use of the cervical collar. These authors conclude that MRI of the cervical spine does not provide clinically relevant information and is not needed.

In 2008, Menaker and colleagues[14] reported on 203 patients with a persistently unreliable neurologic examination and a normal cervical spine CT on admission. MRI of the cervical spine was performed on all of these patients. Eighteen (8.9%) of these studies were abnormal. Two of these patients required surgery and 14 were treated with a cervical collar. Two patients required no treatment. The authors concluded that CT scan missed both stable and unstable injuries in unreliable patients and that a combination of studies was required for clearance of the cervical spine.

The EAST Practice Management Guidelines Committee has reviewed and summarized the available evidence regarding the evaluation of the cervical spine in the obtunded patient.[5] There is no definitive recommendation; this is left to the discretion of each institution. The authors are selective in their use of MRI of the cervical spine in these patients. The study is performed within the first 72 hours after injury is obtained with the use of MRI. If the study is normal, the use of cervical collar is discontinued. In most patients, however, MRI is not used, instead maintaining the cervical collar for an extended time.

SUMMARY

The physician who evaluates an injured patient must first be concerned with identification and treatment of immediate life-threatening injuries. During this time, the cervical spine is protected by immobilization with a semi-rigid cervical collar. "Clearance" of the cervical spine can be accomplished by clinical evaluation if the patient is awake, alert, oriented, free of intoxication, without distracting pain or injury, and has no pain on palpation or active range of motion of the cervical spine. All other patients require radiologic evaluation. Axial CT with sagittal and coronal reconstructions has replaced plain film radiography as the preferred imaging modality to screen for cervical spine injury. Patients who are neurologically intact but have persistent cervical spine tenderness and a normal CT of the entire cervical spine can be evaluated with FE films or MRI, although neither practice is supported by high-quality evidence-based studies. Clearance of the cervical spine in the obtunded patient remains controversial, and a clear recommendation cannot be made.

REFERENCES

1. Hoffman JR, Mower WR, Wolfson AB, et al. Validation of a set of clinical criteria to rule out injury to the cervical spine in patients with blunt trauma. N Engl J Med 2000;343:94–9.

2. Stiell IG, Wells GA, Vandemheen KL, et al. The Canadian c-spine rule for radiography in alert and stable trauma patients. JAMA 2001;286(15):1841–8.
3. Stiell IG, Clement CM, McKnight RD, et al. The Canadian C-Spine Rule versus the NEXUS low-risk criteria in patients with trauma. N Engl J Med 2003;349:2510–8.
4. Duane TM, Dechert R, Wolfe LG, et al. Clinical examination and its reliability in identifying cervical spine fractures. J Trauma 2007;62:1405–10.
5. Como JJ, Diaz JJ, Dunham CM, et al. Practice management guidelines for identification of cervical spine injuries following trauma: update from the Eastern Association for the Surgery of Trauma Practice Guidelines Committee. J Trauma 2009;67:651–9.
6. Mower WR, Hoffman JR, Pollack CV, et al. Use of plain radiography to screen for cervical spine injuries. Ann Emerg Med 2001;38(1):1–7.
7. Gale SC, Gracias VH, Reilly PM, et al. The inefficiency of plain radiography to evaluate the cervical spine after blunt trauma. J Trauma 2005;59(5):1121–5.
8. Brown CV, Antevil JL, Sise MJ, et al. Spiral computer tomography for the diagnosis of cervical, thoracic, and lumbar spine fractures: its time has come. J Trauma 2005;58(5):890–5 [discussion: 895–6].
9. Griffen MM, Frykberg ER, Kerwin AJ, et al. Radiographic clearance of blunt cervical spine injury: Plain radiograph or computed tomography scan? J Trauma 2003;55:222–7.
10. Holmes JF, Akkinepalli R. Computed tomography versus plain radiography to screen for cervical spine injury: a meta-analysis. J Trauma 2005;58(5):902–5.
11. Insko EK, Gracias VH, Gupta R, et al. Use of flexion-extension radiographs of the cervical spine in blunt trauma. J Trauma 2002;53(3):426–9.
12. Schuster R, Waxman K, Sanchez B, et al. Magnetic resonance imaging is not needed to clear cervical spines in blunt trauma patients with normal computed tomographic results and no motor deficits. Arch Surg 2005;140:762–6.
13. Como JJ, Thompson MA, Anderson JS, et al. Is magnetic resonance imaging essential in clearing the cervical spine in obtunded patients with blunt trauma? J Trauma 2007;63(3):544–9.
14. Menaker J, Philip A, Boswell S, et al. Computed tomography alone for cervical spine clearance in the unreliable patient – are we there yet? J Trauma 2008; 64(4):898–904.

Imaging for Blunt Carotid and Vertebral Artery Injuries

Clay Cothren Burlew, MD[a],*, Walter L. Biffl, MD[b]

KEYWORDS

- Cerebrovascular • Carotid artery • Vertebral artery • Injury
- Trauma

Over the past decade, multiple studies have provided the scientific rationale to promote the early identification and treatment of blunt carotid artery injuries (CAIs) and blunt vertebral artery injuries (VAIs), collectively known as blunt cerebrovascular injuries (BCVIs).[1–5] Initially BCVIs were thought to have unavoidable, devastating neurologic outcomes, but several reports suggested that anticoagulation improves neurologic outcome in patients suffering ischemic neurologic events.[6–9] Further study elucidated a latent period of blunt carotid and vertebral injuries; this asymptomatic period, before the onset of stroke, permits early identification of a patient's BCVIs and institution of treatment. Screening protocols, based on patient injury patterns and mechanism of injury, have been developed to identify high-risk patients so that appropriate imaging may be performed early in the postinjury period.[10] Current studies suggest that early antithrombotic therapy in asymptomatic patients with BCVIs reduces stroke rates and prevents neurologic morbidity[1–3,5,9–12]; hence, identification of injuries with appropriate imaging is paramount.

HISTORICAL PERSPECTIVE

BCVIs were first recognized over 30 years ago, but the majority presented with symptoms of neurologic ischemia.[13–18] Crissey and Bernstein[13] postulated 4 fundamental mechanisms of injury: direct blow to the neck, hyperextension with contralateral rotation of the head, laceration of the artery by adjacent fractures involving the sphenoid or petrous bones, and intraoral trauma. The most common mechanism causing CAIs is hyperextension resulting from the stretching of the carotid artery over the lateral articular processes of C1-C3.[19] VAIs are likely a combination of direct injury, which is caused by

The authors have nothing to disclose.

[a] Surgical Intensive Care Unit, Department of Surgery, Denver Health Medical Center, University of Colorado School of Medicine, 777 Bannock Street, Denver, CO 80204, USA

[b] Surgery/Trauma Outreach, Department of Surgery, Denver Health Medical Center, University of Colorado School of Medicine, 777 Bannock Street, Denver, CO, USA

* Corresponding author.

E-mail address: clay.cothren@dhha.org

doi:10.1016/j.suc.2010.10.004
0039-6109/11/$ – see front matter © 2011 Elsevier Inc. All rights reserved.
surgical.theclinics.com

associated fractures of the vertebrae involving the transverse foramen through which the artery courses, and hyperextension-stretch injury, which is caused by the tethering of the vertebral artery within the lateral masses of the cervical spine. Regardless of mechanism, there is intimal disruption of the carotid or vertebral artery. This intimal tear becomes a nidus for platelet aggregation that may lead to emboli or vessel occlusion.

Although the initial focus of BCVIs management was recognizing the injury and treating the devastating neurologic sequelae, subsequent efforts have been directed at diagnosing and treating these injuries during the "silent period," before the onset of stroke. Some patients with BCVIs may present with symptoms of cerebral ischemia within an hour of injury; early identification and treatment in these patients is difficult if not impossible. However, most patients with BCVIs exhibit a latent period between their original injury and the onset of stroke. This time frame range from hours to up to 14 years, but the majority seems to develop symptoms within 10 to 72 hours.[1,2,5,6,18–21] Diagnosing BCVIs during this "silent period" affords the opportunity for treatment before and to prevent neurologic sequelae.

Aggressive screening for BCVIs was initially suggested in the mid-1990s[9,10] after recognizing that specific patterns of injuries were associative.[6,7,22] A recently published report questioned the utility of such an aggressive screening approach,[23] whereas other studies have a screening yield of more than 30% in high-risk populations.[3–5,11] Indications for imaging have been proposed that identify a high-risk population of patients based on injury patterns.[1,3,5,11,19,24,25]

INDICATIONS FOR IMAGING

The initial screening protocol initiated in Denver in 1996 was relatively liberal, in an attempt to include all potential injury mechanisms and patterns.[10] The screening criteria included (1) an injury mechanism compatible with severe cervical hyperextension or rotation or hyperflexion, particularly if associated with displaced or complex midface or mandibular fracture; (2) closed head injury consistent with diffuse axonal injury of the brain; (3) near-hanging injury resulting in cerebral anoxia; (4) seat belt abrasion or other soft tissue injury of the anterior neck resulting in significant cervical swelling or altered mental status; (5) basilar skull fracture involving the carotid canal; and (6) cervical vertebral body fracture or distraction injury, excluding isolated spinous process fracture. A multivariate analysis of injury mechanisms and patterns was performed to identify high-risk factors, and 4 injury patterns were identified that were independent predictors of CAIs: Glasgow Coma Score (GCS) less than 6, petrous bone fracture, diffuse axonal brain injury, and LeFort II or III fracture.[26] Patients with any of these risk factors had a risk of 41% for CAIs. In those with all 4 injuries, the risk of CAI increases to 93%. In this same study by Biffl and colleagues, the only significant risk factor for VAI was cervical spine injury. Subsequent analysis of VAIs by Cothren and colleagues[27] found that nearly all cervical spine injury–related VAIs were associated with subluxations, foramen transversarium fractures, and fractures involving C1-C3. Based on these studies, a high-risk patient population has been identified that should undergo imaging to exclude BCVIs (**Box 1**).[24–26] However, in early series, up to 20% of patients with BCVI had none of these injuries,[26] with screening performed based on clinical suspicion of injury. With the improved accuracy of noninvasive screening modalities, there is a tendency to liberalize screening to capture all injuries, rather than try to restrict screening to the highest-risk groups.[28] These groups may include patients with mandible fractures, those with upper thoracic trauma combined with cranial injuries, and the pediatric population. To date, there have not been any large-scale analyses to determine the yield of such protocols.

Box 1
Denver screening criteria for BCVIs

Signs/Symptoms of BCVIs

Arterial hemorrhage from neck or nose or mouth

Cervical bruit in patients younger than 50 years

Expanding cervical hematoma

Focal neurologic deficit (transient ischemic attack, hemiparesis, vertebrobasilar symptoms, Horner syndrome)

Neurologic examination incongruous with head computed tomographic (CT) scan findings

Stroke on CT scan or magnetic resonance imaging

Risk Factors for BCVIs

High-energy transfer mechanism with

LeFort II or III fracture

Cervical spine fracture patterns: subluxation, fractures extending into the transverse foramen, fractures of C1-C3

Basilar skull fracture with carotid canal involvement/petrous bone fracture

Diffuse axonal injury with GCS less than 6

Near hanging with anoxic brain injury

Clothesline type injury or seat belt abrasion with significant swelling, pain, or altered mental status

---

DIAGNOSTIC IMAGING

A major focus of the recent literature on BCVIs has been the optimal screening diagnostic test. Four-vessel arteriography has long been considered the gold standard to diagnose BCVIs. Undoubtedly, many clinicians question the need for subjecting patients to angiography. Angiography is invasive, labor intensive, and costly; risks include complications related to catheter insertion (1%–2% hematoma, retroperitoneal bleeding, arterial pseudoaneurysm), contrast administration (1%–2% renal dysfunction, allergic reaction), infection, exposure to radiation, and stroke (<1%).[2,5] In addition, if angiography is not available at smaller hospitals, the patient requires emergent transfer for definitive evaluation.

Duplex ultrasonography (US) is widely used for imaging the extracranial carotid arteries for atherosclerotic disease; however, experience in diagnosing BCVIs is limited. In a multicenter review, US had 86% sensitivity for identifying internal carotid artery (ICA) injuries.[6] In that population of patients, the lesions missed by US were located at the base of the skull. Because most CAIs involve the distal ICA at or near the base of the skull, this is conceptually a major weakness of this imaging modality. Likewise, artifact from the bony canal encasing the vertebral artery may obscure a low-grade injury. Furthermore, although US can provide indirect evidence of injuries by detecting turbulence or other blood flow disturbances, these findings are not routinely seen in patients with stenoses less than 60%. In a recent series of over 1400 blunt trauma patients, the overall sensitivity of US was just 39%, with US missing 8 injuries that resulted in stroke.[29] Consequently, US is not recommended for BCVI screening.

Magnetic resonance angiography (MRA) seemed to be an attractive alternative to angiography (**Fig. 1**). MRA is noninvasive, does not require contrast administration, and detects cerebral ischemia earlier than CT scanning. Several reports advocate

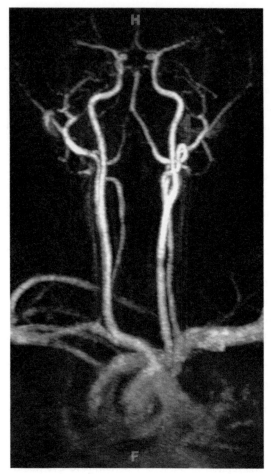

Fig. 1. MRI of the carotid and vertebral arteries.

use of MRA to diagnose BCVIs.[30–32] However, several trials, including those from Denver and Memphis, have documented poor sensitivity and specificity of MRA.[2,33,34] In addition, with issues of timely availability and incompatibility of equipment, MRA is not considered a reliable or optimal screening test for BCVIs.

CT angiography (CTA) has emerged as the preferred screening test for BCVIs. In addition to being a noninvasive imaging modality, most patients undergoing screening for BCVIs have indications for CT scanning of other regions. Hence, imaging can often be accomplished with only one "road trip." With high-speed scanners, the duration of imaging has been markedly reduced, as has the amount of contrast required, with dye loads being less than that used for conventional angiography. In addition, the use of coronal and sagittal reconstructions permits identification of injuries in 3 dimensions, with correlation to associated spine or skull trauma. CTA interpretation may be limited by streak artifacts from foreign bodies, motion artifacts, and beam hardening by dense venous contrast (**Fig. 2**). Optimal identification of injuries may be associated with the experience of the radiologist, with subtle findings otherwise missed (**Fig. 3**). The accuracy of early generation 1- to 4-slice CTA was poor,[2,33] with sensitivities between

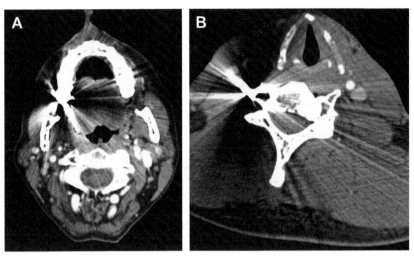

Fig. 2. Streak artifacts from foreign bodies such as dental work (*A*) and bullet fragments from prior penetrating trauma (*B*) may limit CTA interpretation.

47% and 68% and specificity of 67%. BCVI identification improved with the introduction of multidetector-row CTA.[28,35–37]

Four published studies have evaluated the accuracy of 16-slice CTA compared with arteriography. Eastman and colleagues[38] evaluated 162 patients with CTA, of whom 146 agreed to angiography. Reported screening yield was 28%, with an overall incidence of BCVIs of 1.25%. This study reported 100% sensitivity of 16-slice CTA for CAIs, and 96% sensitivity for VAIs, with 1 false-negative CTA of a grade 1 injury. The Harborview group performed arteriography on 82 patients who had had a normal screening CTA and initially found that CTA missed 7 BCVIs, for a negative predictive

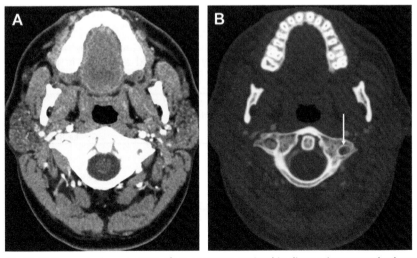

Fig. 3. (*A, B*) Bone windows on CTA often are more optimal in diagnosing a vertebral artery injury (*arrow in B*).

Box 2
Denver grading scale for BCVIs

Grade 1: irregularity of the vessel wall or a dissection/intramural hematoma with less than 25% luminal stenosis

Grade 2: intraluminal thrombus or raised intimal flap is visualized, or dissection/intramural hematoma with 25% or more luminal narrowing

Grade 3: pseudoaneurysm

Grade 4: vessel occlusion

Grade 5: vessel transection

---

value of 92%.[39] However, retrospective review of the CTA images found that the injuries were evident in 6 of the 7 patients and that the seventh patient's abnormality was most likely not traumatic in origin. Although selection bias exists in this study's design, it does illustrate the importance of experience in identifying BCVIs on a CTA; all missed injuries occurred in the first half of the study period. Two studies offer a note of caution in adopting CTA as the preferred imaging modality. Malhotra and colleagues[40] screened 119 patients with 92 undergoing confirmatory angiography; they reported a 43% false-positive and 9% false-negative rate for CTA. However, as in the series of Utter and colleagues,[39] the inaccuracy of CTA seemed to be related in large part to the radiologists' inexperience, as all of the missed BCVIs occurred in the first half of the study period. In the second half of the study, the sensitivity and negative predictive value of CTA was 100%. Each of these studies[39–40] recognizes that injuries in the region of the skull base seem to be the most difficult to identify, underlining the importance of carefully examining this high-risk region. The final study to evaluate CTA and arteriography by Goodwin and colleagues[41] reported the worst results for high-resolution CTA. They report the sensitivity for 16-slice CTA to be 29% and 64-slice CTA to be 54%. The authors acknowledge that the impact of the interpreting radiologist as a contributing factor has not been evaluated in any studies to date. Without quality control it is difficult to understand how best to interpret this study's impact on screening options for BCVIs. Conversely, a preliminary report by Fakhry and colleagues[42] indicates that CTA may be oversensitive in diagnosing BCVIs.

Overall, it seems that 16-slice (or more) CTA is reliable for screening for clinically significant BCVIs but that the accuracy diminishes with fewer detector rows. If CTA is not available, conventional angiography is the gold standard. In patients with

---

Table 1
Stroke rate by blunt cerebrovascular injury grade

	Grade of Injury	Stroke Rate by Grade
CAI	1	3%
	2	14%
	3	26%
	4	50%
	5	100%
VAI	1	6%
	2	38%
	3	27%
	4	28%
	5	100%

a normal CTA but high clinical suspicion or an equivocal CTA, angiography may be warranted to definitively exclude an injury.

INJURY GRADING SCALE

With the recognition of varied luminal irregularities comprising BCVIs (dissection, pseudoaneurysms, occlusion, and transection), was the identification of disparate outcomes.[6,9] An injury grading scale was developed[19] not only to provide an accurate

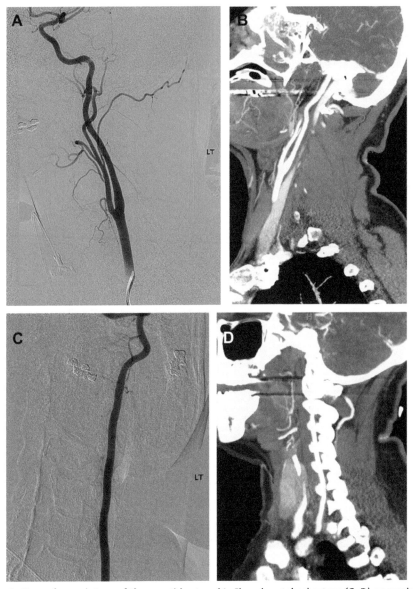

Fig. 4. Normal vasculature of the carotid artery (*A, B*) and vertebral artery (*C, D*) on angiography and CTA imaging.

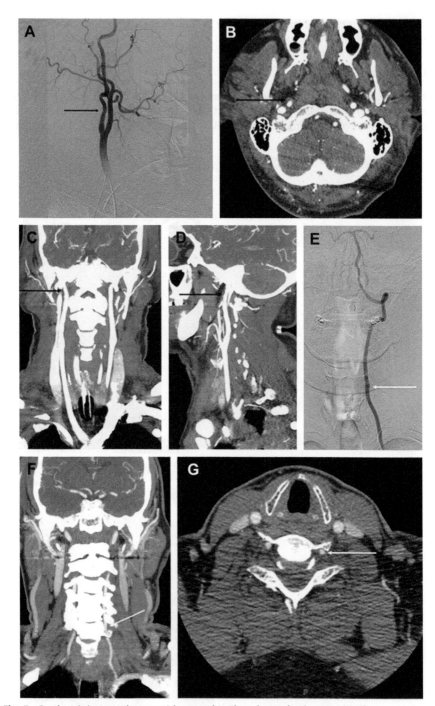

Fig. 5. Grade 1 injury to the carotid artery (*A–D*) and vertebral artery (*E–G*).

description of the injury but also to define stroke risk by injury grade (**Box 2**). Untreated injuries have an overall stroke rate of 21% to 64%[1,10,11]; CAIs have increasing stroke rate by increasing grade, whereas VAIs tend to have a more consistent stroke rate of approximately 20% for all grades of injury (**Table 1**).[2] When reviewing a patient's CTA or angiogram, recognition of normal vasculature is important (**Fig. 4**). A grade I injury is an intimal irregularity or dissection with less than 25% luminal narrowing (**Fig. 5**). Grade 2 injuries are dissections or intramural hematomas with greater than or equal to 25% luminal narrowing, intraluminal clot, or a visible intimal flap (**Fig. 6**). Pseudoaneurysms are defined as a grade 3 injury (**Fig. 7**). A complete occlusion is grade 4 injury (**Fig. 8**), and transection with active extravasation is grade 5 injury (**Fig. 9**).

TIMING OF IMAGING

All patients with indications for screening, and no contraindications to antithrombotic therapy, undergo imaging as soon as possible. For patients who do not undergo CTA of the neck on initial trauma imaging, repeat imaging should be performed as soon as possible. In labile patients, or those at risk for contrast-induced nephropathy, one may delay imaging if the patient has a contraindication to antithrombotics (intracranial hemorrhage, ongoing bleeding, high-grade solid organ injury); identification of an injury when treatment cannot be instituted is not paramount.

Patients with identified BCVIs undergo repeat imaging 7 to 10 days after their initial diagnostic study. The importance of follow-up imaging is particularly salient in patients

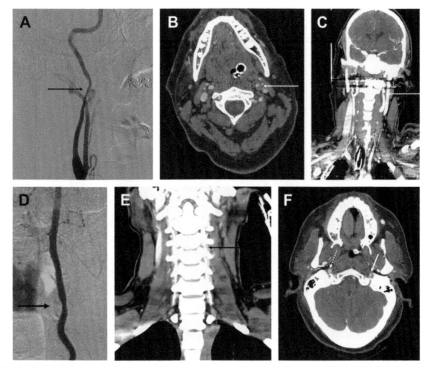

Fig. 6. Grade 2 injury to the carotid artery (*A–C*) and vertebral artery (*D–F*), with luminal narrowing greater than 25%. (*E, F*) Two different patients: normal caliber right vert (*dashed arrow in F*) and narrowed lumen of left vertebral artery (*solid arrow in F*).

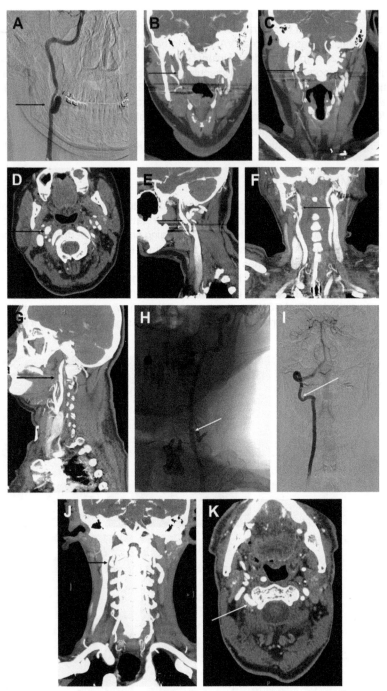

Fig. 7. Pseudoaneurysms of the carotid (*A–G*) and vertebral (*H–K*) artery are classified as grade 3 injuries.

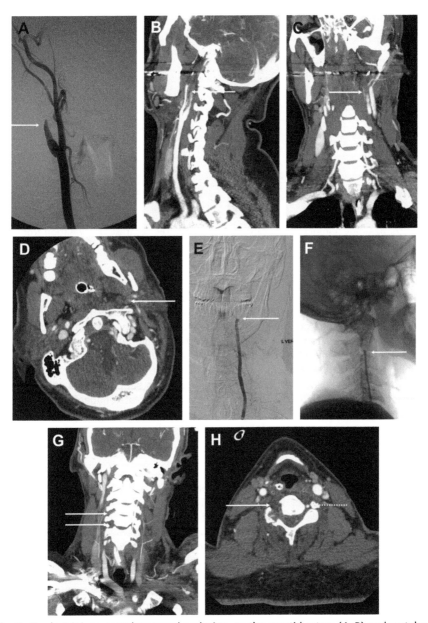

Fig. 8. Grade 4 injury, complete vessel occlusion, to the carotid artery (*A–D*) and vertebral artery (*E–H*). (*C*) Occluded left carotid artery with contrast fading out at the tip of the arrow; contrast within the internal jugular vein is evident just lateral to this. (*D*) Occluded left carotid artery with no contrast seen at the tip of the arrow. (*G*) Occluded right vertebral artery with no contrast seen within the foramen transversarium. (*H*) Occluded right vertebral artery with no contrast seen in the foramen transversarium (*solid arrow*) with a normal appearing left vertebral artery (*dashed arrow*).

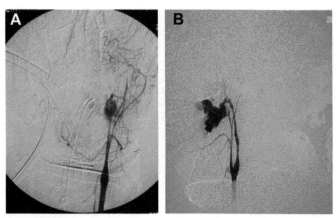

Fig. 9. (*A*, *B*) Grade 5 injury of the carotid artery with free contrast extravasation from the transected vessel.

with grade 1 injuries; more than half of grade 1 injuries completely heal, allowing cessation of antithrombotic therapy.[1,2] Conversely, less than 10% of all grade 2, 3, and 4 injuries heal, with injury progression rates of approximately 12% for all treated BCVIs.[1] Some investigators have advocated an endovascular approach to pseudoaneurysms,[43] hence supporting the use of repeat angiography to diagnose such lesions. The authors' most recent evaluation of endovascular stents in patients with postinjury BCVIs, however, suggests that antithrombotic therapy remains the gold standard treatment.[9] However, other investigators have supported the use of endovascular techniques with appropriate postprocedure antiplatelet agents.[12,44] Patients with carotid or vertebral artery occlusions may not require reimaging, as approximately 80% show no change on follow-up imaging.[1,2]

TREATMENT OF BCVIs

After the recognition that BCVIs were responsible for patients' adverse neurologic events, treatment modalities were debated. The vast majority of these lesions occur in surgically inaccessible areas of the blood vessels, either high within the carotid canal at the base of the skull or within the foramen transversarium. Such a location makes the standard vascular repair approaches, including reconstruction or thrombectomy, challenging if not impossible. Initial therapy for BCVIs was based on anecdotal reports of neurologic improvement with heparinization in patients suffering stroke related to BCVIs.[6,7,9] Subsequently, intravenous heparin was thought to be the treatment of choice for those asymptomatic patients with blunt injuries,[2,4] with a modified protocol to reduce the incidence of bleeding in multisystem trauma patients.[10,19] As a result of the ease of administration, the initiation of antiplatelet agents gained favor.[2,21,45] Although the optimal regimen remains unanswered, there seems to be equivalence between the 2 therapies.[1,2,4,5] Which therapeutic agent is used, must continue to be evaluated in prospective studies. With an attendant permanent neurologic morbidity rate up to 80% and mortality rate up to 40%,[20,46,47] prompt treatment of diagnosed injuries is critical. Patients who are diagnosed early and treated with antithrombotics almost universally avoid stroke.[1,4,5] After initiation of antithrombotics, treatment is empirically continued for 6 months. Comprehensive long-term follow-up beyond the acute hospitalization has not been reported in the literature, as is true in most trauma population studies. The Memphis group has the longest follow-up of patients with CAIs,[44] but this seems to be a selected group. Therefore, whether these injuries heal or persist over the lifetime of the patient is unknown.

SUMMARY

Screening, diagnostic imaging, and treatment of BCVIs have evolved over the past 3 decades. Currently, protocols exist for screening based on injury mechanism and associated injuries. Prompt initiation of antithrombotic therapy after identification of injuries in asymptomatic patients reduces the incidence of stroke. Surgeons caring for the multiply injured should screen for carotid and vertebral artery injuries in high-risk patients.

REFERENCES

1. Cothren CC, Biffl WL, Moore EE, et al. Treatment for blunt cerebrovascular injuries: equivalence of anticoagulation and antiplatelet agents. Arch Surg 2009;44:685–90.
2. Biffl WL, Ray CE Jr, Moore EE, et al. Treatment-related outcomes from blunt cerebrovascular injuries: importance of routine follow-up arteriography. Ann Surg 2002;235(5):699–706 [discussion: 706–7].
3. Cothren CC, Moore EE, Ray CE, et al. Screening for blunt cerebrovascular injuries is cost effective. Am J Surg 2005;190:845–9.
4. Miller PR, Fabian TC, Croce MA, et al. Prospective screening for blunt cerebrovascular injuries: analysis of diagnostic modalities and outcomes. Ann Surg 2002;236:386–95.
5. Cothren CC, Moore EE, Biffl WL, et al. Anticoagulation remains the gold standard therapy for blunt carotid injuries to reduce stroke rate. Arch Surg 2004;139:540–6.
6. Cogbill TH, Moore EE, Meissner M, et al. The spectrum of blunt injury to the carotid artery: a multicenter perspective. J Trauma 1994;37:473–9.
7. Davis JW, Holbrook TL, Hoyt DB, et al. Blunt carotid artery dissection: incidence, associated injuries, screening, and treatment. J Trauma 1990;30:1514.
8. Anson J, Crowell RM. Cervicocranial arterial dissection. Neurosurgery 1991; 29(1):89–96.
9. Fabian TC, Patton JH Jr, Croce MA, et al. Blunt carotid injury: importance of early diagnosis and anticoagulant therapy. Ann Surg 1996;223:513.
10. Biffl WL, Moore EE, Ryu RK, et al. The unrecognized epidemic of blunt carotid arterial injuries: early diagnosis improves neurologic outcome. Ann Surg 1998; 228:462.
11. Miller PR, Fabian TC, Bee TK, et al. Blunt cerebrovascular injuries: diagnosis and treatment. J Trauma 2001;51(2):279–85.
12. Stein DM, Boswell S, Sliker CW, et al. Blunt cerebrovascular injuries: does treatment always matter? J Trauma 2009;66(1):132–43.
13. Crissey MM, Bernstein EF. Delayed presentation of carotid intimal tear following blunt craniocervical trauma. Surgery 1974;75(4):543–9.
14. Batzdorf U, Bentson JR, Machleder HI. Blunt trauma to the high cervical carotid artery. Neurosurgery 1979;5(2):195–201.
15. Perry MO, Snyder WH, Thal ER. Carotid artery injuries caused by blunt trauma. Ann Surg 1980;192(1):74–7.
16. Dragon R, Saranchak H, Lakin P, et al. Blunt injuries to the carotid and vertebral arteries. Am J Surg 1981;141(4):497–500.

17. Welling RE, Saul TG, Tew JM Jr, et al. Management of blunt injury to the internal carotid artery. J Trauma 1987;27(11):1221–6.
18. Mokri B, Piepgras DG, Houser OW. Traumatic dissections of the extracrianial internal carotid artery. J Neurosurg 1988;68(2):189–97.
19. Biffl WL, Moore EE, Offner PJ, et al. Blunt carotid arterial injuries: implications of a new grading scale. J Trauma 1999;47(5):845–53.
20. Krajewski LP, Hertzer NR. Blunt carotid artery trauma: report of two cases and review of the literature. Ann Surg 1980;191(3):341–6.
21. Fabian TC, George SM Jr, Croce MA, et al. Carotid artery trauma: management based on mechanism of injury. J Trauma 1990;30(8):953–61.
22. Parikh AA, Luchette FA, Valente JF, et al. Blunt carotid artery injuries. J Am Coll Surg 1997;185(1):80–6.
23. Mayberry JC, Brown CV, Mullins RJ, et al. Blunt carotid artery injury: the futility of aggressive screening and diagnosis. Arch Surg 2004;139(6):609–12.
24. Biffl WL, Cothren CC, Moore EE, et al. Western Trauma Association critical decisions in trauma: screening for and treatment of blunt cerebrovascular injuries. J Trauma 2009;67(6):1150–3.
25. Bromberg WJ, Collier BC, Diebel LN, et al. Blunt cerebrovascular injury practice management guidelines: the eastern association for the surgery of trauma. J Trauma 2010;68(2):471–7.
26. Biffl WL, Moore EE, Offner PJ, et al. Optimizing screening for blunt cerebrovascular injuries. Am J Surg 1999;178:517–22.
27. Cothren CC, Moore EE, Biffl WL, et al. Cervical spine fracture patterns predictive of blunt vertebral artery injury. J Trauma 2003;55:811–3.
28. Biffl WL, Egglin T, Benedetto B, et al. Sixteen-slice computed tomographic angiography is a reliable noninvasive screening test for clinically significant blunt cerebrovascular injuries. J Trauma 2006;60:745–51.
29. Mutze S, Rademacher G, Matthes G, et al. Blunt cerebrovascular injury in patients with blunt multiple trauma: diagnostic accuracy of duplex doppler US and early CT angiography. Radiology 2005;237:884–92.
30. Friedman D, Flanders A, Thomas C, et al. Vertebral artery injury after acute cervical spine trauma: rate of occurrence as detected by MR angiography and assessment of clinical consequences. AJR Am J Roentgenol 1995;164:443–7.
31. Bok APL, Peter JC. Carotid and vertebral artery occlusion after blunt cervical injury: the role of MR angiography in early diagnosis. J Trauma 1996;40:968–72.
32. Weller SJ, Rossitch EJR, Malek AM. Detection of vertebral artery injury after cervical spine trauma using magnetic resonance angiography. J Trauma 1999;46:660–6.
33. Biffl WL, Ray CE Jr, Moore EE, et al. Noninvasive diagnosis of blunt cerebrovascular injuries: a preliminary report. J Trauma 2002;53:850–6.
34. Levy C, Laissy JP, Raveau V, et al. Carotid and vertebral artery dissections: three-dimensional time-of-flight MR angiography and MR imaging versus conventional angiography. Radiology 1994;190:97–103.
35. Berne JD, Reuland KS, Villarreal DH, et al. Sixteen-slice multi-detector computed tomographic angiography improves the accuracy of screening for blunt cerebrovascular injury. J Trauma 2006;60:1204–9.
36. Bub LD, Hollingworth W, Jarvik JG, et al. Screening for blunt cerebrovascular injury: evaluating the accuracy of multidetector computed tomographic angiography. J Trauma 2005;59:691–7.
37. Schneidereit NP, Simons R, Nicolau S, et al. Utility of screening for blunt vascular neck injuries with computed tomographic angiography. J Trauma 2006;60:209–16.

38. Eastman AL, Chason DP, Perez CL, et al. Computed tomographic angiography for the diagnosis of blunt cervical vascular injury: is it ready for primetime? J Trauma 2006;60:925–9.

39. Utter GH, Hollingworth W, Hallam DK, et al. Sixteen-slice CT angiography in patients with suspected blunt carotid and vertebral artery injuries. J Am Coll Surg 2006;203:838–48.

40. Malhotra AK, Camacho M, Ivatury RR, et al. Computed tomographic angiography for the diagnosis of blunt carotid/vertebral artery injury: a note of caution. Ann Surg 2007;246:632–43.

41. Goodwin RB, Beery PR, Dorbish RJ, et al. Computed tomographic angiography versus conventional angiography for the diagnosis of blunt cerebrovascular injury in trauma patients. J Trauma 2009;67:1046–50.

42. Fakhry SM, Aldaghlas TA, Robinson L, et al. Computed tomographic angiography: false positives in the diagnosis of blunt cerebrovascular injuries. AAST Annual Meeting presentation. Pittsburgh PA, October 2009.

43. Coldwell DM, Novak Z, Ryu RK, et al. Treatment of posttraumatic internal carotid arterial pseudoaneurysms with endovascular stents. J Trauma 2000;48(3):470–2.

44. Edwards NM, Fabian TC, Claridge JA, et al. Antithrombotic therapy and endovascular stents are effective treatment for blunt carotid injuries: results from longterm follow-up. J Am Coll Surg 2007;5:1007–14.

45. Wahl WL, Brandt MM, Thompson BG, et al. Antiplatelet therapy: an alternative to heparin for blunt carotid injury. J Trauma 2002;52:896–901.

46. Martin RF, Eldrup-Jorgensen J, Clark DE, et al. Blunt trauma to the carotid arteries. J Vasc Surg 1991;14:789–95.

47. Fakhry SM, Jaques PF, Proctor HJ. Cervical vessel injury after blunt trauma. J Vasc Surg 1988;8(4):501–8.

Current Use of CT in the Evaluation and Management of Injured Patients

David J. Milia, MD*, Karen Brasel, MD, MPH

KEYWORDS

• Computed axial tomography • CT scan • Trauma

From its beginnings as a time consuming and an inefficient imaging modality with no place in the evaluation of traumatically injured patients, computed axial tomographic (CT) scanners have evolved to yield rapid, highly sensitive images, revolutionizing trauma management protocols. With utility in blunt and penetrating traumas, new applications for this modality are continually being described.

CT FUNDAMENTALS
Technology

The use of CT in blunt trauma was originally reported in the 1980s.[1–3] Long acquisition times and poor resolution limited its use. Since then, newer technology has allowed CT to contribute more and more to the evaluation of injured patients. The 2 biggest advances in CT imaging have been helical scanning and the use of multidetector imaging. Helical scanning, whereby data acquisition occurs simultaneously with patient positioning has had numerous positive effects. The entire series of images can be obtained in 20 to 30 seconds. This property has not only led to reduced scan times and increased resolution but also led to greatly decreased volume of contrast material needed for the same degree of vessel opacification.

The first multidetector CT (MDCT) scanner was developed in 1998. This machine used a 4-slice detector array. Since then, 16-, 32-, and 64- slice MDCTs, and recently, 128- and 256-slice MDCTs are available.[4] Combined with helical scanning, MDCT reduces the scan time further. This reduction allows imaging with a thinner collimation (1–2 mm), yielding higher resolution images more rapidly with reduction of motion artifact from patient movement and cardiac activity. The use of MDCT has allowed for more flexibility in image reformatting and applications such as CT angiography.

The authors have nothing to disclose.
Division of Trauma and Critical Care, Medical College of Wisconsin, 9200 West Wisconsin Avenue, Milwaukee, WI 53226, USA
* Corresponding author.
E-mail address: dmilia@mcw.edu

Surg Clin N Am 91 (2011) 233–248
doi:10.1016/j.suc.2010.10.018
0039-6109/11/$ – see front matter © 2011 Elsevier Inc. All rights reserved.

Contrast

Contrast-induced nephropathy is the third leading cause of hospital-acquired renal failure in the United States.[5] Elderly patients with chronic kidney disease, diabetes, and congestive heart failure are at increased risk. Combined with the hypovolemic state of trauma and the concurrent use of nephrotoxic drugs, elderly trauma patients are thought to be at a very high risk of contrast nephropathy.[6] A study of more than 1000 elderly (age>55 years) trauma patients, however, did not support this fact. There was no statistical difference in the incidence of acute kidney injury (AKI) between patients receiving intravenous contrast and those not receiving it. Approximately 2% of patients in each arm developed AKI. However, the development of AKI was an independent predictor of mortality. These data are consistent with those from studies of cardiac catheterization. Data cite a 1% to 6% incidence in AKI in unselected populations.[7,8] Up to 70% of patients may experience a transient increase in serum creatinine (SCr) levels; however, most of these patients will not develop AKI.[9] High-risk groups including patients with diabetes mellitus and chronic renal insufficiency (SCr>2 mg/dL) have reported rates of AKI up to 50%.[10,11]

Radiation

Patients presenting to the emergency department, trauma patients, and critically ill patients are some of the most frequently imaged patients. The cumulative effective dose for critically ill patients in one study was 30 times the annual radiation dose for the US general population.[12] Tien and colleagues[13] performed a prospective study using dosimeters placed on trauma patients to calculate their exposure. The investigators found the mean dose to be 22.7 mSv (average background for the general US population was 2.4 mSv). They noted that the exposure was not evenly distributed, with the majority of the exposure centering on the neck and thyroid (58.5 mSv). Almost one-fourth of the patients had a greater than 100 mSv exposure to the thyroid (mean 168 mSv for this group), the level above which rates of thyroid cancer increase significantly. The other key finding from this study was that dose estimates predicted cumulative doses to be 25% less than the actual measured doses received by the patients.[13]

The 2 basic radiation-lowering strategies are decreasing the number of studies performed and lowering the ionizing radiation delivered in any given study. Increasing the MDCT from 4 to 16 slice and above has been shown to significantly reduce radiation exposure.[14] In one study on the use of CT scan for diagnosing appendicitis, reducing the energy from 100 mA to 30 mA resulted in no change in the diagnostic utility. The effective reduction in radiation dose to females and males was 5.2 to 1.4 mSv and 7.1 mSv to 2.2 mSv, respectively.[15] Other techniques, such as an adaptive statistical iterative reconstruction (ASIR) algorithm, take advantage of postprocessing software to perform improved noise reduction. Radiation dose reduction is often limited by increases in background noise. ASIR has allowed more than 60% reduction in radiation doses without significant loss in image quality. At present, the only disadvantage of ASIR is its increased processing time (about 30%); however, it is likely that this will be reduced with ongoing improvements in computer software.[16]

IMAGING PROTOCOLS

MDCT has gained an ever-increasing role in evaluating hemodynamically normal patients sustaining traumatic injury causing intra-abdominal hemorrhage. The role of physical examination alone has been studied, and although the negative predictive value is high in patients with a reliable physical examination, a large percentage of patients presenting to the trauma room do not have a reliable examination.[17] Multiple strategies have been developed to help decide which patients will benefit most from CT examinations. Whereas some advocate the liberal use of CT for blunt trauma,[18] others think that a more selective approach is safe and, at the same time, will reduce radiation risk, reduce cost, and expedite care.[19]

An approach using liberal or routine abdominal CT scans finds unexpected injuries in 7.1% to 38% of patients.[19–21] Those advocating this approach cite subsequent changes in management that occur in 11% to 26% of these patients. However, in all studies, most management changes affect disposition and would not likely have affected outcome. Additional procedures are reported in less than 1% of the patients.

An algorithm for selection of patients using physiologic parameters instead of mechanistic ones has been developed for selective approach to the use of abdominal CT (**Fig. 1**). Through multivariate analysis, an algorithm using 9 variables from the physical examination, focused assessment with sonography for trauma (FAST), lab analysis, and chest radiographs was created with a sensitivity of 97%. This algorithm reduces the need for CT over routine scanning by 22% without any compromise in patient safety.[22]

A similar controversy exists with respect to CT of the chest. A routine mechanism-based protocol will find more injuries than a more selective approach. To what level these injuries affect care and, more importantly, outcome is currently debated. More traumatic findings occur in the routine group, with one group showing that these lead to management changes in 7%.[18] As with the abdominal CT studies, most management decisions affected only disposition. There was an additional bronchoscopy, 6 additional chest tube insertions/manipulations, and 2 aortic repairs. It is difficult to tell from the study what effect these measures had on patient outcomes.

Most clinically relevant traumatic chest injuries can be diagnosed using a more selective approach. Age greater than 55 years; abnormal chest physical examination; altered level of consciousness; abnormal examination of thoracic spine; abnormalities in chest, pelvis, or thoracic spine radiograph, abdominal FAST; base deficit greater than 3 mmol/L, and hemoglobin levels less than 6 mmol/L have been suggested as parameters to guide selective use of chest CT.[19] When chest CT was omitted in those with none of the above-mentioned criteria, 13% of injuries were missed, with only 2% being clinically relevant. Others have suggested patients with chest wall tenderness and those with abnormal respiratory effort in addition to an abnormal chest radiograph are candidates for chest CT.[20]

SPECIFIC INJURIES
Abdomen

Originally published in 1988, the American Association for the Surgery of Trauma (AAST) has devised a set of organ injury scales (OISs). Originally graded during operative exploration, the solid organ injury scale has now been defined by radiological (specifically CT) criteria. The first iteration of this report (OIS I for Spleen, Liver, and Kidney) recently underwent validation using entries into the National Trauma Data Bank. This analysis showed successful nonoperative management of spleen, liver, and kidney injuries in 73%, 85%, and 89%, respectively, regardless of the injury grade. Operative intervention did increase with increasing grade, with a notably decreased rate of operative intervention for patients with isolated solid organ injury.

Spleen

Approximately 60% to 80% of patients with blunt splenic injury are currently managed nonoperatively with a success rate approaching 95%.[21,23,24] Early inclusion criteria for

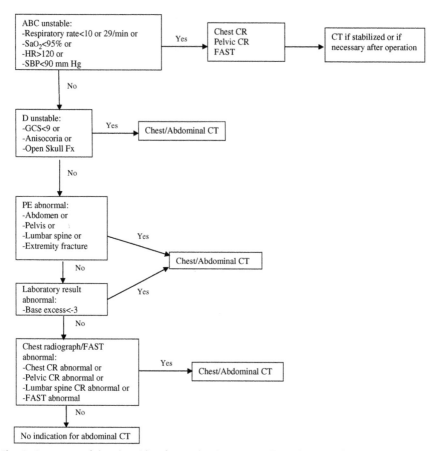

Fig. 1. Summary of the algorithm for a selective approach to abdominal CT scanning as outlined by Deunk and colleagues[22] Inclusion of further imaging (head and cervical spine) is not addressed in this approach. Definitions of abnormal physical examination and radiographic findings are addressed in detail in the original publication. A, airway; B, breathing; C, circulation; CR, conventional radiography; D, disability; FAST, focused assessment with sonography for trauma; Fx, fracture; GCS, Glasgow Coma Scale; HR, heart rate; PE, physical exam; Sao_2, arterial oxygen saturation; SBP, systolic blood pressure. (*Adapted from* Deunk J, Brink M, Dekker H, et al. Predictors for the selection of patients for abdominal CT after blunt trauma; a proposal for a diagnostic algorithm. Ann Surg 2010;251: 518; with permission.)

nonoperative management mandated hemodynamic stability and absence of other associated operative injuries. Failure of nonoperative management correlates with radiological grade of injury and presence of active extravasation (**Fig. 2**).[25] The role of nonoperative management has been extended at some institutions to include transient responders to fluid resuscitation.[26] Critics of this management scheme warn that this practice pattern necessitates timely response by interventional radiology and may prolong the treatment and increase transfusion requirements of patients with a surgically correctable disease.

Hemodynamically normal patients with intraparenchymal splenic pseudoaneurysm or arteriovenous fistula are candidates for arterial embolization. Routine CT surveillance of splenic injury looking for pseudoaneurysm or arteriovenous fistula is debated.[27–29] In one study by Weinberg, splenic pseudoaneurysm was noted in 7%

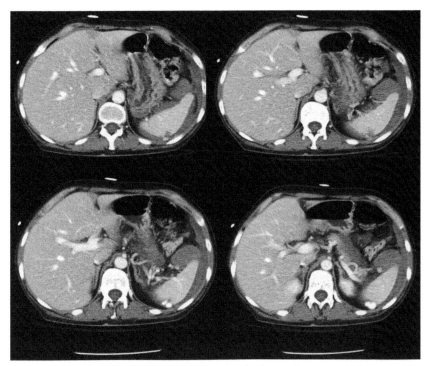

Fig. 2. CT images of a 23-year-old man involved in a high-speed motor vehicle crash. CT scan showing splenic laceration with active contrast extravasation (*blush*).

of patients studied 24 to 48 hours after initial diagnosis. One quarter of these patients had grade I or II injuries, indicating that even patients with low-grade splenic injuries are at risk for complications of nonoperative management.

Liver

Similar to splenic injuries, most blunt hepatic injuries are managed nonoperatively. Most studies document successful nonoperative management rates greater than 90%.[30–34] Hepatic abscess, biloma, delayed hemorrhage, and hemobilia are recognized complications of hepatic trauma.

Fang and colleagues noted, by retrospective review, that patients with intraperitoneal contrast extravasation, hemoperitoneum in 6 compartments, destruction of more than 2 segments, high AAST OIS grade, laceration more than 6 cm deep, and porta hepatis involvement showed a significantly higher likelihood of needing operative intervention.[35] Large hemoperitoneum and contrast extravasation independently predicted the need for operative intervention. Angiography with embolization plays a greater role in hepatic trauma than other solid organ injuries. Angiography can be used primarily in hemodynamically normal patients with active extravasation on CT, as an adjunct to damage control laparotomy, or in the management of delayed complications (eg, hemobilia, delayed hemorrhage, arteriovenous fistula). However, the number of patients requiring therapeutic intervention may be fewer than originally thought. Early reports note therapeutic intervention in 70% to 100% of patients undergoing hepatic angiography.[36] In a study by Misselbeck and colleagues, only 40% of patients undergoing hepatic angiography required embolization.[37] Patients with active extravasation on CT scan and those exhibiting ongoing hemorrhage after an investigation for damage control had higher rates of embolization.

Although the concept of nonoperative management of blunt solid organ injury has been universally accepted, operative exploration remains the standard of care for penetrating solid organ injuries. Traditionally, CT has played a limited role in the management of penetrating injuries. Several groups have questioned this management dictum and shown that carefully selected patients with penetrating solid organ injuries can be managed nonoperatively (**Fig. 3**). Selection of these patients is largely determined by physical examination, vital signs, and findings on CT scan. Using an algorithm that included laparotomy for hemodynamic instability or suspicion of hollow viscera injury and observation for solid organ injury, this method was determined safe. Thirty-nine penetrating trauma patients with 42 injured solid organs were managed nonoperatively.[38] Of these, 2 required operative intervention without adverse consequence for delayed recognition of hollow viscus injuries. Of note, this group relied on delayed laparoscopic exploration for left-sided thoracoabdominal wounds to perform diaphragmatic evaluation and repair, if indicated. Another study from the military reported similar success, adding that physical examination and ultrasonography alone were too unreliable and that CT should be a part of the diagnostic workup if a nonoperative algorithm was going to be used.[39]

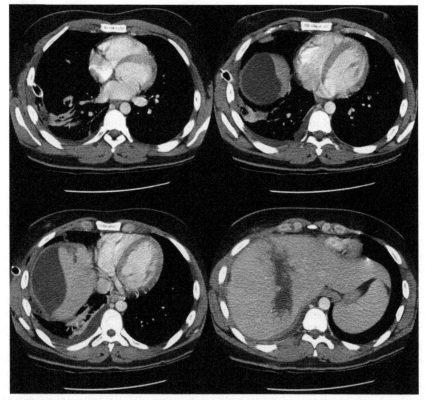

Fig. 3. Selected images from a CT scan of a patient sustaining a gunshot wound to the right upper quadrant. This patient was hemodynamically normal on presentation. Images note a liver laceration without evidence of active extravasation. This patient was managed nonoperatively.

The CT scan seems to be less useful in the evaluation of abdominal stab wounds than in the evaluation of select gunshot wounds. Recent data from the Western Trauma Association Multicenter Trials Group note that in patients sustaining anterior abdominal stab wounds (without evidence of shock or diffuse peritonitis), an evaluation scheme that includes local wound exploration and serial clinical assessments is superior to routine abdominopelvic CT scanning.[40]

Pancreas

Compared with liver and splenic injuries, isolated blunt injuries to the pancreas are rare. The estimated injury rate ranges from 0.2% to 1.3% in patients sustaining blunt trauma.[41] The focus of pancreatic injuries revolves around the suspicion for pancreatic duct injury. CT findings include frank disruption of the main pancreatic duct, peripancreatic fluid, pancreatic enlargement, or alteration of the pancreatic contour (**Fig. 4**). If there is a suspicion, follow-up imaging (CT, MR cholangiopancreatography, endoscopic retrograde cholangiopancreatography [ERCP]) may be necessary.[42] For minor distal pancreatic injuries, CT guided percutaneous drainage offers favorable outcomes. ERCP carries a high morbidity and stricture rate and should be used selectively.[43]

Kidney

Renal injuries may involve simple parenchymal injuries, injuries to the collecting system, or significant renovascular injuries to either the arterial or the venous system. Significant parenchymal injury seen on initial CT should be should be accompanied by an 8- to 10-minute delayed film to evaluate for contrast extravasation indicating damage to the collecting system. Most collecting system injuries can be managed with a combination of endoscopic and percutaneous drainage techniques.

Vascular injuries may involve branches or segmental arteries, evidenced by a wedge infarct on CT or main vessel avulsion with absent cortical enhancement or peripheral enhancement only. Distinguishing between an intimal tear and a vascular avulsion is done by noting the presence of a perirenal hematoma seen with avulsion.

Renal injuries show higher rates of successful nonoperative management than either splenic or hepatic injury. Follow-up CT scan after 24 to 48 hours rarely leads

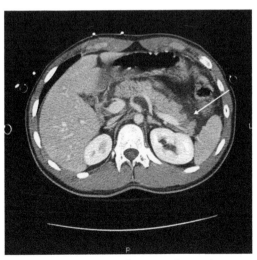

Fig. 4. CT image showing traumatic pancreatic transaction and surrounding peripancreatic edema (*arrow*).

to changes in management.[44] These investigators concluded that renovascular injuries do not warrant routine serial imaging; however, urinary extravasation may require additional imaging for optimal management.

The dictum of mandatory exploration for penetrating renal injury has long been challenged because the success rate for nonoperative management of these patients approaches 50%.[45–47] About 40% of gunshot injuries to the kidney in carefully selected patients (hemodynamically normal, absence of hilar injury) can be managed without operative exploration.[38]

Bowel and Mesentery

Bowel and associated mesenteric injuries are noted in approximately 5% of patients sustaining blunt abdominal trauma (**Fig. 5**).[48] Whereas it is universally accepted that CT excels in the diagnosis of solid organ injury, some controversy exists surrounding its role in hollow viscus injury. The advent of helical and MDCT scanning may change this situation. CT findings consistent with bowel injury include extraluminal air, extraluminal oral contrast (if administered), and moderate (4–5 consecutive CT images) to large (>6 consecutive CT cuts) volumes of free intraperitoneal fluid in the absence of solid organ injury or pelvic fracture. Using these criteria, the sensitivity of diagnosing surgically significant bowel trauma has been reported to be as high as 94% and the accuracy and positive predictive value have been reported to be 86% and 90%, respectively.[49]

CT is slightly less favorable in diagnosing clinically significant mesenteric injuries. Clinically significant mesenteric findings are active extravasation and bowel wall thickening associated with mesenteric hematoma. Mesenteric hematoma alone is not typically regarded as a surgically significant finding. Using similar criteria, the sensitivity of MDCT for detection of mesenteric injury is 96%; however, its use in determining clinically significant findings was only 75%.[50]

Chest

Thoracic aorta

Classically described as a result of significant deceleration, traumatic aortic injury accounts for as many as 20% of fatalities in blunt chest trauma (**Fig. 6**). Estimates suggest that 85% of patients will die immediately. Of the survivors, historical estimates suggest that if left untreated, up to one-third will die within 6 hours of injury and most of

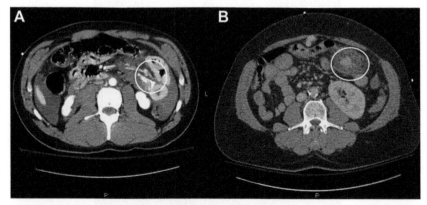

Fig. 5. (*A, B*) Axial sections representing mesenteric injury in a patient sustaining blunt injury from a motor vehicle crash. Both figures note bleeding in the mesentery. (*A*) Image shows a prominent blush in the mesentery of the left colon.

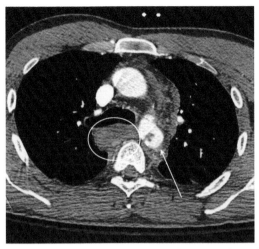

Fig. 6. Axial CT image showing traumatic aortic injury (*arrow*) with mediastinal hematoma (*circle*).

the remaining will die within 4 months.[51] With the increasing sensitivity of CT scans, these numbers have been challenged. Plain radiograph of the chest has a sensitivity greater than 90% in detecting mediastinal hemorrhage and is used as a screening test to determine the need for further evaluation. Classic chest radiograph findings of mediastinal hemorrhage are well documented (**Fig. 7**). The most useful of these findings are obliteration of the aortic knob and mediastinal widening (sensitivity 53%–100% and 81%–100%, specificity 21%–55% and 10%–60%; respectively). Although the exact definition of mediastinal widening has been debated, data support the use of a subjective assessment as an adequate screening measure.[52,53] CT has virtually replaced traditional aortography and transesophageal echocardiography as the gold standard for diagnosis, which was evidenced in a comparison study between 2 similar AAST multicenter prospective studies separated by a decade (1997 and 2007) examining blunt aortic injury.[54] The 2007 study noted a near complete elimination of conventional angiography and TEE, with nearly all patients undergoing CT angiography.

Chest wall
The presence and number of rib fractures on plain radiograph has been used both as a marker for other thoracic injuries as well as an independent predictor of mortality. Additional data suggest that the presence of more than 3 fractured ribs on a radiograph should prompt transfer to a trauma center.[55] These data, however, are not likely applicable to rib fractures diagnosed by CT alone. Thoracic CT is more sensitive than chest radiograph for the detection of fractured ribs and, at the same time, provides detailed information as to the anatomic displacement and number of ribs fractured. Data suggest that although CT has greater sensitivity and anatomic definition, injuries noted on chest radiographs may be a better marker for pulmonary complications.[56] Although outcomes and clinical utility of rib fixation are still being studied, 3-dimensional reconstruction of the thoracic cage may assist in operative planning (**Fig. 8**).

Diaphragm
Blunt diaphragmatic rupture is a rare injury with an incidence reported between 0.8% and 8% in the literature. CT diagnosis has historically been difficult, mainly because of the horizontal orientation of the diaphragm. Helical scanning and the use of MDCTs

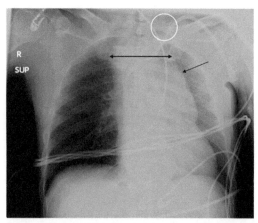

Fig. 7. Chest radiograph with findings of aortic injury. Note the left-sided hemothorax, widened mediastinum (*double-sided arrow*), loss of aortic knob (*single-sided arrow*), and fracture of the first rib (*circle*).

have assisted in the radiographic diagnosis. Using 3- to 5-mm axial sections with 3-dimensional volume-rendered images and multiplanar reconstructions has increased the sensitivity and specificity to 71% and 100%, respectively. Four radiographic signs of diaphragmatic rupture have been described,[57,58] including (1) discontinuity of the hemidiaphragm with a gap in the muscle, (2) herniation of intra-abdominal viscera, (3) rim sign, represented by edges of rupture wrapped around viscera, and (4) dependent viscera sign,[59] which is the loss of posterior support by the diaphragm allowing the involved viscera to lie directly on the posterior ribs.

INCIDENTAL FINDINGS
Masses and Follow-up

With submillimeter resolution and increasing numbers of scans performed, the rate of incidental radiographic findings has increased dramatically. Rates of incidental

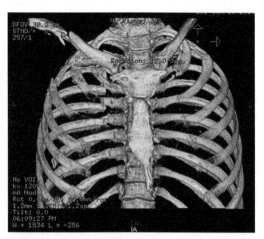

Fig. 8. A 3-dimensional reconstruction of the thoracic cavity. This image shows multiple right-sided rib fractures with significant overlap. This reconstruction assisted in the preoperative planning of this patient's rib fixation.

findings have been estimated between 10% and 50%.[60–62] Whereas some have argued that these findings place undue stress on an already overburdened medical system, studies have shown that a significant portion of these incidental findings represent potentially life-threatening diagnoses. In one series of incidental thyroid masses, out of more than 200 thyroid masses discovered, 118 were biopsied, revealing a 22% malignancy rate. In a series of incidentally discovered adrenal masses, the rate of malignancy for masses greater than 3 cm was nearly 30%.

More recent studies have classified these findings according to the urgency in which they need to be addressed. Among the most common lesions needing attention during admission include pulmonary nodules (7%), adrenal lesions (4%), mediastinal lymphadenopathy (6%), hepatic lesions (4%), and thyroid nodules (3%). Other findings that are less likely to require timely workup include renal/hepatic cysts, inguinal/ventral hernias, and diverticular disease.[63]

Ensuring proper follow-up of these incidental findings has become extremely important, although often difficult in the trauma population. Retrospective chart studies have found that only 49% of patients with clinically significant incidental findings had documented follow-up for these diagnoses.[64] There was no comment on the outcome of these patients and therefore the risks of inadequate follow-up.

Pulmonary Embolus

The incidence of asymptomatic pulmonary embolus (PE) in moderately to severely injured patients is approximately 25%. In 90 asymptomatic trauma patients studied by Schultz and colleagues, 22 had demonstrable clot burden on helical CT of the chest (performed between trauma days 3–7).[65] The emboli in 2 of these patients were present on the presenting trauma CT. Those with PE were older, more severely injured patients. There was no difference in the rate of prophylactic anticoagulation.

The management of patients with small asymptomatic pulmonary emboli is debated. The American College of Chest Physicians (ACCP) guidelines recommend short-term anticoagulation for nonmassive PE.[66] Others, however, think that observation alone is sufficient in asymptomatic patients with minor clot burden. In the aforementioned study, those with minor clot burden (Miller Score 0.25–2.0) were managed expectantly, not placed on systemic anticoagulation, and had no adverse outcomes. Patients with major clot burden (Miller score>4.25) were systemically anticoagulated according to the ACCP guidelines.

Occult Pneumothorax and Hemothorax

Occult pneumothorax (OPTX) is defined as pneumothorax (PTX) diagnosed by CT scan not originally suspected by clinical examination or supine plain film radiograph (**Fig. 9**). According to trauma registries, the incidence is around 5%. The actual incidence, however, varies depending on the frequency with which CTs are obtained and how the plain films are interpreted. Rates of OPTX in trauma patients undergoing CT scans of the chest approach 15%. Studies using radiologist interpretation show far lower incidences than studies with trauma surgeon interpretation (as high as 76%). Subtle radiographic signs, such as the deep sulcus sign, are quoted as the main reasons for missing PTX on initial plain films.

Management of OPTX is controversial, and differences are likely related to physician perceptions and historical dogma rather than to data. Rates of tube thoracostomy between overt and occult PTX vary greatly. One study cites more than 60% chest tube insertion rate for overt PTX as compared with a 30% insertion rate for OPTX, irrespective of patient hemodynamics or respiratory symptoms.[67] Despite data to the contrary, this is thought to be caused by the perception that occult PTXs represent

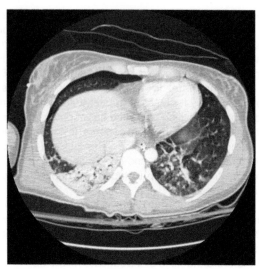

Fig. 9. Contrast-enhanced CT image showing a small anterior PTX. This patient was asymptomatic, and this finding was not evident on chest radiograph.

lesser lung collapses than overt PTXs. This perception has been questioned, and in one study using CT to compare overt and occult PTXs, no statistical difference in size of collapse was noted.[68]

Occult hemothoraces are similarly defined, with rates estimated between 20% and 30%.[69,70] As in OPTX, the true incidence of occult hemothorax is difficult to estimate. Although there is much less information on the natural history and appropriate management, one study noted that patients successfully managed expectantly had smaller hemothroaces (<2 cm) and lower injury severity scores.[71]

SUMMARY

There is no question that CT scanners have changed the way injured patients are evaluated and managed. As resolution is further increased and acquisition times are decreased, more applications will likely be described. It is important, however, to remember no imaging modality can replace sound surgical judgment. Increasing resolution will likely yield even more findings. More research is necessary to understand the clinical significance of these findings. Throughout their lifetime, patients are undergoing increasing numbers of radiological evaluations. As physicians, it is imperative to remember the longitudinal effects of ionizing radiation and subject the patients to only those studies that will have a significant effect on their outcome.

REFERENCES

1. Fabian TC, Mangiante EC, White TJ, et al. A prospective study of 91 patients undergoing both computed tomography and peritoneal lavage following blunt trauma. J Trauma 1986;26:602–8.
2. Kearney PA Jr, Vahey T, Burney RE, et al. Computed tomography and diagnostic peritoneal lavage in blunt abdominal trauma: their combined role. Arch Surg 1989;124:344–7.
3. Federle MP. Computed tomography in blunt abdominal trauma. Radiol Clin North Am 1983;21:461–75.

4. Rogalla P, Kloeters C, Hein P. CT technology overview: 64-slice and beyond. Radiol Clin North Am 2009;47:1–11.
5. Venkataraman R. Can we prevent acute kidney injury? Crit Care Med 2008;36: S166–71.
6. Toprak O. Risk markers for contrast-induced nephropathy. Am J Med Sci 2007; 334:283–90.
7. Mehran R, Nikolsky E. Contrast-induced nephropathy: definition, epidemiology, and patients at risk. Kidney Int 2006;69:S11–5.
8. McCullough PA, Wolyn R, Rocher LL, et al. Acute renal failure after coronary intervention: incidence, risk factors, and relationship to mortality. Am J Med 1997; 103(5):368–75.
9. Davidson CJ, Hlatky M, Morris KG, et al. Cardiovascular and renal toxicity of a nonionic radiographic contrast agent after cardiac catheterization: a prospective trial. Ann Intern Med 1989;110:119–24.
10. Dangas G, Iakovou I, Nikolsky E, et al. Contrast-induced nephropathy after percutaneous coronary interventions in relation to chronic kidney disease and hemodynamic variables. Am J Cardiol 2005;95:13–9.
11. Guitterez N, Diaz A, Timmis GC, et al. Determinants of serum creatinine trajectory in acute contrast nephropathy. J Interv Cardiol 2002;15:349–54.
12. Kim P, Gracias V, Maidment A, et al. Cumulative radiation dose caused by radiologic studies in critically ill trauma patients. J Trauma 2004;57:510–4.
13. Tien H, Tremblay L, Rizoli S, et al. Radiation exposure from diagnostic imaging in severely injured trauma patients. J Trauma 2007;62:151–6.
14. Moore W, Bonvento M, Olivieri-Fitt R. Comparison of MDCT radiation dose: a phantom study. AJR Am J Roentgenol 2006;187:498–502.
15. Keyzer C, Tack D, Maertelaer V, et al. Acute appendicitis: comparison of low-dose and standard-dose unenhanced multi–detector row CT. Radiology 2004;232(1): 164–72.
16. Silva A, Lawder H, Hara A, et al. Innovations in CT dose reduction strategy: application of the adaptive statistical iterative reconstruction algorithm. AJR Am J Roentgenol 2010;195:191–9.
17. Schurink GW, Bode PJ, van Luijt PA, et al. The value of physical examination in the diagnosis of patients with blunt abdominal trauma: a retrospective study. Injury 1997;28:261–5.
18. Brink M, Deunk J, Dekker H, et al. Added value of routine chest MDCT after blunt trauma: evaluation of additional findings and impact on patient management. AJR Am J Roentgenol 2008;190:1591–8.
19. Brink M, Deunk J, Dekker H, et al. Criteria for the selective use of chest computed tomography in blunt trauma patients. Eur Radiol 2010;20:818–28.
20. Traub M, Stevenson M, McEvoy S, et al. The use of chest computed tomography versus chest X-ray in patients with major blunt trauma. Injury Int J Care Injured 2007;38:43–7.
21. Caddeddu M, Garnett A, Al-Anezi K, et al. Management of spleen injuries in the adult trauma population: a ten year experience. Can J Surg 2006;49:386–90.
22. Deunk J, Brink M, Dekker H, et al. Predictors for the selection of patients for abdominal CT after blunt trauma; a proposal for a diagnostic algorithm. Ann Surg 2010;251:512–20.
23. Cogbill TH, Moore EE, Jurkovich GJ, et al. Nonoperative management of blunt splenic trauma: a multicenter experience. J Trauma 1989;29:1312–7.
24. Cooney R, Ku J, Cherry R, et al. Limitations of splenic angioembolization in treating blunt splenic injury. J Trauma 2005;59:926–32.

25. Rajani RR, Claridge JA, Yowler CJ, et al. Improved outcome of adult blunt splenic injury: a cohort analysis. Surgery 2006;140:625–35.
26. Hagiwara A, Fukushima H, Murata A, et al. Blunt splenic injury: usefulness of transcatheter arterial embolization in patients with a transient response to fluid resuscitation. Radiology 2005;235:57–64.
27. Lyass S, Sela T, Lebensart PD, et al. Follow-up imaging studies of blunt splenic injury: do they influence management? Isr Med Assoc J 2001;3:731–3.
28. Thaemert BC, Cogbill TC, Lambert PJ. Nonoperative management of splenic injury: are follow-up computed tomographic scans of any value? J Trauma 1997;43:748–51.
29. Allins A, Ho T, Nguyen TH, et al. Limited value of routine follow-up CT scans in nonoperative management of blunt liver and spleen injuries. Am Surg 1996;62:883–6.
30. Croce MA, Fabian TC, Menke PG, et al. Non-operative management of blunt hepatic trauma is the treatment of choice for hemodynamically stable patients. Results of a prospective trial. Ann Surg 1995;221:744–53.
31. Pachter HL, Knudson MM, Esrig B, et al. Status of non-operative management of blunt hepatic injuries in 1995: a multicenter experience with 404 patients. J Trauma 1996;40:31–8.
32. Malhotra AK, Fabian TC, Croce MA, et al. Blunt hepatic injury: a paradigm shift from operative to non-operative management in the 1990s. Ann Surg 2000;231:804–13.
33. Velmahos GC, Toutouzas K, Radin R, et al. High success with non-operative management of blunt hepatic trauma: the liver is a sturdy organ. Arch Surg 2003;138:475–80 [discussion: 480–1].
34. Christmas AB, Wilson AK, Manning B, et al. Selective management of blunt hepatic injuries including non-operative management is a safe and effective strategy. Surgery 2005;138:606–10 [discussion: 610–1].
35. Fang JF, Wong YC, Lin BC, et al. The CT risk factors for the need of operative treatment in initially hemodynamically stable patients after blunt hepatic trauma. J Trauma 2006;61(3):547–53.
36. Johnson JW, Gracias VH, Gupta R, et al. Hepatic angiography in patients undergoing damage control laparotomy. J Trauma 2002;52:1102–6.
37. Misselbeck T, Teicher E, Cipolle M, et al. Hepatic angioembolization in trauma patients: indications and complications. J Trauma 2009;67(4):769–73.
38. Demetriades D, Hadjizacharia P, Constantinou C, et al. Selective nonoperative management of penetrating abdominal solid organ injuries. Ann Surg 2006;244(4):620–8.
39. Beekley AC, Blackbourne LH, Sebesta JA, et al. Selective nonoperative management of penetrating torso injury from combat fragmentation wounds. J Trauma 2008;64(Suppl 2):S108–16.
40. Biffl B, Kaups K, Cothren C, et al. Management of patients with anterior abdominal stab wounds: a Western Trauma Association multicenter trial. J Trauma 2009;66:1294–301.
41. Buccimazza I, Thomson SR, Anderson F, et al. Isolated main pancreatic duct injuries. Spectrum and management. Am J Surg 2006;191:448–52.
42. Mullinix J, Foley D. Multidetector computed tomography and blunt thoracoabdominal trauma. J Comput Assist Tomogr 2004;28:S20–7.
43. Lin B, Liu N, Fang J, et al. Long-term results of endoscopic stent in the management of blunt major pancreatic duct injury. Surg Endosc 2006;20(10):1551–5.
44. Malcolm J, Derweesh I, Mehrazin R, et al. Nonoperative management of blunt renal trauma: is routine early follow-up imaging necessary? BMC Urol 2008;8:11.

45. Carroll PR, McAninch JW. Operative indications in penetrating renal trauma. J Trauma 1985;25:587–93.
46. Heyns CF, De Klerk DP, De Kock ML. Non-operative management of renal stab wounds. J Urol 1985;134:239–42.
47. Armenakas NA, Duckett CP, McAninch JW. Indication for non-operative management of renal stab wounds. J Urol 1994;161:768–71.
48. Peitzman AB, Arnold SA, Boone DC. Trauma manual. Pittsburgh (PA): University of Pittsburgh Press; 1994. p. 93.
49. Atri M, Hanson J, Grinblat L. Surgically important bowel and/or mesenteric injury in blunt trauma: accuracy of multidetector CT for evaluation. Radiology 2008; 249(2):524–33.
50. Killeen K, Shanmuganathan K, Poletti P, et al. Helical computed tomography of bowel and mesenteric injuries. J Trauma 2001;51(1):26–36.
51. Parmley LF, Mattingly TW, Manion TW, et al. Nonpenetrating traumatic injury of the aorta. Circulation 1958;17:1086.
52. Fisher RG, Chasen MH, Lamki N. Diagnosis of injuries of the aorta and brachiocephalic arteries caused by blunt chest trauma: CT vs aortography. AJR Am J Roentgenol 1994;162:1047–52.
53. Gundry SR, Williams S, Burney RE, et al. Indications for aortography: radiography after blunt chest trauma; a reassessment of the radiographic findings associated with traumatic rupture of the aorta. Invest Radiol 1983;18:230–7.
54. Demetriades D, Velmahos GC, Scalea TM, et al. Diagnosis and treatment of blunt thoracic aortic injuries: changing perspectives. J Trauma 2008;64(6):1415–8 [discussion: 1418–9].
55. Lee R, Bass S, Morris JJ, et al. Three or more rib fractures as an indicator for transfer to a level I trauma center: a population based study. J Trauma 1990; 30:689–94.
56. Livingston D, Shogan B, John P, et al. CT diagnosis of rib fractures and the prediction of acute respiratory failure. J Trauma 2008;64:905–11.
57. Iochum S, Ludig T, Walter F, et al. Imaging of diaphragmatic injury: a diagnostic challenge? Radiographics 2002;22:S103–16.
58. Killeen KL, Mirvis SE, Shanmuganathan K. Helical CT of diaphragmatic rupture caused by blunt trauma. AJR Am J Roentgenol 1999;173:1611–6.
59. Bergin D, Ennis R, Keogh C, et al. The "dependent viscera" sign in CT diagnosis of blunt traumatic diaphragmatic rupture. AJR Am J Roentgenol 2001;177: 1137–40.
60. Paluska TR, Sise MJ, Sack DI, et al. Incidental CT findings in trauma patients: incidence and implications for care of the injured. J Trauma 2007;62(1):157–61.
61. Eskandary H, Sabba M, Khajehpour F, et al. Incidental findings in brain computed tomography scans of 3000 head trauma patients. Surg Neurol 2005;63(6):550–3.
62. Furtado CD, Aguirre DA, Sirlin CB, et al. Whole-body CT screening: spectrum of findings and recommendations in 1192 patients. Radiology 2005;237(2):385–94.
63. Barett T, Schierling M, Zhou C, et al. Prevalence of incidental findings in trauma patients detected by computed tomography imaging. Am J Emerg Med 2009;27: 428–35.
64. Munk M, Peitzman A, Hostler D, et al. Frequency and follow-up of incidental findings on trauma computed tomography scans: experience at a level one trauma center. J Emerg Med 2010;38(3):346–50.
65. Schultz DJ, Brasel KJ, Washington L, et al. Incidence of asymptomatic pulmonary embolism in moderately to severely injured trauma patients. J Trauma 2004;56(4): 727–31.

66. Kearon C, Kahn S, Agnelli G, et al. Antithrombotic therapy for venous thromboembolic disease: American College of Chest Physicians Evidence-Based Clinical Practice Guidelines (8th edition). Chest 2008;133:454S–545S.
67. Ball C, Kirkpatrick A, Laupland K, et al. Incidence, risk factors, and outcomes for occult pneumothoraces in victims of major trauma. J Trauma 2005;59(4):917–24.
68. Ball C, Kirkpatrick A, Laupland K, et al. Factors related to the failure of radiographic recognition of occult posttraumatic pneumothoraces. Am J Surg 2005; 189(5):541–6.
69. Marts B, Durham R, Shapiro M, et al. Computed tomography in the diagnosis of blunt thoracic injury. Am J Surg 1994;168:688–92.
70. Poole G, Morgan D, Cranston P, et al. Computed tomography in the management of blunt thoracic trauma. J Trauma 1993;35:296–302.
71. Stafford R, Linn J, Washington L. Incidence and management of occult hemothoraces. Am J Surg 2006;192:722–6.

Positron Emission Tomography for Benign and Malignant Disease

Anthony Visioni, MD[a], Julian Kim, MD[b],*

KEYWORDS

- Positron emission tomography • Imaging
- Fluorodeoxyglucose

Imaging modalities play an important complimentary role to traditional history, physical examination, and laboratory tests in the diagnosis and management of patient disease. Improved sensitivity and specificity of imaging studies with respect to diagnosis and staging represents an opportunity for advancement of quality of medical care, quality of life, and even cost of medical care. For example, an imaging test that can accurately identify mediastinal lymph node metastases in a patient with primary lung cancer can result in avoidance of mediastinoscopy. In addition, a patient with a solitary pulmonary nodule could be spared a pulmonary wedge resection if accurate diagnostic imaging could confirm benign disease. In both instances, it could be argued that the quality of medical care is improved, the quality of life of the patient is improved, and the cost of medical care of the individual patient is reduced by the introduction of accurate diagnostic imaging. Improved sensitivity, specificity, and predictive value of newer imaging techniques are critical to optimizing patient care.

FUNCTIONAL IMAGING

Functional imaging refers to modalities that combine information about anatomic location and intrinsic tissue characteristics such as metabolic rate. Functional imaging can be applied in conjunction with computed tomography (CT), magnetic resonance imaging (MRI), and ultrasound, and typically uses a radiolabeled substrate that either

The authors have no financial disclosure relative to this manuscript Supported by NIH K23CA109115-04 (JK).
[a] Department of Surgery, University Hospitals Case Medical Center, Case Western Reserve University, 11100 Euclid Avenue Mailstop LKSD 5047, Cleveland, OH 44106, USA
[b] Division of Surgical Oncology, University Hospitals Case Medical Center, Case Western Reserve University, 11100 Euclid Avenue Mailstop LKSD 5047, Cleveland, OH 44106, USA
* Corresponding author.
E-mail address: julian.kim@uhhospitals.org

accumulates or is converted within a tissue differentially based on a unique tissue characteristic. For example, a radiolabeled tracer that binds dopamine receptor can be used in combination with MRI to characterize the changes in the human brain associated with Parkinson disease.[1–3] The ability to add information about tissue function and merge this with anatomic detail has the potential to improve the sensitivity and specificity of the imaging studies compared with traditional contrast-enhanced imaging.

Positron emission tomography (PET) is a method of functional imaging that can be merged or coregistered with traditional studies such as CT or MRI to improve diagnosis of benign versus malignant disease or extent of malignant disease. Current PET uses radiolabeled fluorodeoxyglucose (FDG), which is a glucose analogue that accumulates in tissues that are metabolically active. FDG is labeled with ^{18}F at the 2' hydroxyl position, which prevents the normal degradation during glycolysis and allows the radiolabeled FDG to accumulate within the tissue. Malignant tissues tend to have increased metabolism compared with normal surrounding tissues, which provides an opportunity for differential accumulation of radiolabeled FDG in malignant tissues compared with benign. Thus, [^{18}F]FDG-PET functional information that is coregistered with anatomic imaging such as CT provides the opportunity to identify tissues with increased metabolism, which can help distinguish benign from malignant disease as well as extent or spread of malignancy. These images can alter patient management, as illustrated in **Fig. 1** in which a patient with regional lymph node metastases of melanoma was found to have an incidental bone metastasis on the preoperative staging PET-CT, which led to the use of primary systemic therapy as opposed to radical surgery.

This article provides a review of the use of PET primarily in the management of patients with malignant disease. For each disease, there is a short background about standard treatment and how it can be affected by preoperative imaging. The performance characteristics of PET-CT are reviewed for each disease type with respect to primary diagnosis of malignancy (ie, benign vs malignant tissue), assessing extent of malignant disease in patients with a known diagnosis (ie, staging), and follow-up of patients to determine locoregional or distant recurrence of malignant disease. Data on how PET-CT altered patient management are presented when available, although many studies report only on sensitivity and specificity of imaging findings. The use of PET-CT for radiation treatment planning, for pediatric patients and for benign disease is discussed. The data presented in this article provide the reader with an update on the current status of the use of PET-CT as well ways that the technology may ultimately be used to improve medical care.

USE OF PET-CT IN PATIENTS WITH COMMON MALIGNANCIES
Lung

In 2008, there were more than 200,000 cases of lung cancer diagnosed in the United States, with more than 150,000 deaths. This makes lung cancer the second most commonly diagnosed cancer and the leading cause of cancer-related deaths in both men and women.[4] The use of functional imaging using PET has yielded significant results in the diagnosis and treatment of patients with lung cancer.

Primary diagnosis: solitary pulmonary nodule
Solitary pulmonary nodule (SPN) on routine chest radiograph presents a diagnostic challenge. An SPN is defined as a singe well-defined opacity with normal surrounding lung and no adenopathy. Up to 50% of these SPNs are eventually found to be malignant.[5] Early studies suggested that FDG-PET (without CT) was equal to dynamic

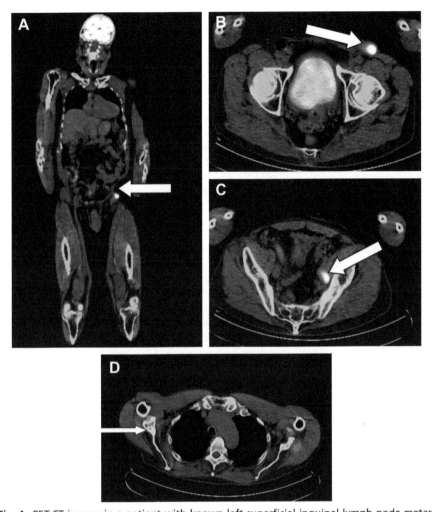

Fig. 1. PET-CT images in a patient with known left superficial inguinal lymph node metastasis. (*A*) Whole-body PET-CT showing hypermetabolic left inguinal lymph node (*arrow*) consistent with metastatic melanoma. (*B*) Coronal view of PET-CT showing hypermetabolic left inguinal lymph node (*arrow*) and showing anatomic relationship of surrounding muscles and blood vessels. (*C*) Coronal view of PET-CT showing a deep iliac lymph node (*arrow*) suspicious for metastasis in the same patient. The large hypermetabolic focus in the central pelvis is the urinary bladder. (*D*) Coronal view of PET-CT showing hypermetabolic focus within the right scapula (*arrow*) in the same patient. The detection of this bone lesion prompted a biopsy and ultimately altered the treatment plan of the patient.

contrast-enhanced CT for differentiating between benign and malignant SPNs.[6] A recent study evaluated PET-CT in 56 patients who had SPNs diagnosed by CT scan.[7] These patients had diagnosis confirmed either by histology or long-term clinical follow-up with repeat CT. After confirmatory testing, 27 of 56 SPNs were diagnosed with malignancies (either primary lung or metastatic), and PET-CT identified 26 true positives, 5 false positives, 24 true negatives, and 1 false negative. This finding corresponds to sensitivity and specificity of 96% and 83%, respectively. The prevalence of malignant SPNs within this study was 48%, which is consistent with previous studies.[5] The positive predictive value (PPV) and negative predictive value (NPV) for PET-CT was 84% and 96%, respectively.

One of the weaknesses of this study was the enrollment of patients with known history of cancer. In another study, 42 patients with no known history of cancer and an SPN were enrolled.[8] These patients had CT, PET, and PET-CT performed, and all patients went on to biopsy for histologic confirmation. Sensitivity and specificity were 97% and 85% respectively. This study had a higher prevalence of malignant SPNs (69%), which corresponds to a PPV and NPV of 94% and 93%, respectively. **Table 1**, includes 2 more studies and shows the operating characteristic for PET-CT to be consistent.[9,10] These studies show the benefit of using PET-CT in the noninvasive diagnosis of SPN. The NPV for all these studies is consistently greater than 90%, which can significantly reduce the need for invasive diagnostic procedures in a proportion of patients.

PET for staging of primary lung cancer

Traditionally, non–small cell lung cancer (NSCLC) requires mediastinoscopy with lymph node biopsy to determine staging and treatment. To reduce the need for mediastinoscopy, PET-CT has been extensively studied for noninvasive staging of mediastinal lymph nodes. In a prospective study by Shim and colleagues,[11] 106 patients with biopsy-proven NSCLC underwent preoperative CT and PET-CT before curative pulmonary resection. Preoperative CT scan accurately identified 69% of mediastinal lymph node metastases, whereas PET-CT accurately identified 84%. In addition, 2 other studies confirm a high specificity and accuracy of preoperative PET-CT in identifying mediastinal lymph node metastases (**Table 2**).[12,13] Taken together, these studies reveal a high NPV of PET-CT for mediastinal lymph node staging in NSCLC, which suggests that patients with a negative PET-CT may be able to proceed directly to curative resection without mediastinoscopy, whereas those with a positive PET-CT may benefit from mediastinoscopy for lymph node biopsy before thoracotomy. In contrast, Carnochan and Walker[14] concluded that PET-CT had a low NPV and was inaccurate in staging patients, therefore mediastinoscopy should continue to be used in all patients for staging.

The ultimate goal of this approach would be to shorten the time to definitive intervention (either surgery or chemotherapy/radiation) and to reduce the number of futile operations. A study by Fischer and colleagues found that PET-CT reduced the number of futile thoracotomies and the number of total thoracotomies, but did not significantly affect mortality.[15] The investigators concluded that PET-CT was able to correctly stage a patient and avoid unnecessary thoracotomy.

PET-CT for locoregional or distant recurrence in patients with lung cancer

For patients with lung cancer, CT is currently the study of choice for the diagnosis of local or distant recurrence. The addition of functional information from PET-CT would

Table 1
Operating characteristics for PET-CT in evaluation of solitary pulmonary nodules

Author	Sensitivity (%)	Specificity (%)	Accuracy (%)	PPV (%)	NPV (%)
Chang et al 2010[10]	88	89	89	84	92
Bar-Shalom et al 2008[7]	96	83	89	84	96
Kim et al 2007[8,71]	97	85	93	94	93
Yi et al 2006[9]	96	88	93	94	92

Table 2					
Preoperative mediastinal lymph node staging by PET-CT					
Author	Sensitivity (%)	Specificity (%)	Accuracy (%)	PPV (%)	NPV (%)
Shim et al 2005[11]	85	84	84	32	98
Tasci et al 2009[13]	72	94	93	49	98
Liu et al 2009[12]	65	97	92	79	90
Carnochan and Walker 2009[14]	52	83	75	53	82

be valuable to differentiate post-therapy fibrosis from malignancy. A study by Keidar and colleagues[16] highlights the benefits of PET-CT for the diagnosis of recurrent lung cancer. This study enrolled 42 patients with suspected recurrence of NSCLC from clinical findings, biochemical markers, or standard imaging and subsequently evaluated them with PET-CT. The study showed promising results with sensitivity, specificity, PPV, and NPV for recurrence of malignancy of 96%, 82%, 89%, and 93%, respectively. Other studies suggest that, despite the high sensitivity for the detection of recurrent lung cancer, the lower specificity from false-positive results mean that PET-CT should not be performed for at least 3 to 5 months after a patient's last treatment.[17,18]

Breast

Breast cancer is the most common cancer in women in the United States and the second most common cause of cancer death.[4] Imaging plays an important role in the diagnosis of primary breast cancer, regional lymph node metastases, and distant metastases.

PET for primary diagnosis of breast cancer

Mammography, ultrasound, and MRI have been shown to be sensitive but lack sufficient specificity in differentiating benign from malignant breast disease.[19] Therefore, many women still undergo invasive diagnostic procedures. Functional imaging has been studied for primary breast cancer diagnosis using whole-body PET-CT, dedicated breast PET-CT, and positron emission mammography (PEM).

A study of 40 women with suspected malignancy on conventional mammography underwent whole-body PET-CT in comparison with MRI mammography.[20] The study reports a sensitivity of 95%, which was not different from MRI, and MRI was better able to characterize the tumor size. Avril and colleagues[19] reports sensitivity and specificity ranging from 64% to 80% and 76% to 94%, respectively, depending on the level of expertise of the interpreting radiologist. In a 2009 study, Bowen and colleagues[21] reported on the feasibility and viability of a dedicated breast PET-CT scanner, but currently no studies provide data to suggest that PET-CT should be routinely used as a screening modality.

PEM is a technique that uses radiolabeled FDG in combination with high-resolution detectors that can be fashioned similarly to standard mammography units. The result is that PEM can detect cancers as small as 5 mm, even in the presence of breasts with significant density on mammography. Several studies indicate that the specificity of PEM is better that mammography. Two preliminary studies indicate that PEM has a sensitivity of 80% to 86% and a specificity of 91% to 100%, a significant improvement compared with conventional mammography.[22,23] One of the major limitations of PET-CT in evaluating breast cancer is decreased sensitivity for small tumors.[24] Although PEM requires a specialized piece of equipment, one advantage is that it may be able to detect smaller tumors than PET-CT, leading to earlier diagnosis.[25] Studies comparing the performance characteristics of PEM versus MRI are in progress, but preliminary results suggest that PEM may provide an alternative to breast MRI with similar diagnostic performance.

PET-CT for axillary staging of patients with breast cancer

One of the most important advances in the treatment of breast cancer has been the surgical management of the axilla. Routine axillary lymph node dissection (AND) is no longer the standard of care for staging of the axilla and has been replaced by sentinel lymph node biopsy (SLNB). Preoperative ultrasound and MRI have been studied to determine whether they can accurately predict sentinel node status, with mixed results. Similarly, studies using PET-CT have not shown this modality to have sufficiently high operating characteristics to warrant replacing SLNB.[26,27] The shortcoming of PET-CT and other imaging studies is the failure to show micrometastases that are detected by SLNB (**Table 3**).[28,29]

Kim and colleagues[30] have shown that PET-CT may identify lymph node macrometastases in some instances, which would allow certain patients to proceed directly to AND rather than have SLNB. Preoperative PET-CT had a PPV of 100% in determining axillary lymph node staging, which the investigators concluded accurately upstages patients and would reduce the number of unnecessary SLNB. Several other studies have concluded that preoperative whole-body PET-CT could be used to evaluate patients for regional lymph node metastasis as well as distant metastasis.[20,24]

They conclude that PET-CT is useful in correctly upstaging patients and, hence, avoiding unnecessary procedures such as SLNB in the presence of axillary lymph node metastases.

PET-CT to determine locoregional or distant recurrence in patients with breast cancer

In a retrospective study, 46 women with increased serum tumor markers were evaluated with PET-CT.[31] Final diagnosis was determined by pathologic evaluation of tissue samples, continued clinical follow-up, or further imaging studies. The investigators report a sensitivity and specificity of 90% and 71%, respectively. Diagnostic accuracy was 83% and the investigators report that the results of PET-CT changed the management of 51% of patients. These findings were similar to another retrospective study that enrolled women with suspected recurrence (**Table 4**).[32] Pan and colleagues[33] performed a meta-analysis comparing MRI, CT, PET (with or without CT), and US for the evaluation of breast cancer recurrence. The study found that MRI and PET had the highest sensitivities (95% and 95.3%, respectively), whereas MRI and US had the highest specificities (93% and 96%, respectively). They concluded that MRI was likely the most useful imaging modality to add to current surveillance techniques. If MRI is contraindicated or inconclusive, the investigators state that PET might be of some usefulness.

Table 3					
Staging of axilla in breast cancer with PET-CT or PET					
Author	Sensitivity (%)	Specificity (%)	Accuracy (%)	PPV (%)	NPV (%)
Taira et al 2009[26]	48	92	–	72	81
Chae et al 2009[27]	49	84	73	–	–
Greco et al 2001[28]	94	86	89	84	95
Schirrmeister et al 2001[29]	79	92	–	–	–

Table 4
PET-CT in breast cancer recurrence

Author	Sensitivity (%)	Specificity (%)	Accuracy (%)	PPV (%)	NPV (%)
Pan et al 2010[33]	95	86	93	95	88
Radan et al 2006[31]	90	71	83	–	–
Veit-Haibach et al 2007[32]	–	–	91	–	–

Prostate

Prostate cancer is the most commonly diagnosed cancer in men and is the second leading cause of cancer-related death. The disease poses significant diagnostic challenges because of the high prevalence of positive screening tests that necessitate an invasive biopsy. Prostate cancer can range from highly aggressive to clinically irrelevant and the treatment (ie, prostatectomy) has significant morbidity.

PET-CT for primary diagnosis of prostate cancer

Current standard of care following abnormal prostate-specific antigen blood testing involves multiple prostate biopsies, which are known to have sampling errors.[34] A reliable imaging technique that could accurately identify aggressive tumors would substantially improve medical care of these patients. However, FDG-PET has significant baseline urinary excretion, which can affect the sensitivity of identifying small malignant lesions within the pelvis. To bypass the urinary excretion issues, studies have shown that [11C]choline can be used as a radioactive substitute for FDG in the detection of prostate cancer.[35,36] In a study by Farsad and colleagues,[37] 36 patients with prostate cancer and 5 controls with bladder cancer all received [11C]choline PET-CT followed by resection of the prostate with subsequent histopathologic confirmation. This study showed that detection of cancer using [11C]choline was feasible, but the high rate of false negatives precluded the use of PET-CT as a first-line test to replace biopsy. They report a sensitivity, specificity, accuracy, PPV, and NPV of 66%, 81%, 71%, 87%, and 55% respectively.

Another area of study involves determining the biologic aggressiveness of known prostate cancer to tailor therapy. Piert and colleagues[38] studied [11C]choline PET-CT in 14 patients with known prostate cancer to determine whether PET-CT could help with treatment planning. The study found that using a ratio of tumor volume to benign background could predict tumors that had aggressive characteristics on final pathology. Although this study was not conclusive, it did provide a framework for future investigations.

PET-CT for staging in patients with prostate cancer

Lymph node metastases in patients with prostate cancer are associated with progressive disease and a decrease in 5-year survival from 85% to 50%.[39] Pelvic lymphadenectomy is currently the gold standard for lymph node staging in prostate cancer, because routine imaging studies (eg, CT, MRI) have not shown sufficient sensitivity. de Jong and colleagues[40] studied 67 patients with biopsy-proven prostate cancer with [11C]choline PET-CT before lymphadenectomy. The investigators found PET-CT to have a sensitivity, specificity, and accuracy in staging pelvic lymph nodes of 80%, 96%, and 93%, respectively. The investigators concluded that PET-CT staging of pelvic lymph nodes could replace pelvic lymphadenectomy in select patients in the future. However, because of the lack of larger confirmatory studies, currently there is little justification for the use of PET-CT for primary diagnosis or staging in patients with prostate cancer.

Colorectal Cancer

Colorectal cancer is a leading cause of cancer in the United States. Although there has been a slight but steady decline in incidence, it remains the third most commonly diagnosed cancer, with the third highest mortality.[4] Imaging studies that could improve the detection of primary colon cancer and malignant polyps using noninvasive approaches would be desirable.

PET-CT for primary diagnosis in patients with colorectal cancer

Colon and rectal cancers are potentially surgically curable if detected at an early stage. Currently, there are several methods being used to screen for colorectal cancer, including fecal occult blood testing, flexible sigmoidoscopy, air-contrast barium enema, and CT colonography (CTC).[41] CTC has the potential to accurately detect cancer and well as improve patient compliance because it is relatively noninvasive.[42] However, CTC continues to have issues that prevent it from widespread screening, including detecting small (<10 mm) and flat/sessile polyps. In an attempt to improve the sensitivity of CTC, PET-CT is currently being developed for the screening of colorectal cancer. In several small feasibility studies, PET-CT colonography was well tolerated by patients and technically feasible, but did not increase the sensitivity or accuracy of CTC.[43–45] Although it seems unlikely that PET-CT will improve on current screening tools for colorectal cancer, several studies have shown that PET-CT colonography is a feasible single-modality study for visualization of primary tumor and the staging of colorectal cancer. Investigators have suggested that this imaging modality might be particularly beneficial to patients with incomplete colonoscopies and those with synchronous lesions.[46,47]

PET-CT for staging of colorectal cancer

Identification of liver metastases in patients with newly diagnosed colon cancer significantly alters patient management and outcome.[48] In patients who have liver metastases, the presence of extrahepatic disease may affect resectability for curative intent. In a study by Sørensen and colleagues,[49] 54 patients with colorectal cancer were evaluated for resection of liver metastasis by their standard protocol. In 19% of cases, treatment plans were altered by imaging information either leading to correctly upstaging or downstaging patients. Studies using preoperative FDG-PET and PET-CT have shown alterations in treatment planning in a similar proportion of patients.[50,51] In a review by Vriens and colleagues,[52] pooled analysis of several studies showed a change in management of colorectal liver metastasis for approximately 10% of patients after PET-CT. This has led some institutions to use PET-CT as a routine part of preoperative work-up of patients with colorectal cancer. However, there are few data to show that PET-CT improves staging information compared with conventional CT or MRI.

PET-CT for locoregional or distant recurrence in patients with colorectal cancer

The current modalities for evaluation of recurrent colorectal cancer include routine clinical examinations, colonoscopy, CT scans, and serum tumor markers. Each is associated with certain limitations; colonoscopy only evaluates for local recurrence, CT does not detect local recurrence well, and serum tumor markers are only 60% to 70% sensitive.[53] PET-CT has been investigated as a single-modality method of detecting recurrence.

Two retrospective studies using PET-CT to evaluate recurrence in patients with colorectal cancer have shown promising results.[54,55] The sensitivity and specificity of PET-CT in detecting colorectal cancer recurrence is between 89% to 95% and 83% to 92%, respectively (**Table 5**). The addition of contrast enhancement to PET-CT may improve the diagnostic accuracy even more.[56] In a review by Vogel and colleagues,[57] the author states that PET-CT seems to be the diagnostic test of choice for evaluation of recurrent colorectal cancer, especially in staging before surgical re-intervention.

Melanoma

Use of PET-CT for staging of patients with melanoma

Yancovitz and colleagues[58] attempted to define the role of imaging for patients with early melanoma. One-hundred and fifty-eight patients with T1b-T3b primary tumors and no clinical evidence of metastases were examined in a retrospective study. A total of 344 preoperative imaging studies (chest radiograph, CT scan, and/or PET-CT) were evaluated. Only 1 of 344 imaging studies (PET-CT scan) corresponded with a confirmed metastatic melanoma. The investigators concluded that, for T1b-T3b tumors with history and physical negative for metastatic disease, the number of false positives and increased costs outweigh the benefits of routine imaging.

The use of FDG-PET to identify regional lymph node metastases to avoid SLNB has also been studied in patients with melanoma. In a study of 55 patients with primary cutaneous melanoma greater than 1.0 mm in thickness, PET scan was performed before SLNB.[59] The study showed that sentinel lymph nodes were positive in 13 patients, only 2 of which were detected by PET. PET scan also showed accumulation in lymph node basin of 5 patients with no tumor positive lymph node (false-positive result). These results have been repeated and lead to the conclusion that FDG-PET cannot replace SLNB for detection of regional lymph node metastases.[60,61]

PET-CT has been shown to be useful for the detection of distant metastases in high-risk patients with melanoma. In a study of patients with T4 tumors or evidence of metastatic disease, Strobel and colleagues[62] showed that PET-CT had a sensitivity and specificity of 98% and 94%, respectively. The accuracy, PPV, and NPV were 96%, 93%, and 99%, respectively. Tyler and colleagues[63] showed a change in management for 15% of patients with stage III melanoma who received a PET scan. Based on these results, PET-CT may be a valuable study for the identification of distant metastasis in patients at high risk with melanoma.

Head and Neck

Primary diagnosis

PET-CT is being increasingly studied for the functional as well as anatomic information it provides for head and neck cancers (HNC). Branstetter and colleagues[64] examined 64 consecutive patients with known or suspected HNC with PET-CT. The investigators showed that PET-CT had a sensitivity and specificity of 98% and 92%, respectively,

Table 5					
PET-CT in colorectal cancer recurrence					
Author	**Sensitivity (%)**	**Specificity (%)**	**Accuracy (%)**	**PPV (%)**	**NPV (%)**
Chen et al 2007[55]	95	83	–	96	77
Votrubova et al 2006[54]	89	92	90	–	–

and was superior to PET or CT alone in the detection of primary tumors. Hannah and colleagues[65] found similar results in an earlier prospective study.

Staging

Early studies using PET without CT showed that PET could be more sensitive and specific for regional lymph node metastases than CT or MRI.[66,67] Schoder and colleagues[68] showed that the sensitivity and specificity of PET-CT was from 87% to 90% and 80% to 93%, respectively, with a diagnostic accuracy between 90% and 96%. These findings are significantly better than those of MRI or CT alone. There was a change in treatment plan in 18% of patients based on PET-CT findings. Although these results were impressive, several studies have found that, in patients with clinically negative nodal status, PET-CT was not sufficiently reliable to be used as an initial study on which to base management decisions.[69,70] Thus, although PET-CT can identify clinically occult lymph node metastases, larger studies are necessary to determine whether PET-CT provides enough NPV to avoid cervical lymph node dissection.

Another potential use for PET-CT at the initial work-up for patients with HNC is to evaluate for second primary tumors and distant metastatic disease. Kim and colleagues[71] enrolled 349 patients with primary HNC and performed whole-body PET-CT for work-up of second primary tumors and distant metastatic disease. Of these patients, 7.4% had distant metastases and 4% had second primary tumors. PET-CT was able to accurately detect these lesions, but also had issues with false-positive results.

In summary, the use of PET-CT in patients with known or suspected HNC continues to evolve. Some investigators recommend only selective usage for evaluation of distant metastases,[72] whereas others use it as a single-modality study to gain information about primary tumors, lymph node status, and distant metastases.[68] **Table 6** shows operating characteristics for various usages of PET-CT in HNC.

Use of PET for locoregional recurrence in patients with HNC

The diagnosis and staging of recurrent head and neck cancer can be difficult because of the frequent alterations in anatomy associated with extensive surgery.[53] Therefore, PET-CT has been studied to determine whether it can overcome the limitations of conventional imaging. A recent prospective study enrolled 91 patients cured of HNC with no clinical evidence of recurrence.[73] These patients were evaluated with

Table 6					
Operating characteristics for various usages of PET-CT in HNC					
Author	Sensitivity (%)	Specificity (%)	Accuracy (%)	PPV (%)	NPV (%)
PET-CT in Identification of Primary Head and Neck Tumor					
Branstetter et al 2005[64]	98	92	94	88	99
Hannah et al 2002[65]	88	100	–	–	–
PET-CT in Detection of Metastatic Head and Neck Lymph Nodes					
Schoder et al 2004[68]	87–90	80–93	90–96	–	–
Hannah et al 2002[65]	82	94	–	–	–
Bailet et al 1992[66]	71	98	–	–	–
Braams et al 1995[67]	91	88	–	–	–
PET-CT for the Detection of Second Primary and Distant Metastases					
Kim et al 2007[8,71]	98	93	93	63	99

whole-body PET-CT to determine its usefulness as an initial modality for the detection of subclinical locoregional disease. Thirty-nine patients had a positive PET-CT and, in 30 patients, recurrence was confirmed. Fifty-two patients had negative PET-CT; and all of these patients remained disease free on clinical examination for 3 months. These results correspond with a sensitivity and specificity of 100% and 85% respectively. These findings are consistent with other studies showing that the sensitivity and specificity for PET (with or without CT) was 83% to 100% and 78% to 98% respectively. Taken together, these studies suggest that PET-CT may be useful in the follow-up of patients with treated HNC for the detection of subclinical recurrence.

USE OF PET FOR RADIATION TREATMENT PLANNING

Radiation treatment planning has become more refined with the use of technology that allows for more precise delivery of radiation to target tissues and minimizes exposures to surrounding tissues. Intensity-modulated radiation therapy uses multiple beams of radiation at various angulations with varying intensity to maximize radiation delivery to tumor and minimize exposure to normal/critical surrounding tissues.[74]

The ability to precisely target lesions and spare surrounding structures has now made precise imaging of the target tumors the rate-limiting step in accurate radiation delivery. CT is the most commonly used modality in radiation therapy (RT) planning. However, there is well-known inter- and intraobserver variability in determining gross tumor volume (GTV) for targeting using conventional CT.[75]

PET-CT is an imaging modality that is being increasingly studied for treatment planning of RT. The goal is to have a reliable imaging study that will accurately depict GTV and reduce the amount of inter- and intraobserver variation.[76] PET-CT has been studied and is gaining widespread use in cancers of lung, head and neck, rectum and anus, uterine cervix, pancreas, and brain, as well as partial breast.[77–82]

Kruser and colleagues[83] provide a robust study showing the benefits of PET-CT for RT planning. This work was a blinded prospective study enrolling 111 patients with various cancers (lung, head and neck, breast, cervix, esophageal, and lymphoma). Patients underwent PET-CT in preparation for RT, and 1 physician who was blinded to PET data designed a treatment plan based on clinical data and CT imaging. The treating physician then designed a second treatment plan based on hybrid PET-CT data. The author found that, in 76/111 patients (68%), treatment plans changed with the inclusion of PET-CT data.

Although there remain several technical limitations, PET-CT is becoming increasingly common in RT planning for various cancers. Ongoing research is showing the feasibility of single-session PET-CT in RT planning, determining the best protocols to reduce variations between institutions, and showing that treatment programs are being changed as a result of this new information. However, more investigation needs to be performed to determine whether any of these advances are having a positive effect on patient morbidity and therapeutic effectiveness of RT.

USE OF PET IN PEDIATRIC PATIENTS

Pediatric malignancies are distinct from cancers in adults because of their relative infrequency, differences in treatment strategies compared with adult malignancies, and prognosis. Although there are many studies examining the role of PET-CT in adults, the evidence for use in pediatrics is sparse. FDG-PET has been studied for many years for use in pediatric brain tumors with good success.[84] However, there is interest in PET-CT for use in pediatric patients as a single-session study in non-CNS malignancies. A recent review by Kumar and colleagues[85] suggests that there may be some role for PET-CT in common pediatric malignancies, including lymphoma, soft-tissue tumors, neuroblastoma, malignant bone tumors, and germ cell tumors.

Tatsumi and colleagues[86] attempted to evaluate the use of PET-CT in various pediatric malignancies. The investigators enrolled 55 patients in whom 151 PET-CT studies were performed for non-CNS tumors. Seventy-one percent were performed for lymphoma and only 16 of 151 studies were performed for initial staging and diagnosis. In posttreatment follow-up, PET-CT had a sensitivity and specificity of 97% and 99%, respectively, compared with 74% and 91% respectively for conventional imaging. The data for use of PET-CT for initial staging and diagnosis was limited by small sample size.

A major concern for the use of PET in the pediatric population is radiation exposure. This concern applies especially to studies that are to be used serially for posttreatment response and surveillance. Murano and colleagues[87] examined the difference in radiation exposure to children with malignancies from current imaging plans compared with PET-CT. This study found that PET-CT had lower doses of radiation compared with current imaging plans such as conventional CT (64–68 mSv compared with 127–169 mSv). At a dose of 100 mSv or greater it is estimated that the risk of a secondary cancer is 1 in 100 individuals.[88] In another study specifically of serial PET-CT in pediatric malignancies, Chawla and colleagues[89] showed that the cumulative radiation dose per patient with PET-CT was 79 mSv (range 6.2–399 mSv). The study showed that most of the radiation dosage came from the CT portion of the study, suggesting that the FDG-PET added little to the total radiation exposure. In summary, although studies are showing that PET-CT may have a role in pediatric malignancies, prospective studies examining specific malignancies are needed to justify widespread clinical use.

BENIGN DISEASE

Although most of the literature on PET-CT has investigated its role in oncology, several investigators are studying the uses of PET-CT for nonneoplastic disease.

Given that FDG uptake occurs preferentially in neoplastic, inflammatory, and infectious processes, one application that is being studied is in patients with fever of unknown origin (FUO). FUO is defined as a recurrent fever of 38.3°C or higher, lasting 2 to 3 weeks, and undiagnosed after appropriate work-up.[90] In a review by Meller and colleagues,[91] sensitivity and specificity of PET in diagnosis of FUO is reported as 81% and 86%, respectively. The investigators report that 25% to 69% of PET scans are helpful in the diagnosis of FUO. Although there is a paucity of research on this specific topic, preliminary studies indicate that PET may be an improvement on the gallium scans currently in use.

Another area in which the use of FDG-PET is being actively studied is in patients with inflammatory bowel disease. Halpenny and colleagues[92] report sensitivities of 59% to 98% and specificities of 50% to 100% for the use of PET-CT in inflammatory bowel disease. The authors discuss monitoring of disease response to therapy, cancer surveillance, and diagnosis of areas of active inflammation all in 1 noninvasive test as the benefits of this modality.

PET-CT is being increasingly applied in cardiology. PET perfusion scans have been studied for use in patients with coronary artery disease. Knaapen and colleagues[93] report sensitivity and specificity from 9 pooled studies to be 90% and 89%, respectively. These results are superior to currently used thallium single-photon emission CT images.

PET is gaining acceptance as a functional study for use in clinical practice in neuro-logic disease. Although not indicated as a primary imaging technique, PET is finding use in conditions such as stroke, epilepsy, dementia, and movement disorders.[94]

SUMMARY

There is evidence to suggest a role for the use of PET-CT in patients with a variety of solid tumors including lung, colorectal, and head and neck. PET-CT is also useful in patients with hematologic malignancies, including lymphoma. PET-CT is quickly becoming a complementary imaging modality for RT treatment planning and is also being considered for use in the pediatric cancer population.

The current literature of the performance characteristics of PET-CT are limited in several important ways. Measurements of sensitivity, specificity, and PPV and NPV are limited in that, in many instances, there is a lack of histologic confirmation. In the instance of lesions that are determined to be PET negative, clinical follow-up of lesions to confirm benign biology are used. In addition, although PET-CT is an imaging modality, the relative endpoint of future studies should be the proportion of instances in which clinical decision making changes as a result of the test. The morbidity and cost of false-positive results are rarely studied and reported in PET-CT studies, and may be the most important factor in determining the cost-effectiveness of this modality. The National Oncology PET Registry is an attempt by insurers as well as Centers for Medicare and Medicaid Services to follow patients who have undergone PET to determine whether medical care and outcomes are improved.

Despite these questions, the development of new probes for use with PET is essentially unlimited. The ability to develop probes that are more sensitive and specific than FDG will only increase the clinical usefulness of functional imaging. Properly controlled studies will yield the results that can show how PET should be incorporated into evidence-based medicine.

REFERENCES

1. Antonini A, DeNotaris R. PET and SPECT functional imaging in Parkinson's disease. Sleep Med 2004;5(2):201–6.
2. Ceballos-Baumann AO. Functional imaging in Parkinson's disease: activation studies with PET, fMRI and SPECT. J Neurol 2003;250(Suppl 1):I15–23.
3. Fukuyama H. Functional brain imaging in Parkinson's disease-overview. J Neurol 2004;251(Suppl 7):vII1–3.
4. Jemal A, Siegel R, Ward E, et al. Cancer statistics, 2008. CA Cancer J Clin 2008; 58(2):71–96.
5. Higgins GA, Shields TW, Keehn RJ. The solitary pulmonary nodule. Ten-year follow-up of Veterans Administration-Armed Forces Cooperative Study. Arch Surg 1975;110(5):570–5.
6. Cronin P, Dwamena BA, Kelly AM, et al. Solitary pulmonary nodules: meta-analytic comparison of cross-sectional imaging modalities for diagnosis of malignancy. Radiology 2008;246(3):772–82.
7. Bar-Shalom R, Kagna O, Israel O, et al. Noninvasive diagnosis of solitary pulmonary lesions in cancer patients based on 2-fluoro-2-deoxy-D-glucose avidity on positron emission tomography/computed tomography. Cancer 2008;113(11): 3213–21.
8. Kim SK, Allen-Auerbach M, Goldin J, et al. Accuracy of PET/CT in characterization of solitary pulmonary lesions. J Nucl Med 2007;48(2):214–20.

9. Yi CA, Lee KS, Kim BT, et al. Tissue characterization of solitary pulmonary nodule: comparative study between helical dynamic CT and integrated PET/CT. J Nucl Med 2006;47(3):443–50.

10. Chang CY, Tzao C, Lee SC, et al. Incremental value of integrated FDG-PET/CT in evaluating indeterminate solitary pulmonary nodule for malignancy. Mol Imaging Biol 2010;12(2):204–9.

11. Shim SS, Lee KS, Kim B-T, et al. Non–small cell lung cancer: prospective comparison of integrated FDG PET/CT and CT alone for preoperative staging. Radiology 2005;236:1011.

12. Liu BJ, Dong JC, Xu CQ, et al. Accuracy of 18F-FDG PET/CT for lymph node staging in non-small-cell lung cancers. Chin Med J (Engl) 2009;122(15):1749–54.

13. Tasci E, Tezel C, Orki A, et al. The role of integrated positron emission tomography and computed tomography in the assessment of nodal spread in cases with non-small cell lung cancer. Interact Cardiovasc Thorac Surg 2009;10(2):200–3.

14. Carnochan FM, Walker WS. Positron emission tomography may underestimate the extent of thoracic disease in lung cancer patients. Eur J Cardiothorac Surg 2009;35(5):781–5.

15. Fischer B, Lassen U, Mortensen J, et al. Preoperative staging of lung cancer with combined PET–CT. N Engl J Med 2009;361(1):32–9.

16. Keidar Z, Haim N, Guralnik L, et al. PET/CT using 18F-FDG in suspected lung cancer recurrence: diagnostic value and impact on patient management. J Nucl Med 2004;45(10):1640–6.

17. Bogot NR, Quint LE. Imaging of recurrent lung cancer. Cancer Imaging 2004; 4(2):61–7.

18. Collins CD. PET/CT in oncology: for which tumours is it the reference standard? Cancer Imaging 2007;7(Special Issue A):S77–87.

19. Avril N, Rose CA, Schelling M, et al. Breast imaging with positron emission tomography and fluorine-18 fluorodeoxyglucose: use and limitations. J Clin Oncol 2000;18(20):3495–502.

20. Heusner TA, Kuemmel S, Umutlu L, et al. Breast cancer staging in a single session: whole-body PET/CT mammography. J Nucl Med 2008;49(8):1215–22.

21. Bowen SL, Wu Y, Chaudhari AJ, et al. Initial characterization of a dedicated breast PET/CT scanner during human imaging. J Nucl Med 2009;50(9):1401–8.

22. Murthy K, Aznar M, Thompson CJ, et al. Results of preliminary clinical trials of the positron emission mammography system PEM-I: a dedicated breast imaging system producing glucose metabolic images using FDG. J Nucl Med 2000; 41(11):1851–8.

23. Levine EA, Freimanis RI, Perrier ND, et al. Positron emission mammography: initial clinical results. Ann Surg Oncol 2003;10(1):86–91.

24. Yang SK, Cho N, Moon WK. The role of PET/CT for evaluating breast cancer. Korean J Radiol 2007;8(5):429–37.

25. Rosen EL, Turkington TG, Soo MS, et al. Detection of primary breast carcinoma with a dedicated, large-field-of-view FDG PET mammography device: initial experience. Radiology 2005;234(2):527–34.

26. Taira N, Ohsumi S, Takabatake D, et al. Determination of indication for sentinel lymph node biopsy in clinical node-negative breast cancer using preoperative 18F-fluorodeoxyglucose positron emission tomography/computed tomography fusion imaging. Jpn J Clin Oncol 2009;39(1):16–21.

27. Chae BJ, Bae JS, Kang BJ, et al. Positron emission tomography-computed tomography in the detection of axillary lymph node metastasis in patients with early stage breast cancer. Jpn J Clin Oncol 2009;39(5):284–9.

28. Greco M, Crippa F, Agresti R, et al. Axillary lymph node staging in breast cancer by 2-fluoro-2-deoxy-D-glucose-positron emission tomography: clinical evaluation and alternative management. J Natl Cancer Inst 2001;93(8):630–5.

29. Schirrmeister H, Kuhn T, Guhlmann A, et al. Fluorine-18 2-deoxy-2-fluoro-D-glucose PET in the preoperative staging of breast cancer: comparison with the standard staging procedures. Eur J Nucl Med 2001;28(3):351–8.

30. Kim J, Lee J, Chang E, et al. Selective sentinel node plus additional non-sentinel node biopsy based on an FDG-PET/CT scan in early breast cancer patients: single institutional experience. World J Surg 2009;33(5):943–9.

31. Radan L, Ben-Haim S, Bar-Shalom R, et al. The role of FDG-PET/CT in suspected recurrence of breast cancer. Cancer 2006;107(11):2545–51.

32. Veit-Haibach P, Antoch G, Beyer T, et al. FDG-PET/CT in restaging of patients with recurrent breast cancer: possible impact on staging and therapy. Br J Radiol 2007;80(955):508–15.

33. Pan L, Han Y, Sun X, et al. FDG-PET and other imaging modalities for the evaluation of breast cancer recurrence and metastases: a meta-analysis. J Cancer Res Clin Oncol 2010;136(7):1007–22.

34. Cookson MS, Fleshner NE, Soloway SM, et al. Correlation between Gleason score of needle biopsy and radical prostatectomy specimen: accuracy and clinical implications. J Urol 1997;157(2):559–62.

35. Hara T, Kosaka N, Kishi H. PET imaging of prostate cancer using carbon-11-choline. J Nucl Med 1998;39(6):990–5.

36. Kotzerke J, Prang J, Neumaier B, et al. Experience with carbon-11 choline positron emission tomography in prostate carcinoma. Eur J Nucl Med 2000;27(9):1415–9.

37. Farsad M, Schiavina R, Castellucci P, et al. Detection and localization of prostate cancer: correlation of (11)C-choline PET/CT with histopathologic step-section analysis. J Nucl Med 2005;46(10):1642–9.

38. Piert M, Park H, Khan A, et al. Detection of aggressive primary prostate cancer with 11C-choline PET/CT using multimodality fusion techniques. J Nucl Med 2009;50(10):1585–93.

39. Danella JF, deKernion JB, Smith RB, et al. The contemporary incidence of lymph node metastases in prostate cancer: implications for laparoscopic lymph node dissection. J Urol 1993;149(6):1488–91.

40. de Jong IJ, Pruim J, Elsinga PH, et al. Preoperative staging of pelvic lymph nodes in prostate cancer by 11C-choline PET. J Nucl Med 2003;44(3):331–5.

41. Bromer MQ, Weinberg DS. Screening for colorectal cancer–now and the near future. Semin Oncol 2005;32(1):3–10.

42. Mulhall BP, Veerappan GR, Jackson JL. Meta-analysis: computed tomographic colonography. Ann Intern Med 2005;142(8):635–50.

43. Gollub MJ, Akhurst T, Markowitz AJ, et al. Combined CT colonography and 18F-FDG PET of colon polyps: potential technique for selective detection of cancer and precancerous lesions. AJR Am J Roentgenol 2007;188(1):130–8.

44. Taylor SA, Bomanji JB, Manpanzure L, et al. Nonlaxative PET/CT colonography: feasibility, acceptability, and pilot performance in patients at higher risk of colonic neoplasia. J Nucl Med 2010;51(6):854–61.

45. Mainenti PP, Salvatore B, D'Antonio D, et al. PET/CT colonography in patients with colorectal polyps: a feasibility study. Eur J Nucl Med Mol Imaging 2007;34(10):1594–603.

46. Veit P, Kuhle C, Beyer T, et al. Whole body positron emission tomography/computed tomography (PET/CT) tumour staging with integrated PET/CT

colonography: technical feasibility and first experiences in patients with colorectal cancer. Gut 2006;55(1):68–73.

47. Kinner S, Antoch G, Bockisch A, et al. Whole-body PET/CT-colonography: a possible new concept for colorectal cancer staging. Abdom Imaging 2007; 32(5):606–12.

48. Bennett JJ, Cao D, Posner MC. Determinants of unresectability and outcome of patients with occult colorectal hepatic metastases. J Surg Oncol 2005;92(1): 64–9.

49. Sørensen M, Mortensen FV, Høyer M, et al. FDG-PET improves management of patients with colorectal liver metastases allocated for local treatment: a consecutive prospective study. Scand J Surg 2007;96:209–13.

50. Ruers TJ, Langenhoff BS, Neeleman N, et al. Value of positron emission tomography with [F-18]fluorodeoxyglucose in patients with colorectal liver metastases: a prospective study. J Clin Oncol 2002;20(2):388–95.

51. Park IJ, Kim HC, Yu CS, et al. Efficacy of PET/CT in the accurate evaluation of primary colorectal carcinoma. Eur J Surg Oncol 2006;32(9):941–7.

52. Vriens D, de Geus-Oei LF, van der Graaf WT, et al. Tailoring therapy in colorectal cancer by PET-CT. Q J Nucl Med Mol Imaging 2009;53(2):224–44.

53. von Schulthess GK, Steinert HC, Hany TF. Integrated PET/CT: current applications and future directions. Radiology 2006;238(2):405–22.

54. Votrubova J, Belohlavek O, Jaruskova M, et al. The role of FDG-PET/CT in the detection of recurrent colorectal cancer. Eur J Nucl Med Mol Imaging 2006; 33(7):779–84.

55. Chen L-B, Tong J-L, Hai-Zhu S, et al. 18F-DG PET/CT in detection of recurrence and metastasis of colorectal cancer. World J Gastroenterol 2007;13(37):5025–9.

56. Soyka JD, Veit-Haibach P, Strobel K, et al. Staging pathways in recurrent colorectal carcinoma: is contrast-enhanced 18F-FDG PET/CT the diagnostic tool of choice? J Nucl Med 2008;49(3):354–61.

57. Vogel WV, Wiering B, Corstens FH, et al. Colorectal cancer: the role of PET/CT in recurrence. Cancer Imaging 2005;5(Spec No A):S143–9.

58. Yancovitz M, Finelt N, Warycha MA, et al. Role of radiologic imaging at the time of initial diagnosis of stage T1b-T3b melanoma. Cancer 2007;110(5):1107–14.

59. Havenga K, Cobben DC, Oyen WJ, et al. Fluorodeoxyglucose-positron emission tomography and sentinel lymph node biopsy in staging primary cutaneous melanoma. Eur J Surg Oncol 2003;29(8):662–4.

60. Crippa F, Leutner M, Belli F, et al. Which kinds of lymph node metastases can FDG PET detect? A clinical study in melanoma. J Nucl Med 2000;41(9):1491–4.

61. Acland KM, Healy C, Calonje E, et al. Comparison of positron emission tomography scanning and sentinel node biopsy in the detection of micrometastases of primary cutaneous malignant melanoma. J Clin Oncol 2001;19(10):2674–8.

62. Strobel K, Dummer R, Husarik DB, et al. High-risk melanoma: accuracy of FDG PET/CT with added CT morphologic information for detection of metastases. Radiology 2007;244(2):566–74.

63. Tyler DS, Onaitis M, Kherani A, et al. Positron emission tomography scanning in malignant melanoma. Cancer 2000;89(5):1019–25.

64. Branstetter BF 4th, Blodgett TM, Zimmer LA, et al. Head and neck malignancy: is PET/CT more accurate than PET or CT alone? Radiology 2005;235(2):580–6.

65. Hannah A, Scott AM, Tochon-Danguy H, et al. Evaluation of 18F-fluorodeoxyglucose positron emission tomography and computed tomography with histopathologic correlation in the initial staging of head and neck cancer. Ann Surg 2002; 236(2):208–17.

66. Bailet JW, Abemayor E, Jabour BA, et al. Positron emission tomography: a new, precise imaging modality for detection of primary head and neck tumors and assessment of cervical adenopathy. Laryngoscope 1992;102(3):281–8.
67. Braams JW, Pruim J, Freling NJ, et al. Detection of lymph node metastases of squamous-cell cancer of the head and neck with FDG-PET and MRI. J Nucl Med 1995;36(2):211–6.
68. Schoder H, Yeung HW, Gonen M, et al. Head and neck cancer: clinical usefulness and accuracy of PET/CT image fusion. Radiology 2004;231(1):65–72.
69. Nahmias C, Carlson ER, Duncan LD, et al. Positron emission tomography/computerized tomography (PET/CT) scanning for preoperative staging of patients with oral/head and neck cancer. J Oral Maxillofac Surg 2007;65(12):2524–35.
70. Schoder H, Carlson DL, Kraus DH, et al. 18F-FDG PET/CT for detecting nodal metastases in patients with oral cancer staged N0 by clinical examination and CT/MRI. J Nucl Med 2006;47(5):755–62.
71. Kim SY, Roh JL, Yeo NK, et al. Combined 18F-fluorodeoxyglucose-positron emission tomography and computed tomography as a primary screening method for detecting second primary cancers and distant metastases in patients with head and neck cancer. Ann Oncol 2007;18(10):1698–703.
72. Quon A, Fischbein NJ, McDougall IR, et al. Clinical role of 18F-FDG PET/CT in the management of squamous cell carcinoma of the head and neck and thyroid carcinoma. J Nucl Med 2007;48(Suppl 1):58S–67S.
73. Abgral R, Querellou S, Potard G, et al. Does 18F-FDG PET/CT improve the detection of posttreatment recurrence of head and neck squamous cell carcinoma in patients negative for disease on clinical follow-up? J Nucl Med 2009;50(1):24–9.
74. Bortfeld T. IMRT: a review and preview. Phys Med Biol 2006;51(13):R363–79.
75. Gregoire V, Haustermans K, Geets X, et al. PET-based treatment planning in radiotherapy: a new standard? J Nucl Med 2007;48(Suppl 1):68S–77S.
76. Gupta T, Beriwal S. PET/CT-guided radiation therapy planning: from present to the future. Indian J Cancer 2010;47(2):126–33.
77. Krengli M, Milia ME, Turri L, et al. FDG-PET/CT imaging for staging and target volume delineation in conformal radiotherapy of anal carcinoma. Radiat Oncol 2010;5:10.
78. Jingu K, Ariga H, Kaneta T, et al. Focal dose escalation using FDG-PET-guided intensity-modulated radiation therapy boost for postoperative local recurrent rectal cancer: a planning study with comparison of DVH and NTCP. BMC Cancer 2010;10:127.
79. Topkan E, Yavuz AA, Aydin M, et al. Comparison of CT and PET-CT based planning of radiation therapy in locally advanced pancreatic carcinoma. J Exp Clin Cancer Res 2008;27:41.
80. Deantonio L, Beldi D, Gambaro G, et al. FDG-PET/CT imaging for staging and radiotherapy treatment planning of head and neck carcinoma. Radiat Oncol 2008;3:29.
81. Coon D, Gokhale AS, Burton SA, et al. Fractionated stereotactic body radiation therapy in the treatment of primary, recurrent, and metastatic lung tumors: the role of positron emission tomography/computed tomography-based treatment planning. Clin Lung Cancer 2008;9(4):217–21.
82. Ford EC, Herman J, Yorke E, et al. 18F-FDG PET/CT for image-guided and intensity-modulated radiotherapy. J Nucl Med 2009;50(10):1655–65.
83. Kruser TJ, Bradley KA, Bentzen SM, et al. The impact of hybrid PET-CT scan on overall oncologic management, with a focus on radiotherapy planning: a prospective, blinded study. Technol Cancer Res Treat 2009;8(2):149–58.

84. Hoffman JM, Hanson MW, Friedman HS, et al. FDG-PET in pediatric posterior fossa brain tumors. J Comput Assist Tomogr 1992;16(1):62–8.
85. Kumar R, Shandal V, Shamim SA, et al. Clinical applications of PET and PET/CT in pediatric malignancies. Expert Rev Anticancer Ther 2010;10(5):755–68.
86. Tatsumi M, Miller JH, Wahl RL. 18F-FDG PET/CT in evaluating non-CNS pediatric malignancies. J Nucl Med 2007;48(12):1923–31.
87. Murano T, Tateishi U, Iinuma T, et al. Evaluation of the risk of radiation exposure from new 18FDG PET/CT plans versus conventional X-ray plans in patients with pediatric cancers. Ann Nucl Med 2010;24(4):261–7.
88. Kleinerman RA. Cancer risks following diagnostic and therapeutic radiation exposure in children. Pediatr Radiol 2006;36(Suppl 2):121–5.
89. Chawla SC, Federman N, Zhang D, et al. Estimated cumulative radiation dose from PET/CT in children with malignancies: a 5-year retrospective review. Pediatr Radiol 2010;40(5):681–6.
90. Petersdorf RG. Fever of unknown origin. An old friend revisited. Arch Intern Med 1992;152(1):21–2.
91. Meller J, Sahlmann C-O, Scheel AK. 18F-FDG PET and PET/CT in fever of unknown origin. J Nucl Med 2007;48:35–45.
92. Halpenny DF, Burke JP, Lawlor GO, et al. Role of PET and combination PET/CT in the evaluation of patients with inflammatory bowel disease. Inflamm Bowel Dis 2009;15(6):951–8.
93. Knaapen P, de Haan S, Hoekstra OS, et al. Cardiac PET-CT: advanced hybrid imaging for the detection of coronary artery disease. Neth Heart J 2010;18(2):90–8.
94. Kumar S, Rajshekher G, Prabhakar S. Positron emission tomography in neurological diseases. Neurol India 2005;53(2):149–55.

Index

Note: Page numbers of article titles are in **boldface** type.

Surg Clin N Am 91 (2011) 267–276
doi:10.1016/S0039-6109(10)00173-8
0039-6109/11/$ – see front matter © 2011 Elsevier Inc. All rights reserved.

surgical.theclinics.com

Moving?

Make sure your subscription moves with you!

To notify us of your new address, find your **Clinics Account Number** (located on your mailing label above your name), and contact customer service at:

Email: journalscustomerservice-usa@elsevier.com

800-654-2452 (subscribers in the U.S. & Canada)
314-447-8871 (subscribers outside of the U.S. & Canada)

Fax number: 314-447-8029

Elsevier Health Sciences Division
Subscription Customer Service
3251 Riverport Lane
Maryland Heights, MO 63043

*To ensure uninterrupted delivery of your subscription, please notify us at least 4 weeks in advance of move.

Printed and bound by CPI Group (UK) Ltd, Croydon, CR0 4YY

03/10/2024

01040458-0008